11/25/05

THE PET LOVER'S GUIDE TO CAT & DOG SKIN DISEASES

About The Pet Lover's Series

Your pets are important members of your family. When they have a medical condition, you want them to get the best care that can be provided. You also want to know everything you can about their condition, including all the treatment options. This series, written by leading veterinary authors, will help you, as a pet owner, understand the causes, diagnosis, treatment, and prevention options for many common conditions your pets may have.

This series provides quality veterinary information, written by the veterinary leaders your veterinarian trusts, but in an easy-to understand manner that allows you to talk with your veterinarian about your pet's condition. **The books in this series are not intended as substitutes for visits to your veterinarian.** Instead, they should be read as a way to get more information about your pet's condition so that you'll know what to do, what to ask, and what to expect when you take your pet to your veterinarian.

THE
PET LOVER'S GUIDE TO CAT & DOG SKIN DISEASES

Karen L. Campbell
DVM, MS, Diplomate, ACVIM, ACVD

Professor and Section Head, Specialty Medicine
Department of Veterinary Clinical Medicine
University of Illinois College of Veterinary Medicine
Urbana, Illinois

SAUNDERS

ELSEVIER

ELSEVIER
SAUNDERS

11830 Westline Industrial Drive
St. Louis, Missouri 63146

The Pet Lover's Guide to Cat and Dog Skin Diseases
Copyright © 2006, Elsevier Inc.

ISBN 13: 978-1-4160-2543-6
ISBN 10: 1-4160-2543-X

Notice

The Publisher

3 4873 00402 3750

ISBN 13: 978-1-4160-2543-6
ISBN 10: 1-4160-2543-X

Publishing Director: Linda Duncan
Senior Editor: Liz Fathman
Developmental Editor: Shelly Stringer
Publishing Services Manager: Patricia Tannian
Project Manager: John Casey
Cover/Book Design Direction: Amy Buxton
Cover/Book Design: Bill Smith Studio

Printed in United States of America

Last digit is the print number: 9 8 7 6 5 4 3 2 1

Working together to grow
libraries in developing countries
www.elsevier.com | www.bookaid.org | www.sabre.org

ELSEVIER   BOOK AID   Sabre Foundation
           International

I want to dedicate this book to pet owners everywhere. I hope that the knowledge you gain from reading this book will help you in working with your veterinarian to provide your pet with relief from any skin afflictions. Be sure to always consult a veterinarian before attempting to treat any disease.

Preface

The skin and hair coat can tell you a lot about your pet and its environment. The appearance of your pet's skin and hair coat reflects the general health of your pet and is also influenced by many environmental factors. It's not at all surprising that skin disease is one of the most common reasons for pet owners to seek veterinary care for their dogs and cats. The diagnosis and treatment of skin diseases can be difficult and frustrating for veterinarians and pet owners. The purpose of this book is to provide insights into the various causes of skin disease, the steps required to arrive at a diagnosis, and the pros and cons of various treatment options.

If you have experienced the frustration of watching your pet suffer from itching, chewing, or hair loss, this book will help you understand what is wrong with your pet and the steps that will be needed to diagnose and treat its disease. Many diseases require a series of diagnostic tests or treatment trials to solve the problem. Understanding the reasons for these tests and trials and the importance of your full cooperation will help you resolve the problem as quickly as possible. **This book is not intended as a substitute for obtaining professional veterinary care, however**. Many diseases look alike, and treating some may require referral to a veterinarian who specializes in dermatology. This book is intended to help readers understand the causes of skin diseases and the "whys" of various tests and treatments. Even if your pet does not have a problem, the information in this book can help you maintain the health of the skin and hair coat.

Karen L. Campbell, DVM, MS
Diplomate, ACVIM, ACVD

Acknowledgments

I have had many excellent mentors throughout my life, starting with my parents—John and Eunice Campbell—and my grandparents (Emery and Hazel Vieten, Carl and Helen Campbell)—who encouraged my love of animals and let me keep a variety of pets on their farms. Dr. Joseph Swink, Jr., inspired me to love the field of veterinary medicine and provided me with a role model in demonstrating compassion and respect for the human-animal bond. Dr. Erwin Small provided me with the opportunity to specialize in veterinary dermatology, a field that I truly enjoy.

I am indebted to my many friends and colleagues in the field of veterinary dermatology who have shared their knowledge and photographs, and to my students who have taught me much more than I have taught them. Special thanks is due to Drs. Adam Patterson and Andrew Lowe, who took extra days of clinic teaching to allow me to concentrate on writing, and to Sandra Grable, CVT, for her assistance with photography.

I appreciate the help of the excellent team of professionals at Elsevier who have been involved in this book. I want to give special thanks to Shelly Stringer, who has worked hard to keep this book on schedule.

Last, but not least, I want to acknowledge the love and support given to me by my family. Thank you for allowing me to take time away from you to work on this project—you are the best!

x

Contents

1 **Introduction to the Skin and Hair Coat of Pets, 1**

Functions of the Skin, 1
Structure of the Skin, 4
Hair Composition and Growth, 7
Glands of the Skin, 9
Anal Sacs, 10
Ears, 11
Nails (Claws), 12
Summary, 12

2 **Care of the Skin and Hair Coat, 13**

Grooming, 13
Bathing, 15
Dental Care, 31
Ear Care, 32
Care of the Nails, 32
Topical Medications, 34
Ectoparasite Control, 34
Summary, 40

3 **Symptoms of Diseases Affecting the Skin and Common Diagnostic Evaluations, 41**

Diagnostic Approaches, 42
Skin Lesions (Primary and Secondary), 56
Alopecia (Hair Loss), 56
Itching (Pruritus), 62
Ear Diseases, 63
Nail Diseases, 64
Summary, 64

4 **Allergies, 65**

Atopy, 67
Contact Allergies, 99
Food Allergies, 102
Parasite-Related Allergies, 111
Miscellaneous Allergies, 114
Summary, 115

5 **Bacterial Infections, 117**

Hot Spots (Acute Moist Dermatitis), 119
Skin Fold Pyoderma, 122
Staphylococcal Pyoderma, 124
Miscellaneous Bacterial Infections, 131
Summary, 140

6 Parasitic Skin Diseases, 141

Fleas, 142
Mange and Other Mite Infestations, 148
Ticks, 167
Miscellaneous Ectoparasites, 170
Summary, 180

7 Hormone-Related Skin Diseases, 181

Adrenal Disorders, 182
Thyroid Disorders, 194
Sex Hormone Disorders, 208
Miscellaneous Disorders, 215
Summary, 224

8 Fungal Infections, 225

Dermatophytes (Ringworm), 225
Yeast Infection (*Malassezia* Infection), 241
Subcutaneous and Systemic Fungal Infections, 248
Fungal-Like Infections (*Pythium* and *Lagenidium* Infections), 254
Summary, 256

9 Immune-Mediated Skin Diseases, 257

Pemphigus Complex, 258
Lupus Complex, 266
Miscellaneous Immune-Mediated Skin Diseases, 272
Medications for Immune-Mediated Diseases, 279
Summary, 282

10 Pediatric, Congenital, and Hereditary Skin Diseases, 283

Acanthosis Nigricans, 284
Acral Mutilation Syndrome, 285
Color Mutant Alopecia and Black Hair Follicular Dysplasia, 287
Congenital Hypotrichosis, 289
Dermatomyositis, 291
Ehlers-Danlos Syndrome, 293
Epidermolysis Bullosa, 295
Follicular Dysplasia, 297
Ichthyosis, 297
Idiopathic Facial Dermatitis of Cats, 298
Juvenile Pyoderma (Juvenile Cellulitis, Puppy Strangles), 299
Lethal Acrodermatitis, 300
Mucinosis, 302
Pattern Baldness, 303
Primary Keratinization Defects (Primary Seborrhea), 304
Sebaceous Adenitis, 306
Zinc-Responsive Dermatoses, 308
Summary, 310

11 Behavior-Related Skin Diseases, 311

Lick Granuloma (Acral Lick Dermatitis), 314
Psychogenic Alopecia and Dermatitis in Cats, 322

Tail Sucking and Biting, 327
Flank Sucking, 328
Self-Nursing, 329
Foot Licking, 329
Anal Licking, 330
Summary, 332

12 Ear Diseases, 333

Diseases Affecting the Earflap, 334
Outer Ear Infections (Otitis Externa), 343
Middle Ear Infections (Otitis Media), 364
Inner Ear Infections (Otitis Interna), 365
Ear Surgery, 367
Summary, 368

13 Skin Tumors, 369

Non-Neoplastic Skin Masses, 370
Tumors of Epithelial Cells, 372
Tumors of the Skin Glands and Hair Follicles, 376
Dermal Tumors, 381
Lymphohistiocytic Tumors, 385
Tumors Derived from Melanocytes, 388
Miscellaneous Tumors, 389
Skin Diseases Associated with Remote Tumors
(Paraneoplastic), 390
Summary, 392

References, 393

Glossary, 397

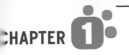

INTRODUCTION TO THE SKIN AND HAIR COAT OF PETS

Your pet's skin and hair coat are of vital importance, not only for beauty but also for life itself. The skin is the second largest body system, after the skeleton, and accounts for almost 25% of the weight of a newborn kitten or puppy and 12% to 15% of the weight of an adult cat or dog. The skin is a dynamic organ with many different functions. It is always producing new cells (called keratinocytes because they're made mainly of proteins known as keratin), hair, and secretions from the glands in the skin. The skin uses up 25% to 30% of an animal's daily intake of protein to support these activities. Because of this constant activity, the skin is prone to injury, diseases, and the effects of poor nutrition.

Functions of the Skin

The skin has a wide range of functions, including the following:

Enclosing barrier: The skin acts as a flexible support and a covering for underlying tissues—such as muscles, organs, vessels—and prevents the loss of water, electrolytes (salts), and cells. Preventing the body from drying out is essential to life on land. The skin covers and protects the body much like a bread wrapper keeps the bread from drying out.

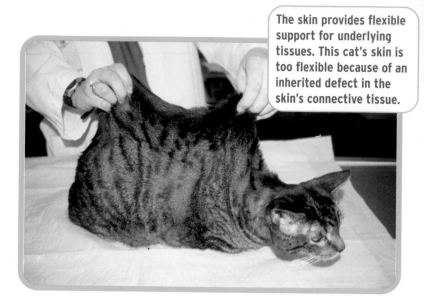

The skin provides flexible support for underlying tissues. This cat's skin is too flexible because of an inherited defect in the skin's connective tissue.

Protection: The skin serves as a physical barrier against most harmful chemicals and organisms. Secretions from the **apocrine** (sweat) and **sebaceous** (oil) **glands** provide a chemical barrier that stops the growth of many **microorganisms**.

Flexibility: The **connective tissue** of the skin stretches to allow movement. This flexibility is essential to your pet's ability to move around and also helps cushion your pet's body against impact, such as that which results from falls or bumps.

*Production of **adnexa***: The hair, claws (nails), and sweat and oil glands are accessory structures produced by the skin (the word *adnexa* is from the Latin *annexa*, meaning conjoined, subordinate, or associated anatomic parts). Adnexa play many important roles in protection and defense.

Temperature regulation: The skin has an extensive blood supply that helps regulate body temperature. Vasoconstriction (narrowing of blood vessels) in cold weather shunts blood away from the skin to lessen heat loss. Vasodilation (widening of blood vessels) directs blood toward the body surface to help cool the body during exercise and in warm environments. The dense hair coats of dogs and cats insulate their bodies from heat gain in hot environments and heat loss in cold ones. Piloerection (the raising of hairs by the contraction of small muscles associated with hair follicles) increases the insulating properties of the hair coat by trapping more air in the pelage (hairy covering). Dogs and cats do have sweat glands, but they don't play much of a role in heat loss through evaporation; in hot environments, however, cats lick their skin and hair coat, depositing saliva that cools the skin as it evaporates.

Vitamin D production: Light reacts with chemicals in the skin to produce the active form of this important vitamin.

Sensory function: The skin has an extensive network of sensory receptors for the perception of pressure, temperature, texture, pain, and itch.

Pigmentation: **Melanocytes** in the lower layers of the skin and in the germinal portion of the hair follicles (where the hairs originate) produce **melanin** pigments that are transferred to the skin cells (keratinocytes) and hair shafts. These pigments provide protection against ultraviolet light and also play a role in camouflage and reproduction (providing "sex appeal").

Storage: The skin and the tissues beneath it store fat and also hold reserves of water, electrolytes, vitamins, and proteins.

Immunosurveillance: The skin provides a mechanical barrier against disease-causing organisms. The skin also plays an active role in immunity through its antigen-presenting cells (cells that recognize and respond to foreign molecules). Antigen-presenting cells of the skin include Langerhans' cells and keratinocytes. **Lymphocytes** and other **white blood cells** respond to harmful substances that reach the dermis (see pages 4 to 6).

Antimicrobial functions: The skin protects the body from bacteria and viruses in various ways. The hairs and outer horny layer of skin (the **stratum corneum**) provide a mechanical barrier. Secretions from the sweat and oil glands produce a chemical barrier. The acidic pH of the skin's surface results in a pH barrier (many disease-causing microorganisms grow best at a neutral or slightly alkaline pH). **Antibodies** produced by lymphocytes and secreted in sweat and serum provide a specific **immunologic** barrier. Finally, resident microflora (the microorganisms that are the normal inhabitants of the skin) compete with the invaders for nutrients and also secrete substances that inhibit the growth of other organisms.

The skin is truly amazing in its many diverse functions!

Structure of the Skin

The skin usually is divided into three layers: the **epidermis**, **dermis**, and hypodermis (subcutaneous tissue).

Canine skin. The skin is divided into three layers: the epidermis, the dermis, and the subcutaneous layer, or hypodermis. Each hair follicle is made up of a single primary hair surrounded by several secondary hairs. Sebaceous and apocrine (epitrichial) glands empty their secretions into the hair follicle.

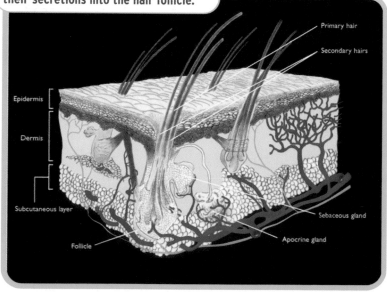

The epidermis is the outermost layer of the skin. Made up of cells called *keratinocytes,* it is just three to five cells thick in dogs and cats. The cells at the bottom of the epidermis are called the **stratum basale**. These cells always are dividing to produce new skin cells. The new cells are pushed up toward the skin's surface. During this migration, they make keratin (tough, fibrous threads of protein). As each keratinocyte reaches the skin's surface, the nucleus falls apart and the cell flattens, forming a horny layer called the *stratum corneum.* The uppermost cells flake off and fall apart. The movement from the stratum basale to the stratum corneum takes 21 to 23 days in normal dogs and cats. This period is referred to as the *epidermal turnover time.* Turnover time is reduced in many diseases, resulting in the production of more skin cells in a shorter period of time and, as a result, visible scales, or dandruff. The skin also responds to injury by becoming thicker. Just as people develop calluses on areas of their skin that are subjected to constant friction, an animal's skin becomes thicker in response to continual rubbing or scratching. The skin of a dog or cat that is constantly scratching will become so thick that it can resemble the bark of a tree.

The epidermis also contains melanin pigment–producing cells called *melanocytes.* These cells increase in number and activity when the skin is irritated, and the skin becomes darker (hyperpigmented). Just as human skin tans when exposed to damaging sunlight, the skin of dogs and cats becomes darker when it is damaged. In some dogs with chronic skin disease, the skin becomes so thick and black that it starts to resemble the skin of an armadillo.

The dermis layer of the skin contains connective tissue, blood vessels, nerves, and a gel-like substance called *ground substance.* The dermis supports and nourishes the skin. The junction between the dermis and epidermis is referred to as the *basement-membrane zone.* It includes fibers and other structures that bind the epider-

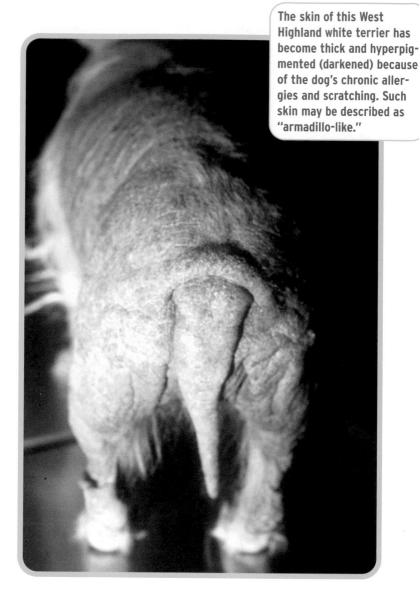

The skin of this West Highland white terrier has become thick and hyperpigmented (darkened) because of the dog's chronic allergies and scratching. Such skin may be described as "armadillo-like."

mis to the dermis. The dermal connective tissue has two types of fibers: **collagen** and elastin. Collagen fibers give the skin the ability to stretch. Elastin fibers are important in making the skin flexible. Ground substance is made up of large molecules containing proteins and carbohydrates that bind large amounts of water.

The hypodermis (subcutaneous tissue) is located between the dermis and underlying muscle or bone. It is made up of connective tissue, fat cells, blood vessels, and nerves. The hypodermis serves as a storage site for fat and supports the overlying dermis and epidermis.

Hair Composition and Growth

Hairs are flexible, elastic, horny fibers that cover the skin of dogs and cats. The part of the hair above the surface of the skin is called the hair shaft. The part below the surface of the skin is the hair root. Dogs and cats have compound **hair follicles**: a single large primary hair surrounded by several smaller secondary hairs that share an opening to the skin surface. Primary hairs are also called *guard hairs*. Secondary hairs form the pet's undercoat. Hair follicles develop at 30- to 60-degree angles to the skin. Overall, they slope toward the tail and the ground to help pets shed water. In 1 year a dog produces 60 to 180 grams of hair per kilogram of body weight; cats produce 30 to 40 grams of hair per kilogram of weight.

Every hair shaft has three parts: a cuticle, a cortex, and a medulla. The cuticle (the outermost layer) consists of cells that overlap like shingles. This overlap is so noticeable in cats that, under a microscope, the profile of their hairs appears jagged. The cortex is made up of tightly packed spindle-shaped keratin cells that form the middle layer of the hair shaft. The medulla, the inner core of a hair, is found only in primary hairs. Cells in the medulla contain spaces filled with air and glycogen (a kind of sugar). Hair roots end in a knoblike bulb that attaches the hair to the dermis in a structure called the *dermal papilla*.

Hair grows in cycles. The growth phase is called the **anagen** phase of the hair cycle. Hair growth originates in the hair bulb. As cells in the hair bulb divide, they push older cells upward, causing the hair shaft to grow longer. Hairs grow an average of 0.1 mm per day. The length that a hair grows is determined mostly by genetics (for example, a poodle's hairs grow continuously for many years) but is also influenced by nutrition, the time of year (because of the seasonal variation in daylight), temperature, and other factors (for instance, many diseases shorten the anagen phase). Once a hair reaches its maximum length, the hair bulb begins to break apart (catagen phase) and the hair enters a resting stage called **telogen**. A new hair bulb forms over the dermal papilla and grows below the level of the older hair. As the new hair grows, it pushes the older hair upward in the skin. As the hair bulb breaks apart, the old hair shaft becomes less firmly attached to the hair follicle, and it may be dislodged by normal wear and tear (for instance, friction during such activities as lying down and getting up, rolling, and rubbing against surfaces).

Normal shedding patterns (in the spring and fall) are determined mainly by changes in the amount of daylight from season to season (known as the *photoperiod*). Dogs and cats that are kept indoors are exposed to extra hours of artificial light throughout the year and may shed year-round.

Each hair follicle has an associated muscle called the *arrector pili muscle*. When this muscle contracts, it straightens the hair follicle from its normal 30- to 60-degree angle to the skin surface, causing the hair shaft to stand up. The arrector pili muscles contract in response to **epinephrine** when the animal is afraid or excited and in displays of dominance or aggression (you've probably seen a dog raising its hackles); the hairs also stand up during cold weather as a way of regulating body temperature (thermoregulation). Hairs in the telogen phase may loosen and fall out when their arrector pili muscles contract, which is why many dogs and cats

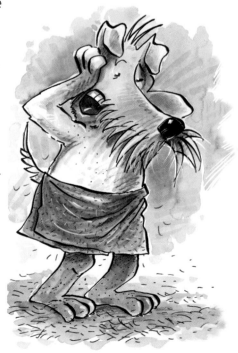

shed so heavily when they go for a ride in the car or visit the veterinarian.

Whiskers, also known as *vibrissae*, are specialized hairs found on the sides of the muzzle, the lower jaw, above the eyes, and, in cats, on the front legs. These hairs, called *tactile hairs*, are important in the sensation of touch. Tactile hairs are surrounded by a blood-filled space that contains many nerve endings for sensory perception.

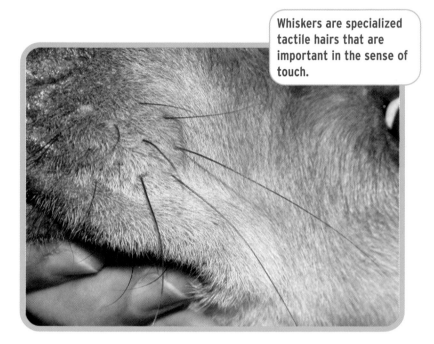

Whiskers are specialized tactile hairs that are important in the sense of touch.

Glands of the Skin

Sebaceous (oil) glands are found with both primary and secondary hairs. These glands produce **sebum**, an oily mixture containing cholesterol, waxes, and fatty acids. The ducts of sebaceous glands empty into the hair follicle, and sebum spreads over the hairs to keep them flexible and shiny. Sebum also spreads over the surface of the skin to help it retain moisture by retarding the evaporation of water from skin cells. Sebaceous glands are largest and most numerous on the chin, the back of the neck, the rump, the top side of the tail, between the toes, and around body openings.

Epitrichial sweat glands are associated with hair follicles. Their ducts empty into the hair follicles. In dogs and cats, these glands also are called *apocrine sweat glands*. Epitrichial sweat glands produce a milky, protein-rich fluid that is believed to have pheromonal (scent) and antimicrobial functions (stopping the growth of microorganisms on skin and hairs). They are not important in thermoregulation because dogs and cats do not sweat in response to high temperatures.

Atrichial sweat glands are found in the footpads of dogs and cats. The ducts of these glands open directly onto the surface of the skin. They are similar to our eccrine sweat glands, and they produce a watery secretion. However, because of their location only on the footpads, they do not play a significant role in cooling in dogs and cats.

Tail glands in cats are large sebaceous glands located along the top surface of the tail. When the tail glands secrete too much oil, a condition called "stud tail" results. The hair in the area mats or becomes thin; the skin becomes greasy with scales and crusts. The tail glands of dogs are located on the top surface of the tail, over the fifth to seventh bones of the tail. Hairs in this region are stiffer and coarser than normal, and secretions from the tail glands may be seen as a waxy yellow deposit on the skin. These secretions are thought to have pheromone (personal scent) activity.

Anal Sacs

The anal sacs are paired structures located between the two layers of sphincters associated with the anus. Each sac has a single duct that opens to the skin surface at the 3 o'clock and 9 o'clock positions around the anus. The walls of the sacs contain many sebaceous glands and a smaller number of atrichial sweat glands. Secretions from these glands accumulate in the anal sacs to form a brownish, oily fluid with a strong odor. The sacs are normally compressed when the animal defecates, causing the expulsion of some of the fluid. These muscles may also contract when an animal is frightened, causing the foul-smelling fluid to be expelled.

When the ducts become plugged, the quality of an animal's feces changes, or the muscle tone of the anal sphincter changes, the sacs may become too full. The secretions of an impacted anal sac are often pasty and dry. Infection may result in inflammation and, eventually, abscess or rupture of the anal sac. Dogs and cats with impacted or infected anal sacs may lick, bite, rub, or scoot upon the area around their anus. Some cats also pull hair out over the base of the tail or on the lower abdomen. Treatment involves manually pressing out (expressing) the contents to relieve the irritation. Infections require veterinary treatment, which includes emptying the anal sacs, instilling an antibiotic solution, and prescribing oral antibiotics.

Ears

The ears of dogs and cats contain structures that are important in sound perception (hearing) and balance. The ear has three main parts: the external ear, the middle ear, and the inner ear. The external ear includes the ear **pinna** (the outer "flap") and the ear canal, which has a vertical portion and a horizontal portion. The pinna funnels sound waves into the ear canal, which ends at the tympanic membrane (eardrum). Vibrations from the sound waves are transmitted through the middle ear to the cochlea of the inner ear, where they trigger nerve impulses that are sent to the brain. Interpretation of these nerve impulses completes the pathway of hearing. The semicircular canals in the inner ear are essential for balance.

The skin lining the ear canal contains many sebaceous and ceruminal (sweat) glands, as well as hair follicles. **Cerumen** (earwax) is made up of shed epithelial cells and glandular secretions.

Nails (Claws)

Claws, or nails, as they commonly are called, are specialized structures that cover the third (distal) bone of each toe. The dermis of adjacent skin is continuous with the periosteum (outer covering) of the distal phalanx (toe bone). The nail has a rich blood supply, which causes profuse bleeding when a nail is trimmed too short. The upper portion of the distal phalanx, which is crescent shaped, is referred to as the *ungual crest*. The epidermis over the ungual crest is called the *coronary band*. It produces the horny layers of the nail. Growth is most rapid over the center portion of the coronary band, causing the nail to curve down as it gets longer. Nails grow 0.1 to 0.2 mm per week.

Claws have important functions in walking, holding objects and climbing (in cats), hunting, and protection (both offensive and defensive). Abnormal nail growth can increase the risk of lameness and infection. Most dogs require regular nail trimming for healthy feet. Healthy cats with access to scratching posts or other suitable materials will keep their claws in good condition on their own.

Many people wonder whether there is a difference between a nail and a claw. By definition, nails are the thin, horny, translucent, relatively flat plate covering the top surface of the far ends of the fingers and toes of humans and primates. Claws are the thickened, rounded, curved horny plates that cover and extend from the far ends of the toes of most other animals. However, the word *nail* is commonly used when referring to the claws of our pets.

Summary

The skin and its associated structures are intricate and complex. Although the end products are mainly the dead proteins found in the stratum corneum and in hairs, the skin itself is a dynamic, active organ that is affected by numerous internal and external factors. The skin has many functions. Perhaps the most important is its role as a barrier, without which life would be impossible. This chapter provides a basis for understanding the remarkable nature of the skin.

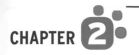

CHAPTER 2

CARE OF THE SKIN AND HAIR COAT

Dogs and cats benefit in several ways from regular grooming. In addition to helping the skin and hair coat stay healthy, grooming strengthens the bond of companionship between you and your pet. Early signs of skin and ear disease can be detected during grooming, allowing you to take action to prevent a mild disease from progressing to a severe one. Pets that are groomed regularly seem to enjoy this attention and usually begin to tolerate less pleasant procedures such as nail trimming and tooth brushing. Many products are available for use on pets' coats, nails, and teeth; learning about these products will help you use them effectively.

Grooming

Dog and cat breeds have many different coat types, each with unique grooming requirements. The equipment needed for grooming includes the following:

- **Brushes**
- **Combs**
- **Scissors**
- **Nail clippers**
- **Nail file**
- **Shampoo**
- **Conditioner**
- **Towels**
- **Ear-cleaning solution**
- **Cotton balls or pads**

13

You should also have **hemostatic** (blood-clotting) powder and a **flea-**preventive preparation on hand. Certain breeds require additional special tools for proper grooming and trimming.

Regular brushing can significantly reduce shedding. Many products to reduce shedding are on the market, but nothing is as valuable as brushing the pet for 10 to 15 minutes twice a week. Brushing removes old, dead hair before it can be shed. Brushing also increases blood flow to the skin, promoting the growth of healthy hair. As you groom your pet, check the skin and hair coat for **parasites,** such as fleas or **ticks**, and any evidence of skin disease (hair loss, excessive scaling, crusts, redness, or bumps).

The amount of grooming that your dog requires depends on its breed. Owners of show dogs should consult someone who can help them learn trimming and grooming techniques specific to that breed. Visit www.petgroomer. com/groomingbasics101.htm to find information on the grooming needs of many different breeds.

In general, breeds with long coats are line-brushed: Spray the hair coat with water, and then part it down to the skin, starting at the neck. Spraying the coat with water before brushing helps reduce damage to the hair. Use a metal pin brush or bristle brush to brush the hair in the direction opposite to the one in which it normally lies, one layer at a time. For each layer, form a new part and brush.

A technique called *hand-stripping* (or *plucking*) is used to groom most terrier breeds. Without hand-stripping, a terrier's coat becomes soft and dull. Hand-stripping removes dead hairs and encourages new growth. It also clears the **hair follicles** of sweat and hair secretions and promotes healthier skin. Shaving or clipping the coat leaves the roots of dead hairs in the skin and often results in red, bumpy skin. Properly performed hand-stripping is not painful to the dog and improves skin condition.

If any mats are too entangled to be brushed out, clip them from the rest of the coat with scissors. Place a

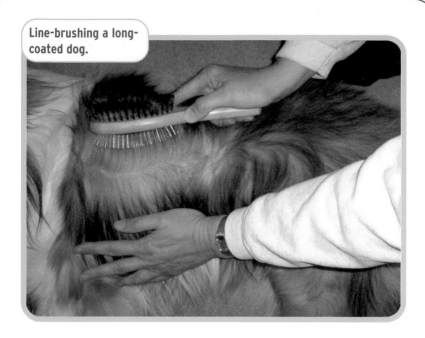

Line-brushing a long-coated dog.

comb under the mat, and cut over the comb to keep from accidentally cutting the skin. Most cats enjoy being brushed, and frequent brushing is a necessity for long-haired cats to prevent matting.

Bathing

The skin surface collects a layer of dead skin cells; secretions from **sebaceous** (oil-producing) and sweat glands; and dirt, bacteria, yeast, pollen, and mold spores from the environment. If not removed by grooming or bathing, the accumulation can cause irritation and increase the risk of skin infection. The bad smells some-times associated with dogs and cats are often caused by bacterial or yeast infections of the skin, ears, or gums.

Where We Stand

Pets with strong body odors should be evaluated by a veterinarian, who can pinpoint the source and recommend preventive and treatment measures.

The frequency with which a pet should be bathed depends on the amount of dirt to which it is exposed and on the animal's overall health, including the condition of its skin and hair coat. Healthy animals that groom themselves (most cats, for instance) or are regularly groomed by their owners seldom need bathing. However, bathing every 2 to 4 days may benefit pets with skin diseases related to **allergies**, infections, skin parasites, or **seborrhea** (greasy, scaly, or thickened skin caused by too much oil production or defects in skin **keratinization**; see page 304).

Getting Ready for a Bath

To prepare your pet for bathing, brush the hair coat and remove any matted hair. Trim or file the nails (see section on nail care later in this chapter). Check between the toes and pads of each foot for foreign objects or matted hair. If mats are not removed before a bath,

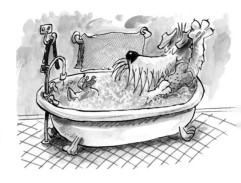

they trap water and become even more knotted, making them more difficult to remove later.

Remember to express the contents of the **anal sacs** (see Chapter 1) before starting your pet's bath so that you can wash away any discharge. You can usually do this by applying pressure with your thumb on one side of the anus and the fingers on the other side, pressing up and forward. (See the section on anal sacs in Chapter 1 for more information.) Be sure to wear a glove, and use cotton pads or gauze sponges to collect the secretions—they have an unpleasant odor! If you find that you can't empty the sacs yourself, you may have to ask your veterinarian to empty them by inserting a gloved finger into the pet's rectum. If your pet's anal glands are impacted, the veterinarian may need to insert a tube and put a lubricating solution into the sacs before they can be emptied.

When to Bathe, What to Use

Myth: Dogs and cats should be bathed only when they get dirty.

Fact: Dogs and cats that keep themselves clean may not need frequent baths for their own health, but bathing with appropriate shampoos does not harm your pet and can actually help cut down on pet-associated **allergies** in people.

Myth: Frequent bathing causes dry skin and dandruff.

Fact: Bathing with a moisturizing shampoo may increase the **hydration** (moisture) of the skin. Bathing with a **keratoplastic** or **keratolytic** shampoo will help control dandruff.

Myth: Human antidandruff shampoos will help treat my pet's dandruff.

Fact: Shampoos for human dandruff that contain tar can kill a cat. Other human dandruff shampoos containing pyrithione zinc can cause blindness in dogs. Always check with your veterinarian before using a medicated shampoo on your pet.

Myth: Dishwashing detergents are excellent for bathing pets.

Fact: Dishwashing detergents strip the natural oils from the skin and hair coat and may leave your pet with dry, irritated skin.

Myth: Baby shampoos are excellent for bathing pets.

Fact: Human skin is more acidic than the skin of dogs and cats. Use a shampoo that is specially formulated for use in dogs or cats.

You also should examine your pet's ears and clean them, if necessary. Many ear-cleaning solutions are oily, and they will leave the pet's head looking dirty unless the residue is removed by shampooing. Place cotton balls or pads in both of your pet's ear canals (gently—don't push) before bathing to keep water and shampoo out.

Shampoos

Veterinarians and pet-supply stores sell a variety of shampoos for both grooming and medicinal purposes. Think about the condition of your pet's skin and hair coat when you pick a shampoo. Consult your veterinarian if your pet has a skin disease. A good shampoo lathers easily, removes soil without stripping away natural oils, rinses quickly, doesn't irritate your pet's skin, and doesn't leave a residue; ideally, your pet's hair is left soft, shiny, and easy to brush or comb. Medicated shampoos have additional purposes, such as reducing oil production; eliminating parasites, bacteria, or fungi; or controlling itching.

What Is in Your Pet's Shampoo, and Why?

Ingredient	Purpose(s)	Cautions
Acetic acid	Kills bacteria and yeast	
Aloe vera	Kills bacteria and moisturizes skin	
Amino acids	Conditions coat (repairs split ends)	
Balsam	Conditions coat, moisturizes skin	

What Is in Your Pet's Shampoo, and Why?—cont'd

Ingredient	Purpose(s)	Cautions
Benzoyl peroxide	Kills bacteria and yeast, cuts grease, flushes hair follicles	Can bleach, dry out, and irritate skin
Biotin	Conditions coat	
Boric acid	Kills bacteria and yeast	
Betadine	Kills bacteria and fungi	May stain skin or fur yellow, can be irritating
Carbaryl	Kills parasites	Can be toxic
Cetyl alcohol	Moisturizes skin	
Chlorhexidine	Kills bacteria and fungi	Can cause deafness if it gets into the middle ear
Citric acid	Antioxidant	
Cocamide diethanolamine	Improves lathering	
Cocamido-propyl betaine	Improves lathering	
Coconut oil	Moisturizes skin	
Collagen	Conditions coat	
D-Limonene	Kills parasites	Some reports of adverse reactions in cats and dogs
Diphen-hydramine	Antihistamine; relieves itching	

What Is in Your Pet's Shampoo, and Why?—cont'd

Ingredient	Purpose(s)	Cautions
Ethyl lactate	Kills bacteria, flushes hair follicles	
Glycerin	Moisturizer, **humectant**	
Hydro-cortisone	Relieves itching and inflammation	May interfere with diagnostic testing for **Cushing's disease**
Keratin	Conditions coat (repairs split ends)	
Ketoconazole	Kills fungi, yeast	
Lactic acid	Moisturizer, humectant	
Lanolin	Moisturizer, **emollient**	
Linoleic acid	Essential fatty acid; moisturizes skin	
Menthol	Relieves itching, fights bacteria (weak)	
Methylparaben	Preservative	Keeps microorganisms from growing in the shampoo
Miconazole	Kills fungi, yeast	

What Is in Your Pet's Shampoo, and Why?—cont'd

Ingredient	Purpose(s)	Cautions
Oatmeal	Relieves itching, moisturizes skin	
Oils (mineral, almond, peanut, corn, cottonseed, sunflower, sesame seed)	Moisturizers; emollients; sources of essential fatty acids	
p-Aminobenzoic acid	Sunscreen	
Polyvinylpyrrolidone	Film-forming conditioner	
Pramoxine	Relieves itching; topical anesthetic	
Propylene glycol	Moisturizes; humectant	
Pyrethrin	Kills parasites	Triggers allergies in some animals (e.g., those that are allergic to chrysanthemums)
Quaternium-15	Preservative	Keeps microorganisms from growing in the shampoo
Salicylic acid	Keratolytic, keratoplastic	Works well with sulfur; both sulfur and salicylic acid are ingredients in many **antiseborrheic** shampoos

What Is in Your Pet's Shampoo, and Why?—cont'd

Ingredient	Purpose(s)	Cautions
Selenium sulfide	Kills fungi, yeast	Not for use in cats; can cause severe irritation
Sodium laureth sulfate	Detergent cleanser	Milder than sodium lauryl sulfate
Sodium lauryl sulfate	Detergent cleanser	Irritating to some dogs and cats
Stearalkonium chloride	Coat conditioner	
Stearyl alcohol	Moisturizer	
Sulfur	Keratolytic, keratoplastic; kills bacteria and fungi, relieves itching	Smelly and likely to stain when applied as a dip, but not as a shampoo
Tars	Keratolytic, keratoplastic; removes oils, relieves itching	Not for use in cats; can be irritating and may leave a yellow stain
Triamcinolone	Relieves itching and inflammation	Potent corticosteroid; may cause **iatrogenic** (medication- or treatment-caused) **Cushing's disease**
Triclosan	Kills bacteria and viruses	
Urea	Moisturizer; humectant	
Vitamin E	Antioxidant	

Human skin is different from the skin of dogs and cats. Human **epidermis** is three times thicker than that of dogs and cats, and our cells require more time to mature. The pH of our skin averages 5.5; cats and dogs have average skin pH readings of 6.7 and 7.5, respectively. For this reason, human pH-adjusted shampoos are too acidic for dog and cat skin and may cause irritation if they're used often.

Most shampoos do not have a soap base. Soap leaves a residue of calcium and magnesium salts on the hair unless special agents are used in the rinse water. Vinegar, which dissolves soap deposits, was once a popular (but smelly) rinse to get hair squeaky clean when soap shampoos were used. Modern shampoos contain detergents with synthetic lathering and wetting agents. On the labels of most shampoos, you will find the detergents sodium lauryl sulfate or sodium lauryl ether sulfate (sodium laureth sulfate). Detergent-based shampoos remove natural oils from the hair and skin, but moisturizing agents are added to balance this drying effect. Moisturizers added to shampoos include glycerol, glycerol esters, lanolin, lanolin derivatives, fatty alcohols, propylene glycol, and various fatty acids and oils.

"Dry" shampoos: Dry shampoos are absorbent powders that you work into your pet's hair coat and then brush out. They can be used to spot-clean dirty areas, but they tend to dry out the coat and worsen static-electricity problems. Dry shampoos shouldn't be used for routine bathing because they don't clean the skin and hair coat as well as a shampoo-and-water bath.

Antiseborrheic shampoos: **Seborrhea** is the term used to describe overproduction of oil, which may lead to scales (dandruff) or a greasy, oily hair coat. Seborrhea can develop because of a hereditary disease of the epidermis (called primary **keratinization defects**) or of the **sebaceous** glands. Seborrhea may also result from a variety of other skin diseases (**allergies**; bacterial or fungal skin infections; **ectoparasites**, such as fleas or mites; skin cancer) or environmental conditions (low humidity, harsh shampoos). The two principal properties of antiseborrheic shampoos are **keratolytic** and **keratoplastic** activity. A keratolytic agent helps soften and dissolve the stratum corneum (outermost layer of skin cells), making it easier to remove scales during a bath. A keratoplastic ingredient slows the production of new skin cells, which helps decrease the amount of scales that are formed. Shampoo ingredients with keratolytic action include salicylic acid, sulfur, tars, benzoyl peroxide, lactic acid, and propylene glycol. Ingredients with keratoplastic activity include tars, salicylic acid, and sulfur. Many antiseborrheic shampoos contain more than one active ingredient to increase effectiveness. Do not use a human dandruff shampoo on your pet without first checking with your veterinarian. The main cause of human dandruff is a yeast called *Malassezia furfur* (formerly known as *Pityrosporum ovale*). Some dogs and cats with dandruff do have a lot of yeast on their skin, but others do not and would not benefit from the use of an antiyeast shampoo. Pyrithione zinc, a keratoplastic agent found in some human dandruff shampoos, can damage the retina in cats and dogs, causing blindness. Never use a shampoo containing tar on a cat; tar can cause seizures, coma, and even death in cats.

Antibacterial shampoos: Dogs and cats with bacterial skin infections benefit from regular bathing with an antibacterial shampoo. Examples of shampoo ingredients with antibacterial activity include benzoyl peroxide, chlorhexidine, sulfur, ethyl lactate, triclosan, and **iodophors**. Benzoyl peroxide and ethyl lactate are preferable for dogs and cats with folliculitis (infection of the hair follicles) because these agents flush debris from the hair follicles. Iodophors should not be used in cats, and they often cause allergic reactions in dogs.

Antifungal shampoos: **Fungal** skin infections in dogs and cats may involve **dermatophyte** (**ringworm**) or **yeast** (***Malassezia***) organisms. Shampoo ingredients that kill both dermatophytes and yeast include ketoconazole, miconazole, chlorhexidine, sulfur, and iodophors (which, as previously mentioned, are often irritating and should not be used in cats). Ingredients that kill yeast but not dermatophytes include selenium sulfide and benzoyl peroxide. Contact time is particularly important when you are treating fungal skin infections: The shampoo must stay on the skin for at least 10 minutes to kill these organisms.

Antiparasitic shampoos: Shampoos help kill ectoparasites (external parasites such as fleas or mites) on an animal and also remove flea feces that might otherwise serve as a food source for developing fleas in the environment. Shampoo ingredients with antiparasitic activity include sulfur, pyrethrin, pyrethroids, carbamates (carbaryl), D-limonene, and lindane. Lindane can be toxic, especially in cats. Longer-acting products are needed to control most ectoparasites (see the section on ectoparasite control later in this chapter).

Antipruritic shampoos: **Pruritus** (excessive itching) is a sign of many skin diseases—ectoparasites, allergies, infection, irritation, skin cancer, and behavioral disorders (anxiety, boredom, **obsessive-compulsive disorder**). Antipruritic shampoos can help relieve the itching. The choice of shampoo depends on the cause of the itching. Antipruritic ingredients in shampoos include the following:

- **Hydrocortisone (a corticosteroid)**
- **Diphenhydramine hydrochloride (an antihistamine)**
- **Colloidal oatmeal**
- **Pramoxine hydrochloride (a topical anesthetic)**
- **Menthol (a cooling agent)**
- **Tars (which are toxic in cats)**
- **Sulfur**

Bathing Techniques for Dogs

The ideal water temperature for bathing your pet is 95° to 100° F. Wet the entire hair coat thoroughly (a spray nozzle makes wetting and rinsing much easier). Diluting the shampoo beforehand with 5 to 10 parts water helps in distributing the shampoo over the hair coat. You can rub the lather into a short-haired dog's coat, but squeeze it through the hair of a longer-coated dog to avoid matting. Use a washcloth to clean around your pet's face. Be careful not to get soap in your pet's eyes or ears (as previously mentioned, you should gently plug the ears with cotton). If you're using a medicated shampoo, leave it in contact with the skin for 10 minutes before rinsing it off. Rinsing the coat thoroughly is important because any shampoo left on the skin can cause irritation. As you rinse, pay special attention to the groin, the underside of the tail, and the feet, where residue often collects. Squeeze excess water from your pet's coat with your hands, then blot with a towel. Gently brushing the hair coat as it dries will remove tangles and help fluff the coat. If you use a hair dryer, keep the heat setting low to avoid damaging the hair or irritating the skin.

Bathing Techniques for Cats

Cats are usually meticulous groomers and do not require bathing as often as dogs. However, bathing may benefit cats with skin disease and those that do not groom themselves because of other health problems. Bathing your cat can also help lessen human allergic reactions by decreasing the amounts of allergen on the cat's hair coat and in your home. Washing your cat once a month in plain warm water can reduce the amount of allergen on your cat by as much as tenfold.

It's best to start a bathing program while your cat is still a kitten, when it will be much more cooperative. An older cat may do better when placed on a grate that provides a surface to grip during the bath. Many cats respond well to being held gently but firmly by the scruff of the neck. You can also use a cat-bathing bag, which will help you restrain the feet and claws while allowing you to lather and rinse the cat. If the cat objects to this handling or tries to bite or scratch, you may not be able to bathe the cat at home. A professional groomer or veterinarian may have better luck and can tranquilize the cat, if necessary, for the safety of the handler.

How to Bathe Your Cat at Home

Bathing a cat at home may seem like a martial art, but many cats tolerate baths quite well if you make the right preparations and provide tender, loving care. Bathing is easier if you start bathing your cat when it is still a kitten.

- **First, put your cat in a carrier or close it in the bathroom so that it can't hide.**
- **Get everything together that you will need:**

1. Shampoo: Fleas, dry skin, or allergies may necessitate a medicated shampoo, but always check with your veterinarian before selecting a shampoo. Read the instructions on the bottle carefully, and *use only products that state on the bottle that they are safe for cats!*
2. Towels for drying
3. Blow dryer
4. Shower hose attachment with a nozzle, or one that attaches to the faucet
5. Bland eye ointment (ask your veterinarian; opinions differ regarding whether to use this)
6. Toothbrush
7. Nail-trimmer
8. Cat brush or comb
9. Timer or watch for medicated baths

10. A bath mat and a grate or screen that fits on the bottom of the tub or sink or one that can be leaned against the side
11. Flea comb
12. Rubber gloves
13. Plastic cup (for diluting shampoo and pouring water)
14. Scissors for removing mats

- **Brush your cat thoroughly. Remove any mats (if scissors are required, slide a comb under the mat to protect the skin from accidental cuts). Trim the claws. *If your cat tries to bite or scratch, stop the bath.* Getting the cat bathed is not worth a trip to the hospital!**

- **Put the bath mat and grate or screen in the tub. Apply eye ointment to each eye (optional). Practice putting your cat in the tub and holding it there. Many cats do best with minimal restraint; be firm but gentle. Holding the scruff of the neck, close to the head, usually works well.**

- **Wet the entire hair coat. Most cats prefer being sprayed with water beginning at the tail and moving toward the head. Other cats prefer being placed in a tub with a few inches of water already in the bottom and then having water poured over them from a cup; do whatever works best for you and your cat. Getting wet is often the part of the bathing process that the cat likes least.**

- **Once the cat is wet, mix a small amount of shampoo in a cup of water and pour it over the cat (or better yet, prepare this diluted shampoo solution ahead of time). Use your hands to work lather throughout the cat's hair coat. You can use a washcloth or a toothbrush to clean around the face. When using a medicated shampoo, allow for a full 10 minutes of**

How to Bathe Your Cat at Home—cont'd

contact time for best results. This is a good time to comb the cat with a flea comb.

- Rinse the cat thoroughly. Don't forget the underside of the tail and between the front and rear legs.

- Use a towel to blot the cat dry. You can try slowly introducing a hair dryer set on a low speed and a low heat setting. If the cat doesn't tolerate the hair dryer, let the cat air dry. Air-drying takes much longer, so make sure that the cat stays in a warm room until it dries completely.

- Be especially good to your cat for the rest of the day. Baths are exhausting!

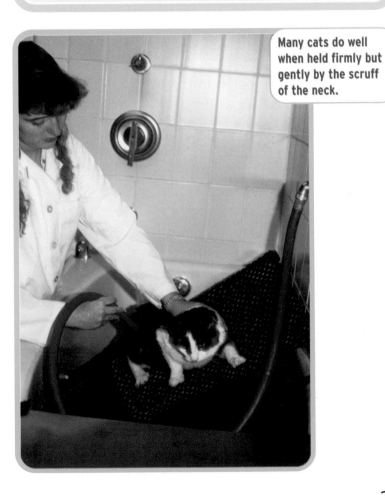

Many cats do well when held firmly but gently by the scruff of the neck.

When wetting down your cat, start at the tail and work up to the head. If your cat is frightened by the sprayer, use a plastic cup to pour water over it. As with dogs, you'll find it easier to lather your cat if you first dilute the shampoo with 5 to 10 parts water. After lathering, rinse the cat thoroughly to remove all shampoo, and blot the coat dry with a towel. Some cats tolerate a hair dryer on a low setting. Once the cat is dry, brush the coat to remove any hairs that were loosened by the bath.

Hair Conditioners

Myriads of hair conditioners are sold for use in dogs and cats. These products can reduce static electricity, moisturize the skin and hair coat, improve the appearance of the hair coat, reduce shedding, and, in the case of medicated conditioners, deliver medication to the skin.

Cationic surfactant conditioners: Conditioners with cationic surfactants (look for stearalkonium chloride on the label) leave a positively charged film on negatively charged hair shafts, eliminating static electricity and flyaway hairs. They also coat the outer layer of the hair, making the coat softer and shinier.

Film-forming conditioners: Some conditioners contain ingredients (look for polyvinylpyrrolidone or PVP on the label) that coat the hair shaft, filling in surface defects and restoring coat softness and shine. Film-forming conditioners also have a positive charge and will neutralize negative charges on hair shafts to eliminate static electricity.

Protein-based conditioners: Protein conditioners contain amino acids and fragments of proteins. They can penetrate a damaged hair shaft to repair split ends. The protein in hair conditioners often comes from animal sources (eggs, placenta, collagen, keratin, milk).

Emollients: Emollients coat the hair and skin surface, hold moisture, and make the coat appear glossy. Check the label for lanolin, lanolin derivatives, oils (mineral, coconut, almond, peanut, corn, cottonseed, sesame seed, sunflower seed), and petroleum derivatives. Linoleic acid (an essential fatty acid) applied to the skin can improve the barrier function of the epidermis, preventing loss of water through the skin.

Humectants: A humectant is a chemical that attracts and binds water. Check the label for ingredients such as lactic acid, glycerin, propylene glycol, and urea. Humectants are most effective when used as after-bath rinses or with water sprays.

Medicated coat conditioners: Medicated conditioners provide greater long-term benefits than medicated shampoos. The active ingredients, which are the same as those in shampoos, can kill bacteria and fungi or relieve itching. Some of these products are intended to be rinsed off after several minutes of contact; others, usually in the form of lotions or sprays, are meant to be left on the coat.

Dental Care

Periodontal disease is one of the most common health problems of dogs and cats. Gum disease begins with a buildup of **plaque** on the surface of the teeth. Bacteria thrive in plaque, causing bad breath, infection, and bleeding gums. Plaque binds calcium and phosphorus to form hard deposits on teeth called **tartar** or **calculus**. Pockets form in the tissues around the teeth, weakening the attachments holding the teeth in place and eventually resulting in tooth loss. A good home dental program will help prevent periodontal disease in dogs and cats.

Dogs and cats will usually allow you to brush their teeth if you are patient in introducing them to the process. Start by rubbing your pet's mouth several times a day, praising the animal when it lets you rub its teeth. After a few days, introduce a soft toothbrush, ribbed finger cot, or wet gauze sponge into the mouth, and rub it on the teeth. Next, use a chicken- or malt-flavored pet toothpaste to gently brush the teeth. Regularly check your pet's mouth for gum inflammation or tooth disease, and consult your veterinarian if you see signs of these conditions.

Ear Care

Normal ears don't require much care beyond the occasional removal of wax from the outer part of the ear canals and the inner surfaces of the ear flaps. Use a gauze cotton square or cotton ball dampened with rubbing alcohol or an ear-cleaning solution designed for pets. Talk to your veterinarian if you notice an odor or discharge in the ear, if your pet seems to be having ear pain, or if your pet is scratching or rubbing its ears. Remember to gently plug the ear canals with cotton balls or pads before each bath to keep out shampoo and water.

Care of the Nails

Most dogs require regular trimming of the nails to keep them short. Nails that are allowed to grow without regular trimming may curve under and eventually cut into the paw pads. Long nails force a dog's weight back onto the heel of the foot, causing the toes to splay. Eventually, the foot breaks down, resulting in lameness. If you start trimming your dog's nails when it is still a puppy, it will learn early in life to tolerate the procedure without struggling. The nails should be kept short enough that they don't touch the ground when the dog is standing squarely. To achieve this ideal nail length, some dogs require weekly trimming. You should also trim the **dewclaws**. Trimming can be performed at home with specialized scissors, guillotine cutters, or a grinding tool (battery or electric; for example, a Dremel grinder*). Because the "quick," or blood line, grows out with the nail (see Chapter 1), be careful when trimming a very long nail to prevent pain and bleeding. The quick is most visible in white nails, so if your dog has a white nail, trim it first and use its length to help determine how much to trim from the darker nails. If you cut your dog's quick, use a styptic pencil containing silver nitrate to seal the blood vessels. The quick will recede after you've trimmed the nail, allowing you to trim more from the nail every few days until it is at its correct length. Visit www.vetmed.wsu/ClientED/dog_nails.htm to see instructions for nail-trimming procedures and accompanying photographs. The term "show cut" refers to extremely short nails; take care not to trim the nails too short because the base of the nail holds the end of the third phalanx, the last bone of the toe. Cutting into this bone will cause your dog pain and may result in a bone infection that can necessitate amputation of the toe.

Most cats keep their nails short and in good condition through regular use of a scratching post. Many types of scratching posts are available: wood, carpet, and rope. You can entice your cat to use a scratching post by rubbing it with catnip or tying a favorite toy or string to the post. To keep your cat from scratching the furniture, cover the items with a thick layer of plastic or double-sided sticky tape. If the cat continues scratching the furniture or does not use a scratching post at all, keep its nails short by trimming them. Cats' nails are trimmed much in the same way described for dogs, with one extra step: Before trimming the nail, extend it by putting pressure on the toe pad. Visit www.catscratching.com/htmls/article.htm for instructions and pictures.

*Inclusion or omission of a company or brand name does not imply endorsement or otherwise by the authors or publisher.

Another way to keep your cat from scratching furniture or other objects is to glue a plastic cap (Soft Paws is one brand) on each nail. Declawing is a permanent solution to destructive scratching, but discuss possible complications with your veterinarian before having this surgery performed on your cat.

Topical Medications

Many topical medications are available for use in dogs and cats. Seek the guidance of your veterinarian because improper use can slow healing, cause resistant strains of organisms to develop, and cause **toxicity** in your pet.

Ectoparasite Control

Many kinds of parasites affect the skin of cats and dogs (see Chapter 6). You should monitor your pet carefully for evidence of skin parasites. Fleas are the ectoparasites that most commonly affect dogs and cats. In most areas, a flea-prevention program is recommended to protect pets from these pests. Many pesticides are available for use on pets and in their environment, but you should always check with a veterinarian who is familiar with all of the pet species in your household before you choose a particular flea remedy. Certain chemicals used in canine flea treatments are toxic to animals such as cats, rabbits, birds, reptiles, amphibians, and fish.

Antiparasitic agents are available as collars, shampoos, cream rinses, dips, powders, sprays, and spot-treatment products. Others are given orally or by injection. Each type of product can be highly effective when used according to directions. Be careful not to administer an overly large dose, and never use the product in a species for which it is not approved.

The following table lists pesticides commonly used in pets.

Antiparasitic Agents and Pest Control Management for Dogs and Cats

Active Ingredients	Uses	Comments
Methyl-carbamate	Up to 6-month protection from adult fleas	Cholinesterase inhibitor; should not be used in combination with other cholinesterase inhibitors
Carbaryl	Found in over-the-counter flea powders	Cholinesterase inhibitor; should not be used in combination with other cholinesterase inhibitors
Phosmet	Kills adult fleas, *Sarcoptes* and *Cheyletiella* mites, lice, and ticks; *not for cats!*	Organophosphate and a potent cholinesterase inhibitor; should not be used in cats or in combination with other cholinesterase inhibitors
Chlorpyrifos	Kills adult fleas, *Sarcoptes* and *Cheyletiella* mites, lice, and ticks; *not for cats!*	Organophosphate and a potent cholinesterase inhibitor; should not be used in cats or in combination with other cholinesterase inhibitors

Antiparasitic Agents and Pest Control Management for Dogs and Cats—cont'd

Active Ingredients	Uses	Comments
D-Limonene	Volatile citrus oil; provides some activity against adult fleas	Adverse reactions reported in both cats and dogs
Pyrethrins	Active against adult fleas and ticks; provides some activity against *Cheyletiella* and *Otodectes* (ear mites)	Derived from chrysanthemums, causes allergies in some pets
Permethrin	Useful against adult fleas and ticks; also active against *Sarcoptes* and *Cheyletiella* mites; spot-treatment formulations highly toxic to cats	Kills quickly; may also repel mosquitoes; concentrations > 0.05% toxic to cats
Rotenone	Active against adult fleas and *Otodectes*	Botanical product; low toxicity, rapid action, little residual effect

Antiparasitic Agents and Pest Control Management for Dogs and Cats—cont'd

Active Ingredients	Uses	Comments
Fipronil	Active against adult fleas, ticks, lice, and *Cheyletiella* and *Sarcoptes* mites	Has >30-day residual activity; not removed by most shampoos; toxic to rabbits
Imidacloprid	Active against adult fleas for 30 days	May be removed by bathing
Nitenpyram	Active against adult fleas	Given orally; rapid onset of action but effective only for a few hours
Selamectin	Active against adult fleas, the American dog tick, *Otodectes* and *Sarcoptes* mites, heartworms, and some intestinal parasites	May also have activity against *Notoedres*, *Cheyletiella*, and lice; active for up to 30 days

Antiparasitic Agents and Pest Control Management for Dogs and Cats—cont'd

Active Ingredients	Uses	Comments
Amitraz	Active against ticks; *Demodex, Sarcoptes, Cheyletiella, Oto-dectes,* and *Notoedres* mites; approved for use only in dogs and for the treatment of *Demodex* (dip) and prevention of ticks (collar).	Monoamine oxidase inhibitor; may interact adversely with other medications; many side effects; not approved for use in cats
Methoprene	Effective against immature fleas	Mimics activity of insect juvenile growth hormones, keeping fleas from maturing
Pyriproxyfen	Effective against immature fleas	Mimics activity of insect juvenile growth hormones, keeping fleas from maturing; prolonged residual activity
Lufenuron	Effective against immature fleas; given once a month orally	Prevents formation of chitin; (covering of adult fleas). Fleas feeding on pet produce eggs that do not hatch and inability of larvae to mature into adults

Antiparasitic Agents and Pest Control Management for Dogs and Cats—cont'd

Active Ingredients	Uses	Comments
Sulfur	Active against *Sarcoptes*, *Otodectes*, feline *Demodex*, fur mites, chiggers, and lice	Natural parasiticide (kills parasites); quite safe but foul-smelling substance that may cause yellow staining
Ivermectin	Approved only for heartworm prevention in pets; in higher doses, active against mites and lice	High incidence of adverse reactions (including death) reported in collies and related breeds when treated with high doses of ivermectin
Milbemycin	Oral form approved only for heartworm prevention; an ear formulation approved for treatment of *Otodectes* (ear) mites; high doses effective against *Demodex*, *Sarcoptes*, *Notoedres*, and *Cheyletiella* mites and lice	Safer than ivermectin for collies, but reports of adverse reactions in some dogs when used in high doses

Summary

A beautiful, well-groomed pet is a source of pride for its owner. The amount of care needed to keep the hair coat beautiful and the skin healthy varies according to the pet's breed and overall health. Pets benefit from regular brushing and care of their teeth, ears, and nails, and most enjoy this extra attention. Taking the time to care for the skin and hair coat helps keep dogs and cats free of skin diseases.

CHAPTER 3

SYMPTOMS OF DISEASES AFFECTING THE SKIN AND COMMON DIAGNOSTIC EVALUATIONS

Disorders of the skin and hair coat are caused by various internal and external factors. Because the skin can respond in only a limited number of ways to disease and injury, different diseases often resemble one another and are difficult to distinguish without the skill of a veterinarian who specializes in the diagnosis and treatment of skin diseases. The American College of Veterinary Dermatology oversees rigorous training programs and the board certification of specialists in veterinary dermatology. Veterinarians who have become board certified in veterinary dermatology are called *diplomates of the American College of Veterinary Dermatology (ACVD).* Check the ACVD web site for more information and a membership list: www.acvd.org.

Where We Stand

Regardless of whether you ask a specialist or a general practitioner to evaluate your pet with skin disease, a systematic approach is important in determining the correct diagnosis and treatment.

Diagnostic Approaches

The systemic approach to diagnosing a skin disorder involves several steps. The first is to obtain a complete history of the patient. Next, the veterinarian performs a thorough physical examination. After performing the physical examination, the vet will make a list of all the problems identified in the history and physical examination. The possible causes for each problem (compiled in a list called the **differential diagnosis**) are then evaluated. This evaluation usually involves a series of diagnostic tests. The results of these tests either support ("rule in") or eliminate ("rule out") the possible causes of a disorder. In some cases, diagnostic tests are necessary to narrow the number of possible causes and arrive at a **definitive** (final) **diagnosis.**

History

A detailed history is one of the most important ways to diagnose a skin problem correctly. The history should start with the pet's background. An animal's age, breed, and sex, referred to as the animal's **signalment**, may provide important clues about the cause of a problem. Many skin diseases are especially common in particular breeds or in animals of certain ages. You may hear your veteri-

The Systematic Approach to Dermatology

Steps in the systematic approach are as follows:

1. History: The veterinarian will take a complete history, including information about the pet's relatives, your family members, animals in contact with your pet, environmental factors (e.g., amount of time spent indoors/outdoors, activities, bedding, furniture, flooring), diet (including treats), appetite, elimination habits, activity level, first symptoms, progression of signs, previous diseases, previous treatments and responses, and current treatments.

2. Physical examination: The veterinarian will perform a thorough physical examination and a thorough dermatologic examination.

3. Listing of problems: The problem list will include abnormalities found in the history or on the physical examination.

4. Formulation of differential diagnoses: A list is made of possible causes for each problem on the problem list.

5. Correlation: The veterinarian evaluates the history and physical examination findings to prioritize the differential diagnoses, ranking them from the most likely to the least likely cause of each problem.

6. Screening diagnostic tests: Testing is performed to obtain results that support ("rule in") or eliminate ("rule out") the possible diagnoses for each problem. Common tests used in dermatology include trichograms, skin and ear cytology, skin scrapings, fungal and bacterial cultures, blood tests, urine tests, skin biopsies, allergy tests, diet trials, and a variety of treatment trials.

The Systematic Approach to Dermatology—cont'd

7. **Narrowing of differential diagnosis:** The results of each test are evaluated and used to rule in or rule out the possible causes of each problem. More tests are performed, and their results are evaluated until the veterinarian identifies a definite cause (definitive diagnosis).

8. **Evaluate options for treatment:** Your veterinarian may suggest a variety of options for treating the condition. You should discuss the advantages and disadvantages of each of these options with the vet.

9. **Make recommendations for follow up:** Because many dermatologic diseases require long-term management, it is important to schedule appointments for re-evaluation of the problem at the intervals recommended by the veterinarian.

narian use the terms *breed predisposition* or *relative risk* in referring to diagnostic clues in the signalment. For example, collies and Shetland sheepdogs are more likely than other breeds to have the hereditary skin disease **dermatomyositis**; Akitas and standard poodles are predisposed to the hereditary disease **sebaceous adenitis**. Dogs younger than 1 year of age are predisposed to juvenile-onset demodicosis (see Chapter 6); dogs older than 10 years are more likely than younger ones to have metabolic diseases (see Chapter 7) and cancers (see Chapter 13). Persian cats are predisposed to ringworm (see Chapter 8); Basset Hounds are predisposed to yeast infections (see Chapter 8.)

Symptoms that seem unrelated to your pet's skin disease may provide important clues to a veterinarian. For example, a dog that is losing hair and drinking and urinating much more than usual probably has **Cushing's disease**, but a cat with hair and weight loss that persists despite an increased appetite probably has **hyperthyroidism**.

It is important for you to give your veterinarian information about the events that occurred around the time you first noticed a skin lesion. For example, was the pet boarded? (It could have been exposed to **ectoparasites** or **ringworm**.) Which came first, the itching or the rash? (If the itching came first, the pet may have an **allergy**; if the rash came first, the problem may be caused by an infection.) The site on the body where symptoms first appeared can provide clues to the cause of the problem. Dogs with fleas usually begin chewing at the back and the rear legs, but dogs with environmental allergies usually begin chewing on their feet and also may rub their faces.

Your pet's bedding and other environmental factors can cause allergies or make your pet susceptible to certain parasitic infections. For example, one type of parasite, *Pelodera strongyloides*, is associated with straw bedding (see Chapter 6). Your veterinarian also will need to consider your pet's regular diet when designing a restrictive diet to help diagnose food allergies (see Chapter 4).

A list of previous treatments and the pet's response to them can be helpful. For example, many allergy symptoms improve after treatment with corticosteroids, but symptoms caused by a fungal infection worsen after this treatment. You should keep records of your pet's previous medications and any diagnostic tests and results because this information can help your veterinarian assess your pet's current problem.

Physical Examination

A pet with a skin disease should receive a full physical examination. Many skin diseases are caused by underlying medical diseases. Abnormalities found during a general physical examination can help identify underlying problems such as liver disease or cancer.

Dermatologic Examination

Next, the veterinarian will perform a thorough examination of every part of your pet's skin. The veterinarian will look for the following important features of the skin problem:

- **Distribution (lesions all over the body, in one place, or in several places; the same on both sides of the body, or asymmetric?)**
- **Progression (is the initial lesion a papule that progresses to a pustule and then to a crust?)**
- **Shape (are the lesions individual, or are they growing together; single or grouped; appearing as rings, lines, arcs, or in a snake-track pattern?)**
- **Depth (superficial, deep, ulcerated, or elevated)**
- **Consistency (solid, fluid-filled, soft, hard, thickened, or atrophied)**
- **Color (red, yellow, white, grey, black)**
- **Consistency (dry, moist, greasy, oozing, bleeding, purulent)**
- **Identification of primary lesions (see section on lesions later in this chapter)**
- **Identification of secondary lesions (see section on lesions later in this chapter)**
- **Careful evaluation of areas of alopecia (broken-off hairs, new hair growth; the ease with which hairs epilate, or pull out)**

Examination for Parasites

Fleas, **lice**, **ticks**, and chiggers often can be seen during a careful examination of the pet's skin and hair coat. A flea comb (see Chapter 6) may be used to remove these parasites for identification. You also can use a clear piece of **acetate tape** to catch parasites. The tape is placed under a microscope for further identi-

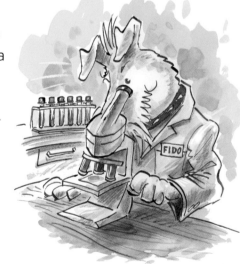

fication of the parasites (for example, head shape is used to distinguish biting lice from sucking lice, but the heads are so tiny that magnification is required.)

Many other parasites are too tiny to be seen without a microscope. Several of these parasites are not only tiny but also live below the surface of the skin. For example, some species (e.g., *Sarcoptes scabiei, Notoedres cati, Demodex gatoi*) tunnel in the superficial layer of the skin; others (e.g., *Demodex canis, Demodex cati, Pelodera strongyloides*) live inside the **hair follicles**. To find these mites, the veterinarian must perform **skin scrapings**. Because parasites are responsible for a variety of skin lesions, a skin scraping should be performed in most cases of skin disease.

The technique used to obtain skin scrapings varies according to the parasite that the veterinarian is trying to find. A few drops of mineral oil are placed on a glass slide. A scalpel blade is then moistened with the oil (mineral oil also may be placed directly on the pet's skin) and used to gently scrape the surface of the skin until it bleeds slightly. When searching for parasites that live in hair follicles, the veterinarian will gently squeeze the skin during the scraping to help bring the mites out of the follicles. When looking for *Sarcoptes* mites, the veterinarian makes multiple scrapings; sometimes as many as 25 are required to find a single mite. In many cases, the veterinarian will recommend a treatment trial to rule out *Sarcoptes* as a cause of skin disease (see Chapter 6).

The veterinarian obtains ear swabs using a long, cotton-tipped applicator stick (similar to the cotton-tipped swabs that people use) to collect debris from the ear canals. The veterinarian will mix the debris with mineral oil on a glass slide and observe it under a microscope to detect ear mites (*Otodectes cynotis*).

Some parasites are identified with a test called *fecal flotation*. The eggs of intestinal parasites are found in feces; feces also might contain mites or other parasites that the pet has ingested while grooming and passed through the digestive tract.

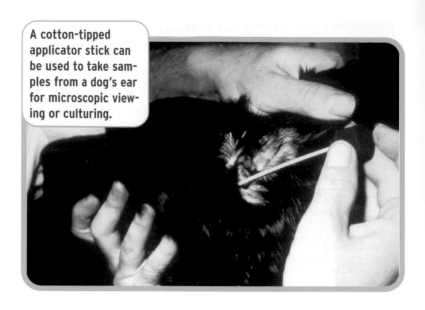

A cotton-tipped applicator stick can be used to take samples from a dog's ear for microscopic viewing or culturing.

Examination for Fungi/Yeasts

Several kinds of fungi cause diseases that affect the skin, ears, and hair of cats and dogs (see Chapter 8). Yeast are fungi, single-celled organisms that reproduce by budding. They are found in many superficial infections of the skin and ears (yeast occasionally causes infections of other body tissues, too). Yeast organisms are tiny and must be viewed under a microscope. The veterinarian can check a skin infection for yeast by pressing a glass slide to the skin surface, placing a piece of clear acetate tape on the skin, and then transferring the tape to a glass slide or taking a swab of the skin (or ears) and rolling it on a glass slide. The slide is then stained and examined under a microscope. Yeast appear as small round or budding cells that resemble miniature snowmen or footprints. The veterinarian can diagnose a yeast infection of deeper tissues by obtaining samples of those tissues using a biopsy instrument or a fine-needle aspirate (FNA). Fine-needle aspirates involve placing a needle in the tissue, often with a syringe attached to apply suction to help suck cells from the tissue into the needle. Next, an empty syringe is filled with air and attached to the syringe, and the air is quickly expelled through the needle and onto a glass slide. Cells in the needle are pushed out onto the glass slide and can be stained for identification under the microscope.

Dermatophytes, fungi that infect **keratin**, are found in hairs, claws, and the surface layer of skin. They cause circular areas of hair loss that often is called *ringworm* but is more correctly named *dermatophytosis* because the problem is caused by a dermatophyte fungus and not a worm. The species of dermatophytes that most commonly infects cats and dogs is *Microsporum canis*. About 50% of the strains (types) of *M. canis* produce a substance in hairs that glows apple-green or yellow under ultraviolet light. Your veterinarian will use a specialized ultraviolet light with a magnifying lens to screen your pet for *M. canis* infection. This specialized light, basically a black light, is called a **Wood's lamp**. If hairs glow apple-green, they are plucked and examined under a microscope or placed on a culture plate for confirmation of the infection because some medications and scaly-crusted material can give a false-positive reaction. Because not all dermatophyte species or even all strains of *M. canis* produce fluorescence, additional tests are used in diagnosing dermatophyte infections.

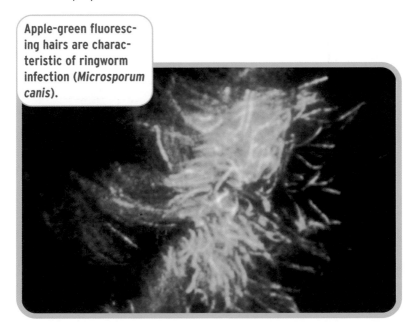

Apple-green fluorescing hairs are characteristic of ringworm infection (*Microsporum canis*).

The veterinarian can pluck hairs and observe them under a microscope to identify dermatophyte spores around the hairs and dermatophyte hyphae (elongated forms of the organisms) in the hair shafts. The hairs usually are placed in several drops of potassium hydroxide (KOH) on the slide to help show the spores and hyphae in a procedure called a *KOH prep*. Unfortunately, even with the help of KOH, the spores and hyphae are difficult to see without special stains. In most cases, a fungal culture also is required to identify the organisms.

Fungal cultures for the identification of dermatophyte infections use a specialized type of culture medium called **dermatophyte test medium** (DTM). Hairs are plucked from around areas of hair loss or obtained by brushing the pet with a sterile toothbrush. Then the hairs are placed on the DTM, and the culture plate (or bottle) is watched for fungal growth. Dermatophytes growing on DTM form a white, fluffy colony and cause the DTM to change from yellow to red. The change in growth and color may require 1 to 4 weeks, although usually it takes 10 to 14 days. The colonies produce spores called **macroconidia**, which can be examined under a microscope to identify the species of dermatophyte growing on the cul-

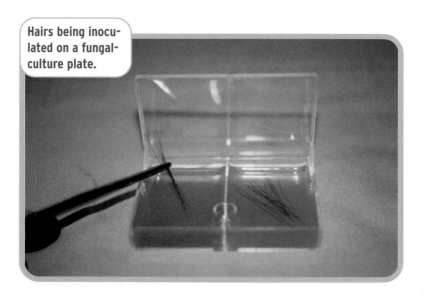

Hairs being inoculated on a fungal-culture plate.

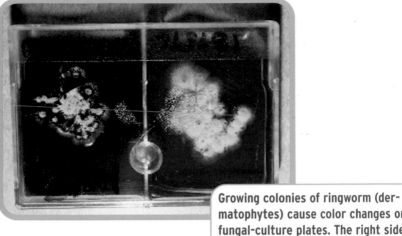

Growing colonies of ringworm (dermatophytes) cause color changes on fungal-culture plates. The right side of this plate contains dermatophyte test medium that has changed from yellow to red as the colony has grown.

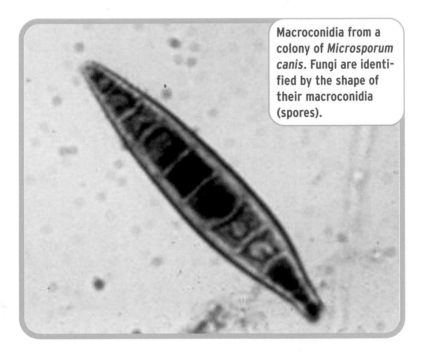

Macroconidia from a colony of *Microsporum canis*. Fungi are identified by the shape of their macroconidia (spores).

ture. Knowledge of the particular species is important in determining the source of the infection (see Chapter 8).

Examination for Bacteria

Bacteria often are involved in skin and ear infections (see Chapter 5). **Cytologic examination** of material from the skin surface or from **exudates** in the ears is used to screen for bacterial infections. Four techniques are commonly employed in obtaining material for cytologic examination:

- **Pressing a glass slide onto the surface of the skin lesion; debris on the skin surface sticks to the glass. This is called a direct impression smear.**
- **Using a piece of clear acetate tape and pressing it onto the skin surface. Superficial skin cells and surface debris stick to the tape, which is then pulled off the skin and placed on a glass slide.**
- **Rolling a cotton-tipped swab on the skin surface or in the ear canal; the swab is then rolled on a slide, leaving the material there.**
- **FNA, which we've already discussed (page 48).**

Once material is on the glass slide, it is stained and examined under a microscope. Different stains can be used to identify different kinds of bacteria. **Diff-Quick** stains turn all bacteria blue. **Gram's staining** separates bacteria into groups, **Gram-negative** and **Gram-positive**. **Acid fast staining** can help identify certain strains of bacteria as being acid-fast or nonstaining with acidic stains.

In some cases, the veterinarian will perform a **microbiology culture and susceptibility test**. Samples are obtained from skin lesions or the ears with a swab, needle aspiration, or tissue biopsy. These samples are sent to a laboratory, where the bacteria are grown on special culture plates. The laboratory performs a series of tests to identify the species of bacteria causing the infection and to determine the types of antibiotics that will be most effective in killing each type of bacteria.

Examination of Masses

Masses may be caused by infections (bacterial, fungal, or parasitic), foreign bodies, cysts, and benign or malignant tumors. Determining the cause of a mass generally involves cytologic examination or biopsies and sometimes bacterial and fungal cultures. The veterinarian may take samples for cytologic examination using a direct-impression smear or an FNA.

Skin Biopsies

Skin biopsies can be helpful in diagnosing the cause of a skin lesion. The veterinarian will probably recommend a skin biopsy when any of the following six criteria are present:

- **The history, physical examination, and laboratory tests have not led to a definitive diagnosis.**
- **The lesions suggest an immune-mediated disease (see Chapter 9).**
- **The lesions suggest a neoplastic disease (e.g., cancer; see Chapter 13).**
- **The lesions are unusual or appear serious.**
- **The skin condition has not responded to what the veterinarian thought was the appropriate therapy.**
- **A deep-tissue sample is needed for bacterial or fungal cultures.**

Most skin biopsies can be obtained with just a local anesthetic. General anesthesia usually is necessary for samples from areas around the eyes, lips, nose, or feet. General anesthesia also may be needed if the dog or cat is especially nervous or hard to restrain. If more than one kind or stage of lesion is present, several samples should be obtained. Most skin biopsies are taken with a special skin-biopsy punch, which removes a piece of tissue the diameter of a pencil. The hole that remains after the biopsy is taken is closed with a stitch or two. In some cases, the veterinarian will recommend taking a larger elliptical piece of skin instead of using a punch for the biopsy. Small masses may be removed completely; this is called an **excisional** biopsy. The samples are sent to a laboratory, where thin slices of the tissue are cut, placed on a glass slide, and stained for evaluation by a **pathologist** (usually a veterinarian with extensive training in the microscopic evaluation of various tissues). The microscopic evaluation of a biopsy sample is called **histopathology**.

Allergy Testing

Dogs and cats may develop allergies to a wide variety of substances in the foods they eat, the environment around them, the medications they are given, or parasites that infest their skin or internal organs. The preferred diagnostic test for food allergies is called a **restrictive diet trial** (see Chapter 4). Testing for environmental allergies may include skin-allergy testing, allergen-specific serum IgE blood tests, patch tests, and avoidance followed by **provocative exposure** (see Chapter 4).

Hormone Testing

Dogs and cats can develop a variety of hormonal deficiencies, excesses, or imbalances. These are called **endocrine** disorders or **endocrinopathies**. Some hormonal disorders affect the skin and hair coat. **Hypothyroidism** is a fairly common endocrine disorder in dogs. A reduced production of thyroid hormones causes hair growth to fail, with a symmetric alopecia (hair loss) on both sides of the body. Hyperadrenocorticism, or Cushing's disease, is another common endocrine disorder in dogs; it is caused by excessive amounts of corticosteroids. Skin changes in hyperadrenocorticism include thinning of the skin, alopecia, easy bruising, frequent skin infections, and, in some cases, calcified areas of skin (referred to as **calcinosis cutis**). Hyperthyroidism, the most common endocrine disorder in older cats, can cause alopecia and abnormally long claws. Your veterinarian can diagnose hypothyroidism or hyperthyroidism by measuring the level of thyroid hormone in circulation. The vet may need to run a series of blood tests and obtain an abdominal ultrasound to diagnose hyperadrenocorticism (see Chapter 7).

Immunologic Testing

Dogs and cats are affected by several types of immunologic problems. **Immunodeficiencies** may result in recurrent bacterial or fungal infections or in generalized **demodicosis**. A hyperactive immune system may result in allergies. In some cases, the immune system becomes misdirected and starts attacking parts of the animal's own body, resulting in an **autoimmune** disease or **immune-mediated disease** (see Chapter 9). Tests to evaluate the function of the immune system include the following:

- **Complete blood count (with particular attention paid to the numbers of the various kinds of white blood cells)**
- **Immunoglobulin quantitation (in which levels of the various classes of antibodies produced by the pet are measured)**
- **Lymphocyte blastogenesis test (which measures the reactivity of the pet's lymphocytes) and neutrophil-function tests (to determine whether one of the kinds of white blood cells is effective in killing microorganisms)**

Tests to find autoimmune or immune-mediated diseases include the following:

- **Specialized blood tests (for example, the antinuclear antibody test, or ANA)**
- **Urine electrophoresis (to evaluate any proteins being excreted in the urine)**
- **Skin biopsies (to identify changes that indicate a given disease)**

Specialized tests also can be performed to detect antibodies against various parts of the skin. Chapter 9 contains additional information about these tests.

Treatment Trials

If other tests have not shown a diagnosis, the veterinarian can use a treatment trial to help determine the cause of a pet's skin disease. For example, the best way to prove that fleas are the cause of skin disease is to start a program of flea treatment and prevention. If symptoms such as itching and skin rash disappear after fleas are eliminated, it can be assumed that fleas were the cause, and no more diagnostic testing is needed. Another common example of a treatment trial is the use of a **scabicide** to find out whether a dog has **sarcoptic mange** (see Chapter 6). Sometimes more than one problem is present at the same time. For example, a pet may have a food allergy *and* a bacterial skin infection. A treatment trial with antibiotics to eliminate the bacterial infection is needed before the severity of the food allergy can be assessed. More than one treatment may be administered at the same time. For example, the pet may be started on antibiotics and a restrictive diet trial. The veterinarian will check the skin disease after the pet finishes antibiotic treatment and then recommend "challenge feeding" the pet its original diet to determine the role food allergies played in the skin disease (see Chapter 4 for more information on feeding trials for the diagnosis of food allergies).

Skin Lesions (Primary and Secondary)

Skin lesions are classified as being primary or secondary:

- **Primary lesions develop as a direct result of the underlying disease and may be a good indication of specific diseases.**
- **Secondary lesions may be caused when the pet scratches, chews, or rubs, resulting in skin trauma, or they may represent the last stage of a primary lesion that is healing. These lesions are rarely a sign of a particular disease, but they may help the veterinarian chart the progression of a disease.**

Alopecia (Hair Loss)

Alopecia may result from a lack of hair growth or may occur when hairs break off or stop growing. Because alopecia has many causes, a variety of diagnostic tests may be necessary. These tests may include skin scrapings, skin cytology, trichogram (hair plucks), fungal (DTM) cultures, antibiotic treatment trials, blood tests (hormone assays), and skin biopsies.

A trichogram involves plucking hairs so that the veterinarian can examine their structure. Hairs are firmly grasped with tweezers or a **hemostat**, then firmly pulled from their follicles. The hairs are placed on a glass slide

Primary Skin Lesions*

Lesion	Definition	Associated Diseases
Bulla	A fluid-filled elevation in the skin more than 1 cm wide	Immune-mediated diseases, hereditary defects in the dermal-epidermal junction (epidermolysis bullosa), burns
Calcinosis	Deposition of mineral salts in a tissue; is called "calcinosis cutis" when in the skin	Hyperadrenocorticism or idiopathic (calcinosis circumscripta)
Comedo	A dilated hair follicle filled with solidified cells and sebum	Acne, vitamin A-responsive dermatosis, Schnauzer comedo syndrome, hyperadrenocorticism, demodicosis, dermatophytosis
Cyst	A nodule containing fluid or semisolid material	Acne, epidermal inclusion cyst, follicular cyst
Folliculitis	Inflammation of the hair follicles	Bacterial infections, dermatophyte infection, demodicosis
Macule	A distinctive flat lesion where the skin has changed color	Pigmented nevus, lentigo, purpura, petechia, vitiligo

*These conditions develop as a direct result of a disease.

Primary Skin Lesions—cont'd

Lesion	Definition	Associated Diseases
Papule	A small, firm elevation of the skin, often pink or red, caused by inflammation	Allergies, insect bite or sting, early stage of a bacterial infection
Patch	An isolated flat change in skin color that is more than 1 cm wide	Ecchymosis (bleeding in skin) also possible after skin irritation; vitiligo
Plaque	A flat-topped, solid elevation of the skin more than 0.5 cm high; persists days or weeks	Eosinophilic plaques (allergic reaction pattern of cats)
Pustule	A small, pus-filled elevation in the skin	Bacterial infections, immune-mediated diseases
Telangiectasia	Small, dilated superficial blood vessel	Associated with Cushing's disease, dermatomyositis, and cutaneous lupus erythematosus
Tumor	A firm swelling in the skin that may extend into deeper tissues	Chronic or severe inflammation (granulomas) or neoplasia (cancer)
Vesicle	A small, fluid-filled elevation in the skin	Immune-mediated diseases, viral infections
Wheal	A flat-topped elevation in the skin caused by edema that disappears within minutes or hours	Allergies, hives, insect bites or stings

Secondary Skin Lesions*

Lesion	Definition	Associated Diseases
Crust	A collection of cell debris, dried weeping serum, inflammatory cells, or blood	May follow injury to the skin or as a regressing stage of a ruptured pustule, vesicle, or bulla
Epidermal collarette	A circular layer of peeling epidermal scales	Develops after the rupture of a pustule, vesicle, or bulla
Erosion	An area of partial loss of epidermis; does not extend through the full thickness of the skin	Scrapes or other localized damage to skin
Excoriation	Linear erosions caused by scratching	Any itch-causing disease
Fissure	Vertical split in the epidermis and dermis	May develop in excessively thickened areas of skin, nose, or footpads
Fistula	An abnormal passage between a structure and the body surface or between two structures	Often appears as a track draining to the skin surface after rupture of a hair follicle
Furunculosis	Severe inflammation surrounding a ruptured hair follicle	Usually associated with severe folliculitis in which hair follicles rupture

*These lesions are produced by trauma to the skin or are the end stage of a regressing primary lesion.

Secondary Skin Lesions—cont'd

Lesion	Definition	Associated Diseases
Hyperpigmentation	Darkening of the skin caused by an increase in melanin pigment	Any chronic dermatitis; hormone imbalances
Hyperkeratosis	An increased thickness of the horny layer of skin	Any chronic dermatitis; hormone imbalances
Lichenification	Thickening and hardening of the skin, usually from chronic irritation or friction	Chronic allergic dermatitis, chronic *Malassezia* dermatitis
Scale	Accumulations of the stratum corneum (horny layer of skin)	Result of chronic irritation to the skin, nutritional deficiencies or imbalances
Scar	An area where damaged skin has been replaced with fibrous connective tissue	Healing stage of ulcers and cuts or tears of the skin
Ulcer	A full-thickness loss of skin	Severe trauma or damage to the skin

Causes of Alopecia in Dogs and Cats

Cause	Hairs Growing?	Examples of Diseases in This Category
Congenital defects in hair-follicle development	No	Localized: ectodermal defects Generalized: breeds prone to hair loss
Itching disorders with self-induced loss of hair	Yes	Allergies (environmental, dietary, parasitic); psychogenic
Infections involving the hair follicles	Yes	*Staphylococci, Demodex,* dermatophytes
Inflammation around hair follicles (immune-mediated)	Variable	Alopecia areata, sebaceous adenitis, dermatomyositis, postinjection alopecia (rabies vaccine)
Abnormalities in hair follicles (atrophic or distorted)	Variable	Color-dilution alopecia, black hair follicle alopecia, recurrent flank alopecia (focal follicular dysplasia), alopecia X, pattern baldness, dermatomyositis, postinjection alopecia (rabies vaccine), neoplastic alopecia
Endocrine diseases	No	Hypothyroidism, hyperadrenocorticism, sex-hormone imbalances, pituitary dwarfism, alopecia X?
Miscellaneous	Variable	Telogen defluxion, anagen defluxion

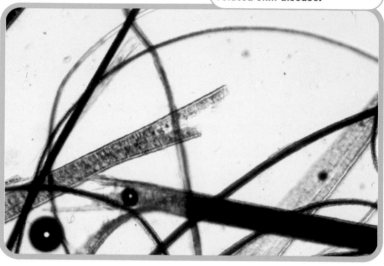

and examined under a microscope. The hair shafts are evaluated for fraying or breaking (which shows that the pet is chewing off the hairs or that the hairs are breaking because they are unusually fragile), excessive clumping of **melanin** (a feature of **color-mutant hair dysplasia**), or evidence of dermatophytes (**spores** or fungal **hyphae** around or inside the hair shafts). The ends of the hairs are examined to see whether the hair is **anagen** (growing) or **telogen** (nongrowing) hair. A telogen hairs has a clubbed root end; an anagen hair often has a hook at its end.

Itching (Pruritus)

Pruritus is defined as an unpleasant sensation within the skin that causes the desire to scratch. **Itching** is a sensation that results from the stimulation of nerve endings in the skin; it is signaled by scratching, chewing, and rubbing at the affected area. Excessive itching and scratching can cause real damage to the skin and hair coat. Pruritus has many causes in animals. The mnemonic **PAIN** can be used to remember possible contributors to itching:

Parasites: fleas, mites, lice, flies, and other ectoparasites (see Chapter 6)

Allergies: environmental, food, drug, or parasitic allergens (see Chapter 4)

Inflammatory (**I**nfections, **I**rritants, **I**mmune-mediated diseases): bacterial and fungal infections, topical irritants, and immune-mediated diseases (see Chapters 5, 8, and 9)

Neurogenic, **N**eoplastic: includes obsessive-compulsive disorders, problems associated with nerve damage, and pruritus associated with certain skin tumors (see Chapters 11 and 18)

Ear Diseases

The skin lining the ear canal may be affected by the same diseases that cause lesions in other areas of the skin. In addition, the warm, moist, dark environment inside the ear canal encourages the growth of bacteria and yeast. Therefore it is not surprising that many dogs and cats are affected by ear disease. Factors that contribute to ear disease are classified as predisposing, primary, or perpetuating (see Chapter 12). Symptoms of ear disease include the following:

- **Black, red, brown, or yellow exudate in the ear**
- **Head-shaking; scratching or rubbing of the ears**
- **Loss of hearing**
- **Pain when the ears are touched**
- **An offensive smell coming from the ears; redness of the ear flaps**
- **A blood-filled pocket on the inside of the ear pinna (aural hematoma)**
- **Holding one side of the head lower than the other**
- **Circling or rolling in one direction**

For more information on ear diseases, see Chapter 12.

Nail Diseases

The horny covering of the **nail** is analogous to the **stratum corneum** of the skin (see Chapter 1). Because the nails grow only about 1 mm per week, recovery from diseases that affect the nails is very slow. Common problems of the nails include trauma, bacterial infection, fungal infection, immune-mediated skin diseases (including one that involves only the nails–**symmetric lupoid onychodystrophy**; see Chapter 9), and neoplastic diseases (e.g., cancers). Symptoms of nail disease include the following:

- **Pain (reluctance to walk)**
- **Swollen toes**
- **Softening (onychomalacia) and splitting (onychorrhexis, onychoschizia) of the nails**
- **Pus around the base of the nails (paronychia)**
- **Abnormal growth of the nails (onychodystrophy)**
- **Sloughing of the nails (onychomadesis)**

The diagnosis of nail disorders may involve cytology, cultures (bacterial and fungal), X-rays, and biopsies (in some cases, the toe must be removed for **histopathologic** evaluation).

Summary

Disorders of the skin and related structures (hair, nails, and ears) can produce many symptoms. Some of these disorders are life-threatening, and others are merely cosmetic. A systematic approach is required to sort through the possible causes of each symptom and arrive at the definitive diagnosis. In this chapter, we've discussed the steps involved in a systematic approach to diagnosing dermatologic diseases, reviewed the diagnostic procedures that are commonly used in veterinary dermatology, and covered the differential diagnoses of the most common symptoms of dermatologic disease.

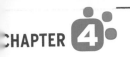
ALLERGIES

Dogs and cats can suffer from allergic reactions to many different substances, including **pollen, mold,** mites, and dust in the environment, the foods they eat, and parasites. If a particular substance always triggers an allergic reaction, the affected animal (or person) is said to have an allergy to that substance. Signs and symptoms of allergies in people include "hay fever" (sneezing, sinus congestion), asthma (coughing, wheezing), increased tear production (watery eyes), itchy skin, rashes, **hives,** vomiting, and diarrhea. The most common symptom of allergies in dogs is severe itching. Other signs in dogs may include recurrent ear infections, recurrent skin infections, foot chewing, face rubbing, red eyes, hives, vomiting, and diarrhea. Cats may overgroom, resulting in a bald belly, or may show intense itching, or various bumps and crusts may develop on their skin.

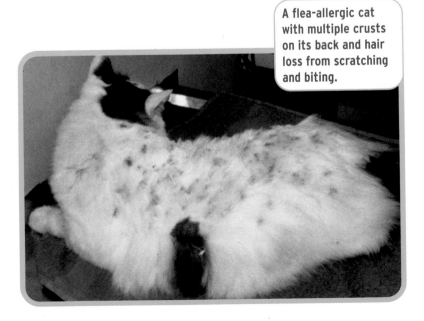

A flea-allergic cat with multiple crusts on its back and hair loss from scratching and biting.

An **allergy** is defined as an altered state of reactivity. The **immune system** is primarily responsible for protecting the body from harmful substances. A substance that can trigger a reaction of the immune system—an **immune response**—is called an **antigen.** Antigens usually are proteins present in substances found in the environment, in foods, or within bodies of parasites. These substances may be harmless in nonallergic animals but can cause problems in allergic animals because their immune system "overreacts" to certain antigens. In allergic animals the immune system makes special **antibodies** called **immunoglobulin E** (IgE). A different IgE antibody is formed for each antigen. The IgE antibodies then bind (attach) to specialized cells known as **mast cells.** Mast cells are most numerous in the skin of dogs and cats (and in the nose and respiratory tract of people). Inside mast cells are granules containing **hist-amine** and many other chemicals that can cause intense **inflammation** (redness, heat, swelling, and pain) in body tissues. When a mast cell coated with IgE comes in contact with the IgE-specific antigen (the one that caused that particular IgE antibody to be formed), degranulation occurs—the cell lets its granules "dump" their contents. During degranulation, histamine and other inflammatory substances are released into the surrounding tissues, producing redness, heat, swelling, and pain (or itching).

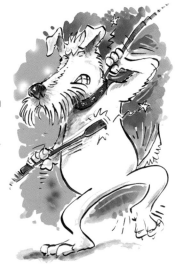

Allergies affect 10% to 25% of dogs and 5% to 15% of cats; therefore, many pet owners have had personal experience in dealing with an allergic pet. Many animals suffer from more than one type of allergy, so identifying **allergens** (anything that can set off an allergic reaction) is not simple, and effective treatments may be hard to find. If your pet is allergic, you should seek guidance from your veterinarian or a specialist in veterinary dermatology.*

Atopy

Definition

The term **atopy** is derived from a Greek word meaning "uncommon" or "out of the way"—in animals or people with atopy, reactions to antigenic substances are especially rapid or severe. This condition is a **familial** predisposition (inherited tendency) to develop IgE antibodies, with resulting allergy to environmental antigens. The antigens may be inhaled (the main route of exposure in people), absorbed through the skin (**percutaneous** absorption—the most common route of exposure in animals)—or ingested.

Inheritance

The predisposition to develop IgE antibodies is hereditary. In humans, if both parents have atopy, there is an 80% probability that their children also will be affected; this drops to 60% if only one parent has atopy. The risks are similar in dogs, and many breed predispositions are recognized. The following breeds are generally at high risk of developing atopy:

- **Boxer**
- **Golden Retriever**
- **West Highland White Terrier**
- **Dalmatian**
- **Chinese Shar-Pei**
- **Cairn Terrier**
- **Scottish Terrier**
- **Lhasa Apso**
- **Boston Terrier**
- **Sealyham Terrier**
- **Wire-Haired Fox Terrier**
- **Cocker Spaniel**
- **Bulldog**

*The American College of Veterinary Dermatology (ACVD) is a group of veterinarian specialists who have completed rigorous training in veterinary dermatology and allergies. For more information and for the location of an ACVD board-certified veterinarian near you, visit http://www.acvd.org.

- American Staffordshire Terrier
- German Shepherd Dog
- Pug
- Irish Setter
- English Setter
- Miniature Schnauzer

The incidence of disease in a given breed varies with areas of the state, country, and world because of differences in gene pools in different regions. Atopy can develop in dogs of any breed and in mixed-breed dogs. Breed predispositions have not been established for cats.

Age at Onset

Clinical signs of atopy in dogs usually develop between the ages of 6 months and 3 years. Signs sometimes are seen in dogs as young as 3 months, but this is uncommon because IgE antibody levels at this age usually are not yet high enough to trigger mast cell degranulation. When allergies develop at a very young age, additional allergies are likely to develop over the lifetime of the affected animal. After several seasons of exposure to allergens, however, development of new allergies in a dog is rare unless it moves into a new environment. Age predispositions have not been defined for cats.

Clinical Signs in Dogs

The initial signs of atopy may be very mild. These may include foot licking, face rubbing, redness of the ears, and scratching or licking at the **axillae** ("armpits") and the underside of the abdomen (the belly). Over time, these symptoms become more severe, and additional areas of the body become affected. The inflammation caused by mast cell degranulation, and made worse by the dog's scratching and licking, creates a warm, moist environment that encourages the growth of bacteria and **yeasts**. Large numbers of bacteria or yeast increase the inflammation of the skin, which increases the growth of the organisms and causes more inflammation—a vicious circle. Additionally, the inflamed skin absorbs more antigens from the environment, worsening the situation. In many dogs, a strong "body odor" and "ear odor" develop with growth of organisms on the skin and in the ears. The skin gradually becomes thickened and darker. Constant scratching and biting may result in extensive hair loss. In areas where the dog licks, white hairs will become stained a reddish brown by **porphyrins** in saliva.

Hair loss, skin thickening (lichenification), and hyperpigmentation (darkening) involving the axillae ("armpits") and front legs of a West Highland White Terrier with chronic allergies.

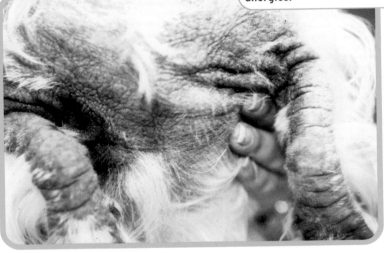

Reddish brown staining of the axilla ("armpit") of a Dalmatian. The staining is from porphyrins in saliva deposited during chronic licking of this area.

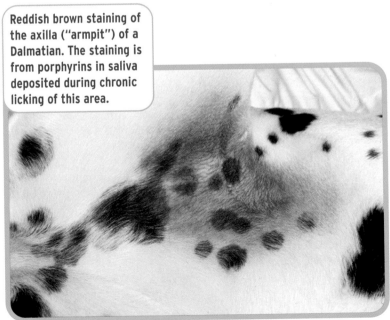

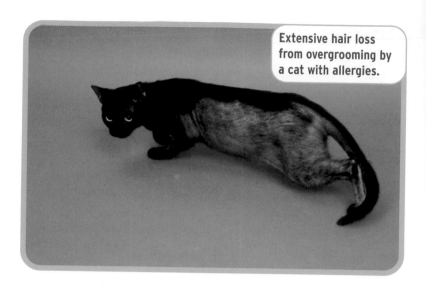

Extensive hair loss from overgrooming by a cat with allergies.

Clinical Signs of Atopy

Signs in Dogs

Pruritus—biting, scratching, chewing, licking

Hair loss

Hyperhidrosis (sweating)

Affected areas: feet, face, axillae (armpits), ventral abdomen/groin, ears

Secondary infections: bacterial and/or yeast infections of skin and/or ears

Secondary skin changes: hyperpigmentation (darkening), lichenification (thickening)

Signs in Cats

Pruritus—biting, scratching, chewing, licking (overgrooming)

Hair loss (bald belly or thighs)

Miliary dermatitis

Indolent ulcer

Eosinophilic plaque

Eosinophilic granuloma

Clinical Signs in Cats

Allergies in cats produce several types of disease:

- **Alopecia (hair loss)**
- **Scratching—especially of the head and neck regions**
- **Miliary dermatitis (scattered crusted skin bumps)**
- **Lip ulcers (indolent ulcers, rodent ulcers)**
- **Eosinophilic plaques**
- **Eosinophilic granulomas**

A cat's tongue has tiny barbs that catch on hairs and pull them out during grooming. Many owners do not recognize when a cat is overgrooming because cats do much of their grooming in private (when no one is watching). Because self-grooming is a normal feline behavior and does not appear to be self-destructive, it is not as alarming as scratching and chewing. But a cat that is overgrooming can pull out so much hair that the belly or thighs become bald. One way to confirm that the cat is pulling its hair out while grooming is to check for hair in its stool (feces). Another method to confirm that hair loss is due to overgrooming is to prevent the cat from grooming by putting it in a "body suit" or a cone-shaped collar (Elizabethan collar). Some cats with allergies exhibit itching and scratching; the face and neck are often affected.

Miliary dermatitis is a skin reaction to allergies that results in small **papules** (pinpoint-sized bumps) that become crusted. If your cat has miliary dermatitis, running your hand over its back will feel like there are millet seeds in its fur (*miliary* means "millet-like"). In other cats with allergies, ulcerations may develop on the upper lip. These are called **indolent ulcers** or "rodent ulcers." Another possible skin reaction in cats is formation of **eosinophilic plaques**—red, raised lesions that contain a type of white blood cell with granules that stain red with eosin dye—hence the name **eosinophil** ("eosin lover"). Eosinophils are the white blood cells responsible for protecting the body from parasites; they also are attracted to areas of skin where mast cells degranulate, so they are found in the skin of animals with allergies. Formation of

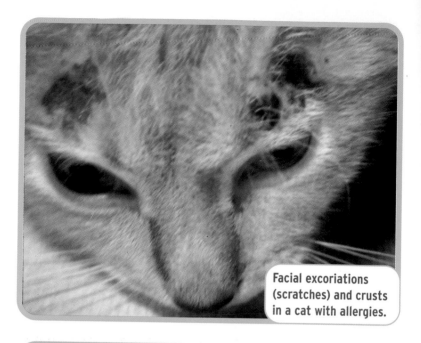

Facial excoriations (scratches) and crusts in a cat with allergies.

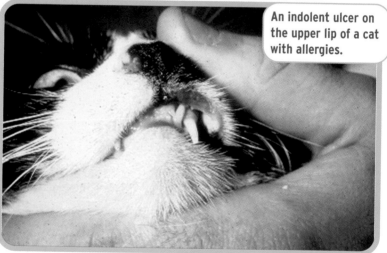

An indolent ulcer on the upper lip of a cat with allergies.

eosinophilic granulomas (skin nodules composed of large numbers of eosinophils) also may occur. All of these patterns of skin reactions can be found in association with atopy, but also with flea allergies and food allergies in cats.

Seasonality

Numerous allergenic pollens, molds, and other particles are present in the environment. Pollens and molds are found in highest concentrations from spring to fall, so allergies often begin during these months. Approximately 75% of dogs have seasonal exacerbation (worsening) of symptoms associated with allergies. Over time, the symptoms tend to worsen and may eventually become a problem year-round.

An interesting finding is that in the northern hemisphere, atopy is more common among puppies born during the months of May, August, and December. These puppies have increased exposure to pollens during their first 4 months of life: those born in May to grass pollens, those born in August to weed pollens, and those born in December to tree pollens.

General Characteristics of Allergens

Allergens are complex particles containing many different molecules, not all of which cause allergic reactions. Significant allergens have two important properties: They can trigger IgE production, and they can reach the site where mast cells are located (in the dermis of cats and dogs, in the respiratory tract of humans). Thus, allergens must be antigenic (capable of triggering an allergic reaction), dispersible (typically wind-borne), absorbable (of a size that can penetrate the skin or be inhaled), and present in sufficient amounts in the environment (must be a source for exposure).

Characteristics of Allergens

- Small enough particle size to be absorbed through skin, digestive tract, or respiratory tract
- Present in the environment
- Plentiful supply (e.g., wind-pollinating plants generally produce largest amounts of pollens)
- Ability to produce an IgE immunological response

Important Allergens Affecting Dogs and Cats

Danders
- Cat
- Cow
- Dog
- Feathers
- Horse
- Human
- Mouse
- Sheep (wool)

Environmental Allergens
- Cotton linters
- Cottonseed
- House dust
- House dust mites (Dermatophagoides)
- Pyrethrum (from chrysanthemums and in some flea-control products)
- Kapok
- Tobacco smoke

Insect Allergens
- Ants
- Flies
- Mosquitoes
- Moths
- Roaches

Grass Allergens
- Alfalfa
- Bermuda grass
- Bluegrass
- Corn
- Johnson grass
- Orchard grass
- Redtop
- Rye grasses
- Timothy
- Sweet vernal

Important Allergens Affecting Dogs and Cats—cont'd

Tree Allergens

- Birch
- Elm
- Juniper
- Maple
- Mulberry
- Oak
- Pecan
- Pine
- Sawdust/wood dust

Weed Allergens

- Cocklebur
- Dandelion
- Dock
- English plantain
- Goldenrod
- Lamb's quarters
- March elder
- Pigweed
- Ragweed
- Sorrels
- Western water hemp

Molds

- Alternaria
- Aspergillus
- Botrytis
- Cephalosporium
- Cladosporium
- Curvularia
- Fusarium
- Helminthosporium
- Hormodendrum
- Mucor
- Penicillium
- Phoma (Acremonium)
- Pullularia
- Rhizopus
- Smuts (grass, grain)
- Stemphylium

Pollens as Allergens

Pollen is essential for the reproduction of seed plants. Pollen is spread from one flower to another by wind, insects, or a combination of both. Wind-driven pollination is less effective, so plants that depend on this type of pollination produce the most pollen (a single tree may produce millions of pollen grains). Although some pollen will reach the target flower, most pollen ends up on the ground. Dogs and cats walking through yards and fields are exposed to massive amounts of pollens. Pollen often is released a few hours after sunrise and becomes airborne by mid-day. Wind-blown pollens can travel for hundreds of miles, although the concentrations will be highest near the pollinating plant. Although pollination seasons usually are short, pollen particles continue to be recirculated by wind for long periods.

Trees

Trees begin pollinating very early in the year. Some conifers (cone-bearing trees—usually evergreens) pollinate in the winter, and most deciduous trees (the ones that drop their leaves in autumn) begin pollinating before leaf development begins in the spring. Conifers produce large quantities of pollens. Pollen grains from pines, spruces, true cedars, black hemlock, and golden larch are large, so these trees rarely cause allergies in people. But these pollens may be more allergenic in dogs and cats because of the different routes of exposure (through the skin in pets versus inhalation in humans). Junipers, red cedar, mountain cedar, and ornamental yews produce pollen with smaller grains that can be allergenic in both people and pets. Deciduous trees that produce allergenic pollens include:

- Maples
- Oaks
- Willows
- Poplars
- Aspens
- Cottonwoods
- Hickories
- Pecans
- Walnuts
- Butternuts
- Hazelnuts
- Elms
- Ashes
- Olive trees
- Maples
- Box elders
- Mulberries

Insect-pollinating trees such as apple and peach trees are not important causes of allergies because little pollen reaches the ground.

Grasses

There are over 4500 species of wind-pollinating grasses. In temperate regions of the United States, the peak pollen season is from mid-May to mid-July. Bluegrass, rye grasses, orchard grass, timothy, Johnson grass, and redtop are common causes of allergies in pets living in the northeastern two thirds of the United States. Bermuda grass is an important cause of allergies in the southern states and along the Pacific coast. Owners should remember that "grass allergies" are to the grass *pollen* and not to the grass itself—so mowing the yard before seedheads are produced will protect your pet from "true" grass allergies (but not from molds and tree pollens, which often are found in high concentrations on grass leaves).

Weeds

Weeds typically are small plants that grow wild and produce enormous quantities of pollen. Some families of weeds include over 20,000 species, so it is easy to understand why these plants can be important in causing allergies. Ragweed is the major cause of hay fever in humans and also can cause allergies in dogs and cats. Other weeds commonly associated with allergies include:

- English plantain
- Lamb's quarters
- Mugworts
- Pigweed
- Western water hemp
- Sorrels
- Sagebrushes
- Marsh elder
- Cocklebur
- Asters
- Goldenrod
- Sneezeweed
- Dog fennel
- Russian thistle
- Kochia (burning bush)
- Dandelions

Note that dandelions are not a common source of allergy for humans, as the pollen grains are large and rarely inhaled. Dogs and cats may be more susceptible, however, because of their close contact with dandelion pollen on the ground. Many cultivated flowers, including chrysanthemums, dahlias, and marigolds, are primarily insect pollinated, so they typically do not cause allergies unless the pet has close contact with them (such as when a cat or dog likes to sleep in flowerbeds).

Molds as Allergens

Molds are found almost everywhere in the environment—both indoors and outdoors. Outdoor molds are most abundant during the summer; however, indoor molds are present throughout the year. *Penicillium*, *Aspergillus*, and *Rhizopus* are common causes of "mildew" in houses and also are found in soil and on plants, breads, cheeses, and damp surfaces. *Alternaria* is one of the most allergenic molds. It grows on plants and plant materials (vegetables, grains, and fruits). *Pullularia* grows on decaying vegetation and is abundant in grass clippings; it also can grow on damp wood, paper, and paint and in caulking compounds. *Cladosporium* produces large numbers of **spores** and is found on decaying plants, damp wood, leather, rubber, cloth, and paper products. *Curvularia* grows on grasses. Many dogs and cats suspected of having "grass allergies" are allergic to *Curvularia* and not to the grass itself. *Epicoccum* grows on grasses and other plant materials including vegetables and fruits. *Helminthosporium* grows on grasses and cereal grain plants (such as wheat and oats). *Stemphylium* grows on vegetable plants, decaying plant material, and damp paper, canvas, and textiles. *Mucor* grows in organic debris and thrives on animal waste (feces). *Phoma* grows on damp paper (books, magazines) and some plants. Some researchers believe **mold spores** are weak allergens; others believe mold spores are important causes of allergies in dogs and cats.

Danders as Allergens

Animals and humans constantly shed hair and dead skin cells (danders) into the environment (see Chapter 1).

Danders are proteins with multiple antigenic molecules. Animal danders often are contaminated with saliva, serum (the liquid part of blood), or urine, any of which can serve as an additional source of allergens. Hairs are too large to be absorbed through the skin or respiratory tract; however, they are often coated with saliva and occasionally with serum or urine, which may flake off from hairs and be absorbed. Many people are allergic to proteins found in the saliva of cats. Also, some dogs are allergic to cats, and vice versa. On average, one person produces 5 grams (about 1 teaspoon) of dander per week. Thus, pets are exposed to large amounts of human dander; in some instances, allergy to the owner's skin may develop. Wool is irritating, and many reactions to sheepskin and wool result from irritation, rather than from true allergy.

House Dust and Allergies

House dust contains numerous allergenic substances including bacteria, animal danders, human dander, molds, insect body parts and feces, plant fragments, food particles, fabric fibers and dust, and mites. More than 35 species of mites have been found in house dust; however, *Dermatophagoides* species are the most important. Mites feed on epidermal debris (skin flakes) from people and animals (skin renews itself every 3 to 4 weeks, so tremendous numbers of dead skin cells constantly flake off into the environment). Mites also feed on food particles and other organic materials in the environment. The highest concentrations of house dust mites are typically in bedrooms on mattresses, on upholstered furniture, and in rugs. House dust mites thrive at humidities over 60% and temperatures of 77° to 86° F. The main allergen is thought to be proteins found in mite feces—a single house dust mite excretes as many as 20 fecal particles per day. Over 250,000 mite fecal particles may be found in 1 gram (about 1/4 teaspoon) of house dust!

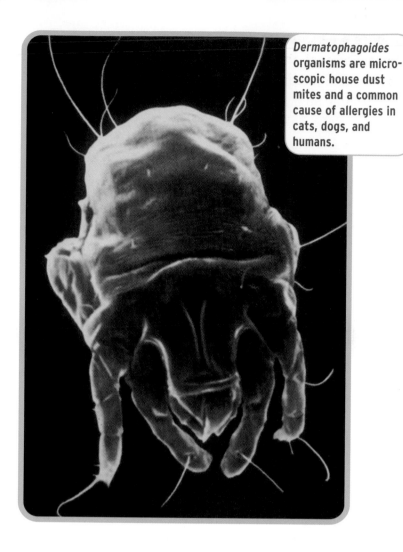

Dermatophagoides organisms are microscopic house dust mites and a common cause of allergies in cats, dogs, and humans.

Other Environmental Allergens

"Cotton linters" are particles that form as cotton and other fabric break down and are occasionally a cause of allergic skin reactions. Kapok is a fiber from the seeds of the kapok tree. It is found in the stuffing of some toys, pillows, sleeping bags, mattresses, life jackets, cushions, and furniture. Cottonseed is found as a contaminant in the stuffing of some mattresses and furniture. Allergies to kapok and cottonseed have become less common with the increased popularity of synthetic fibers. Tobacco smoke is irritating and also can be allergenic to certain pets. Proteins from the bodies and eggs of cockroaches and other insects can be allergenic. Many other insects produce a venom that is allergenic following bites or stings. Sawdust and other wood particles also are responsible for allergic reactions in some pets.

Diagnosing Atopy

Atopy cannot be diagnosed using a laboratory test. Instead, the diagnosis of atopy is based on (1) a suggestive patient history, (2) typical clinical signs, and (3) exclusion of other possible causes of itching and skin inflammation.

Important clues from a patient's *history* include:

- **Symptoms beginning between 6 months and 3 years (in dogs)**
- **A familial history of atopy or breed predisposition**
- **Symptoms that are seasonal (versus nonseasonal for food allergies)**
- **Itching that is alleviated by treatment with corticosteroids**
- **A typical distribution (face, ears, feet, armpits, groin)**

Suggestive *clinical signs* include the following:

- **Itching—typically the first sign, manifested as rubbing, licking, chewing, or scratching, sometimes resulting in brownish saliva stains on the feet or "hot spots" (see Chapter 5)**
- **Perioral inflammation (involving the lips and muzzle)**
- **Inflammation of the ear pinnae (ear flaps)**
- **Recurrent bacterial and/or yeast infections of the feet, skin, and/or external ear canals (see Chapter 5)**
- **Moist skin from increased sweating (hyperhidrosis)**
- **Self-induced hair loss (alopecia)**
- **Lip ulcers (cats)**
- **Miliary dermatitis (cats)**
- **Eosinophilic plaques (cats)**
- **Eosinophilic granulomas (cats)**

Other causes of itching that must be ruled out include fleas and other external parasites (ectoparasites) (see Chapter 6), food allergies, and inflammation secondary to bacterial or yeast infections (see Chapter 5).

By now you may be thinking, "But I thought there *are* tests for allergies!" There are indeed several types of tests available for "allergy testing" of dogs and cats. But

Criteria to Diagnose Atopy

Familial history or breed predisposition

Onset of signs between 6 months and 3 years

Involvement of face, feet, ears, axillae, and/or groin

Itching that is relieved with corticosteroid therapy

Rule out other causes of pruritus:

- **Fleas/flea bite hypersensitivity**
- **Food allergy**
- **Sarcoptic mange**
- **Contact allergies and irritants**
- **Bacterial and yeast infections**

Symptom severity initially varies with season

Allergen-specific reactions on intradermal skin allergy test or on serum IgE tests

these tests are not intended for use in "diagnosing" atopy; instead, they are performed to identify the allergens most likely to be responsible for clinical signs in your pet. Steps can then be taken to avoid exposure to allergens that are identified as "likely offenders" or to **desensitize** the pet through allergen-specific **immunotherapy**.

The reason "allergy tests" cannot be used for the diagnosis of atopy is that many normal dogs and cats—and those with diseases such as sarcoptic mange (see Chapter 6)—will have positive reactions to one or more of the antigens (allergens) used in the tests and could be inaccurately diagnosed as having atopy when they actually do not.

The two general types of tests used for identifying relevant allergens (those responsible for causing clinical signs in the affected animal) are intradermal skin allergy tests and serum (blood) allergy tests.

Intradermal skin tests (IDSTs) are considered the best tests for identifying relevant allergens. In an IDST, small amounts of a weak solution of allergens are injected directly into the dermis of the skin (see Chapter 1). Allergen molecules bind (attach) to any allergen-specific IgE on mast cells in the skin. This binding triggers the mast cells to degranulate, resulting in a "wheal and flare" reaction (seen as a raised welt–the "wheal"–within an area of reddened skin–the "flare"). The selection of allergens to use in a test is based on which ones are most common in a given geographical area; a typical test includes 50 to 70 individual allergens. Your pet's fur must be shaved to allow the injections to be given and for best visibility of the reactions. Most pets are sedated for the injections (would *you* want to lie quietly for 70 injections?).

Where We Stand

The diagnosis of atopy is based on a review of the animal's history and clinical signs, followed by tests to rule out other causes of itching and skin inflammation. Intradermal skin allergy testing and serum IgE allergy testing should be used only as aids to identify allergens to be avoided and to guide the selection of allergens for use in immunotherapy. The intradermal tests are the most specific because they demonstrate allergens that cause inflammation in the target tissue (skin).

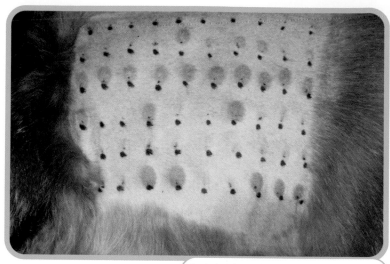

An intradermal skin allergy test in a cat with multiple allergies. The hair coat is shaved so that any reactions are visible. This cat also was given a dye that causes skin with positive reactions to turn blue.

Corticosteroids and antihistamines must be discontinued for several weeks before intradermal skin testing. Interpreting IDSTs (deciding what the results mean) requires skill and experience, so many veterinarians refer patients to a specialist (see http://www.acvd.org).

Serum testing is simpler for both pet owners and veterinarians: A blood sample is taken and mailed to a laboratory specializing in pet allergy testing. Serum allergy tests are designed to detect allergen-specific IgE in the pet's blood. Several different tests are used for serum testing, including the **radioallergosorbent test** (RAST), **enzyme-linked immunosorbent assay** (ELISA), and **Western blot** analysis. Differences also exist between laboratories performing these tests. The detecting system may use special antibodies or special kinds of IgE, or the allergens used may come from different sources or may be combined into groups for the tests. So the results of tests from one laboratory often are very different from those of another. In addition, the results may not match IDST results in the same animal—because IgE may be present in the blood but not on mast cells in the skin. Only the IgE present on mast cells in the *skin* produces skin disease; this is the reason the IDST is best for identifying relevant allergens. However, serum IgE tests may detect potential allergies early in their development (before they would "show up" in an IDST and before they become clinically important) and may still be helpful in managing an animal with atopy (particularly if strategies can be developed to minimize exposure to the allergen.)

Positive test reactions that seem to make little sense are more common than you might think—a cat born and raised indoors in Alaska may have a positive reaction to sagebrush, found only in the Southwest. In such cases, the allergy may be to a closely related allergen (ragweed and dandelion, for example, may cross-react); in other cases, the reaction is a "false positive" (due to impurities or to human error, or to other, often unexplained factors). The interpretation of test results—both for serum tests and for IDSTs—requires careful review of the pet's history (seasonality of signs compared with seasonal peaks in pollen or mold spore production) and of the likelihood that the allergen is present in the pet's environment.

Strategies for Managing Atopy

The goals of treating a dog or cat with atopy include relieving the pet's discomfort, healing any skin lesions, and preventing—or at least minimizing—the recurrence of clinical signs. A time-honored principle of medicine warns: "Above all, do no harm." This is especially important in dealing with allergies—no treatments or medications that may cause problems more serious than the original one should ever be used. Virtually all medications have potential side effects. Some side effects are predictable, and others occur in an unpredictable pattern. So in selecting a treatment for your pet, you and your veterinarian must decide whether probable benefit from the treatment outweighs possible harm from that treatment.

Discomfort associated with allergies is primarily a result of inflammation in the skin, causing the pet to lick, bite (chew), scratch, or rub the affected areas. An important concept to understand is that inflammation in the skin can have many possible sources, with each source contributing to inflammation in an additive fashion. This is referred to as a "summation effect." For example, a pet may be allergic to ragweed, beef (a food allergy), fleas (parasite allergy), and staphylococci (bacterial allergy) and also may have dry skin. The flea infestation and the staphylococcal infection each may produce some inflammation, aside from the allergy. All of these factors work together to aggravate the inflammation in the skin.

Advantages and Disadvantages of Treatment Options for Atopy

Therapy	Advantages	Disadvantages
Topical shampoos/ conditioners	Remove antigens from skin surface, thereby reducing allergen load; remove bacteria and yeasts, thereby reducing recurrence of skin infections	Time-consuming, difficult for some owners; dogs with thick hair coats may be hard to clean and slow to dry; many cats dislike getting wet
Fatty acid supplements	May improve skin and hair coat condition, may lessen inflammation in the skin; few side effects	Some pets dislike taste; may require up to 12 weeks to see improvement; less than 25% response rate
Antihistamines	Few side effects; may help pet sleep better	Large number of products available may be confusing, variable efficacy; some products may predispose dogs to seizures or have interactions with other drugs; must be given multiple times daily

Advantages and Disadvantages of Treatment Options for Atopy—cont'd

Therapy	Advantages	Disadvantages
Corticosteroids	Highly effective in decreasing skin inflammation and itching	Numerous side effects; may have decreased efficacy with prolonged use
Cyclosporine	Highly effective in decreasing skin inflammation and itching	Fewer side effects than with corticosteroids; may cause vomiting and diarrhea when started, proliferation of gum tissue (gingival hyperplasia); may increase risk of developing infections and cancer; expensive
Allergen-specific immunotherapy	Low incidence of side effects; the only therapy directly targeted at cause of disease	Slow onset of action (requires months for improvement); does not work in all pets; requires injections to be given at frequent intervals; some pets have an increase in itching when treatment is started

Another important concept is the **pruritic threshold** ("pruritic" is another word for "itchy"). Each animal has a threshold of **tolerance** for skin discomfort. Below this level or threshold, no clinical signs are apparent; above this threshold, the pet begins to lick, chew, scratch, or rub. The pruritic threshold can be affected by many factors. Nervous animals tend to itch sooner than placid (calm) ones. Nutrition, other diseases, stress, temperature, humidity and other environmental factors all can affect the threshold. Multiple stimuli added together can easily push an animal over its pruritic threshold. Treating and eliminating one or more of these stimuli may put the animal below its pruritic threshold.

The stimulus that sends the animal over its pruritic threshold can be thought of as the famous "straw that broke the camel's back." It often is referred to as the "flare factor" because it is the one that is associated with the appearance of clinical symptoms (even though it may not be the only problem present). For some animals, a bacterial or **yeast** infection will be the "flare factor," and treating the infection will soothe the discomfort. For other animals, fleas will be the flare factor, and use of flea control measures will stop the itching. In still other cases, multiple treatments (against infections, fleas, dry skin, and environmental allergens) will be required before the pet can be made comfortable.

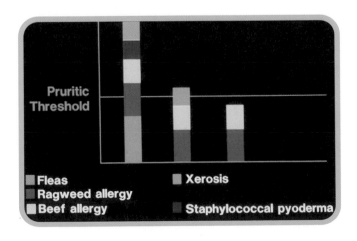

Pruritic Threshold

■ Fleas   ■ Xerosis
■ Ragweed allergy
■ Beef allergy   ■ Staphylococcal pyoderma

Topical therapies have an important role in relieving discomfort, healing lesions, and preventing reoccurrences. Because the main route of exposure to allergens is percutaneous (through the skin), frequent bathing or even rinsing with water will remove allergens before they have a chance to cause inflammation in the skin. You can visualize your dog or cat as a dust mop that is constantly picking up allergen-containing debris from the environment. Water removes that allergen-containing debris. Use of a medicated shampoo (see Chapter 2) will increase allergen removal. Your veterinarian can guide you in selecting the most appropriate medicated shampoo for your pet—these may include shampoos with moisturizers, topical anesthetics, topical **antihistamines**, topical **corticosteroids**, topical **antiseptics**, or topical antifungal agents. The soothing effects will last longer if the shampoo is followed with application of a medicated cream rinse or leave-on conditioner.

A number of diets are marketed as being helpful for pets with allergies. Some of these diets are designed for pets with food allergies (discussed later in the chapter); however, others are designed to lessen symptoms of other allergies. One of the chemical pathways leading to inflammation uses fatty acids of the omega-6 family. Fatty acids of the omega-3 family block the enzymes involved in the actions of omega-6 fatty acids and can lessen inflammation in the skin. The major sources of omega-3 fatty acids are flaxseed meal/oil and fish oil. Diets with ratios of omega-6 to omega-3 fatty acids between 10:1 and 5:1 are considered optimal for promoting healthy skin and helping to reduce skin inflammation. Nutritional supplements containing omega-3 fatty acids also can be used to decrease inflammation in skin.

Antihistamines are widely used to treat human allergies. Many of these medications also are helpful for cats and dogs with allergies. Finding the best antihistamine for your pet may require a series of trials. Variability in individual responses is why there are so many antihistamines from which to choose. A couple of weeks may be needed for antihistamines to work. So you should try each kind for a minimum of 2 weeks before switching your pet to another one. Antidepressants can relieve anxiety and raise the pruritic threshold; some antidepressants also have antihistamine activity. Examples of antihistamines and antidepressants used in dogs and cats are chlorpheniramine (Chlor-Trimeton), diphenhydramine (Benadryl), clemastine (Tavist), hydroxyzine (Atarax), trimeprazine (Temaril), cetirizine (Zyrtec), doxepin (Sinequan), loratadine (Claritin), and amitriptyline (Elavil). Consult a veterinarian to decide which of these may be most appropriate for your pet and what doses to use.

Oral corticosteroids such as **prednisolone**, methylprednisolone, and **prednisone** are very effective in controlling inflammation. Corticosteroids inhibit mast cell degranulation, block the production of many substances involved in inflammation, and prevent the migration of white blood cells into tissues. These medications may be required to break an itch-scratch-itch cycle and to prevent self-inflicted damage to the skin in animals with severe allergies. Unfortunately, corticosteroids have a number of possible side effects including increases in thirst, urination, likelihood of infections, and appetite; liver enlargement; thinning of the skin; weakening of blood vessels; and many more. The risk of side effects can be minimized by giving these medications orally (by mouth) at the lowest dose and longest interval that controls signs (e.g., small dose given by mouth every 2 to 3 days). Injectable forms of corticosteroids should be avoided in dogs because of the high risk of adverse side effects.

With some cats, it is almost impossible to give medications by mouth (although some creative pharmacies may offer fish-flavored syrups and pastes that many cats will eat). Sometimes a steroid injection must be given to stop the itching. Animals on long-term treatment with corticosteroids (for longer than 2 months) should have blood tests and urine cultures on a regular basis (every 3 months or as recommended by the prescribing veterinarian), to detect any adverse effects and secondary infections.

Cyclosporine is a medication approved in 2003 for the treatment of atopy in dogs. Cyclosporine prevents **lymphocytes** (a type of white blood cells) from producing inflammatory substances, slows down processes involving antigens, and reduces mast cell degranulation. It is as good as corticosteroids in relieving discomfort and reducing itching and cutaneous inflammation in most dogs with atopy. Cyclosporine has fewer side effects than corticosteroids. The most common side effect is vomiting or diarrhea (this occurs in approximately 25% of patients but is severe enough to require discontinuing use in only about 5%). Other side effects include gingival hyperplasia (thickening of the gums, especially around the teeth), increased risk of infections, and wartlike lesions in the mouth or on the skin. Cyclosporine may be linked with development of cancer, but the risk is considered to be very low. Cyclosporine is expensive, and most veterinarians recommend its use only when other therapies (such as regular bathing, flea control, topical antipruritic agents, allergen avoidance, oral antihistamines, and desensitization) have failed to soothe the pet's **pruritus** (itching).

Relieving the pet's discomfort, to reduce licking, chewing, scratching, and rubbing, will help lesions to heal. In

Side Effects of Corticosteroids

Organ System Affected	Signs
Skin	Thinning (may become susceptible to tearing, especially in cats), increased susceptibility to bruising, increased susceptibility to infections, calcinosis cutis (calcium deposits in skin), comedones (blackheads), hair loss (may be generalized)
Urinary	Polyuria (increased urine production), polydipsia (increased thirst), increased susceptibility to bladder and kidney infections, protein loss in urine
Pancreas/blood sugar	Elevations in blood sugar, insulin antagonism, may predispose to type 2 diabetes mellitus, pancreatitis
Gastrointestinal tract and liver	Predisposes to ulcers, vomiting, diarrhea, liver enlargement, increases in liver enzymes
Muscles	Weakness, loss of muscle mass (wasting), pendulous abdomen (sagging belly)
Adrenal glands	Atrophy
Respiratory	Panting, increased risk of blood clots in lungs (thromboembolism)
Cardiovascular	Increased blood pressure, may increase risk of congestive heart failure
General	Increased appetite (polyphagia), obesity

Where We Stand

Corticosteroids are hormones that are required for life and are produced by specialized glands called adrenal glands. The amount of corticosteroid present in the blood regulates the activity of adrenal glands. When corticosteroids are given as medications to dogs and cats, the adrenal glands "shut down" and will atrophy (shrink), and eventually the animal becomes dependent on the medications. Adrenal atrophy can be avoided by giving corticosteroids every other day, because the adrenal glands resume production of corticosteroids on the days the medication is not given. The goal of corticosteroid therapy should be to give the lowest possible dose every other day.

Where We Stand

Corticosteroids are highly effective in preventing type I allergic reactions and are useful in the management of pets with atopy. But corticosteroids have numerous side effects, and the benefits must be weighed against the risks for each patient. Injectable corticosteroids should not be used for the management of atopy in dogs—once an injection is given, you cannot take it back. Oral corticosteroids are much safer than injectable forms, and risks can be minimized when a low dose is given every other day.

some cases it may be necessary to prevent the animal from biting and chewing itself by using a cone (Elizabethan collar) or body suit. In many animals with atopy, secondary bacterial and/or yeast (especially *Malassezia*) infections develop in their skin and/or ears. These pets require treatment with antibacterial products (antibiotics given orally for 3 to 6 weeks plus topical antiseptic shampoos and/or lotions or creams used as directed by a veterinarian) or antifungal (anti-yeast) products (oral antifungals for 30 days plus topical antifungal shampoos and/or lotions/dips or creams). Cats with indolent ulcers, eosinophilic plaques, or eosinophilic granulomas often require treatment with corticosteroids to heal these lesions.

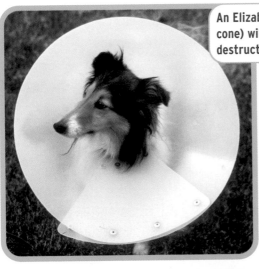

An Elizabethan collar (plastic cone) will prevent self-destructive chewing.

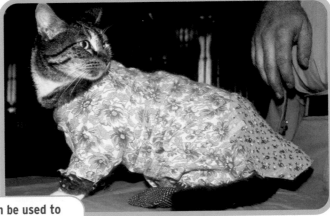

A body suit can be used to protect the pet's skin from self-destructive chewing and scratching.

Several strategies can be used to prevent recurrence of clinical signs and lesions associated with allergies. The best strategy is to avoid the allergen or minimize exposure to it. So the first step in allergen avoidance is intradermal skin allergy testing and/or serum IgE allergy testing, to identify the allergens causing problems. If the pet is allergic to tobacco, the owner should make the home smoke-free. If the pet is allergic to wool, the owner should remove wool-containing rugs, blankets, sweaters, socks, and coats from the home and also avoid using shampoos or other products containing lanolin. If the pet is allergic to feathers, the owner should remove all feather pillows, comforters, sleeping bags, and similar products from the house. If the pet is allergic to kapok, the owner should remove all products containing kapok fibers from the house (these may include stuffed toys, throw pillows, cushions, nonsynthetic furniture, and other similar items.) Regular cleaning and replacement of air filters with HEPA filters (high-efficiency particulate air filters) and the use of HEPA air cleaners and HEPA-filtered vacuum cleaners will help keep the home air free of many airborne allergens.

Many procedures can help control house dust mites within a home. House dust mites are most numerous in bedrooms, because their main food source is human dander, which accumulates in dressing areas and in bed sheets and mattresses. Keeping pets out of bedrooms can help minimize their exposure to house dust mites. Removing carpets, upholstered furniture, bookcases, and nonwashable items from the bedroom is helpful in decreasing accumulations of house dust and mites. Using micropore or plastic encasings for mattresses, box springs, and pillows will keep mites from accumulating in these items. Wet-mopping floors twice weekly can help remove dust and mites. Washing bedding (human and pet), stuffed toys, and curtains weekly at temperatures above 130° F or more will kill house dust mites. Using HEPA air cleaners and filters helps remove mites from air circulating in rooms. Using dehumidifiers also helps, because mites' survival is decreased when the relative humidity is below 50%. Upholstered furniture in the house should be covered with micropore washable slip-covers or treated with benzyl benzoate (Acarosan, made by Bissell) to kill house dust mites. Allersearch ADS Spray (made by National Allergy Supply, Inc.) containing 3% tannic acid can be used on carpets and furniture to neutralize dust mite and animal dander allergens. The levels of house dust mite antigens in rooms can be measured using a Mite-T-Fast Dust Mite Detection Kit (also made by National Allergy Supply, Inc.)

Molds are microscopic fungi that live on organic matter—plant and animal. Molds thrive in warm and humid environments and release large numbers of allergy-causing spores. Outdoors, they are found in shaded areas, in woodpiles, under porches, in lawn thatch, on plants, and in barns. Make these areas off limits to pets, and keep pets indoors when grass is being mowed and during

Control of House Dust Mites

- **Remove carpets.**
- **Remove sources of clutter.**
- **Cover mattresses, box springs, pillows, and upholstered furniture with micropore or plastic casings/covers.**
- **Wash bedding (pet and human) and curtains weekly with hot water (hotter than 130° F).**
- **Wet-mop floors twice weekly.**
- **Use dehumidifiers to keep humidity below 50%.**
- **Use HEPA air cleaners, filters, and vacuum cleaners (discard used filters in sealed bags).**
- **Monitor mite antigen concentrations (using Mite-T-Test or a similar product); if levels are high, treat home with miticides (such as Acrosan).**

the harvest season of grains and other crops. Indoors, molds are most numerous in basements, bathrooms, humidifiers, garbage, and soil of houseplants, and on damp carpets, paper, fabrics, and leather. Strategies to minimize the exposure of indoor pets to molds include keeping the pet out of basements, bathrooms, laundry rooms, crawl spaces, and garages. Move plants outdoors or to rooms off limits to pets. Firewood should be stored outside. Clean and disinfect humidifiers every week. Keep garbage outside, and throw away food before mold grows on it. Remove mildew from bathrooms, kitchens, and other damp areas. Remove any mildewed carpets or rugs. Clean surfaces with chlorine bleach solutions. Use HEPA room air filters.

Pollen concentrations vary in different seasons and at different times of the day. Useful information about pollens can be found at the Internet sites http://allerdays.com/regional.html and http://www.claritin.com/pollen/pollen.cgi. Exposure to pollens can be minimized by not allowing pets in fields and flowerbeds, keeping grass cut short so that it does not pollinate, and keeping pets indoors during peak pollen times (typically in early morning and at dusk). Using air conditioners during summer months and HEPA filters year-round will help reduce pollen levels in the home. Regular bathing and rinsing of feet when the pet comes in from outdoors also will reduce the pollen "load" on its skin.

When all of these strategies do not succeed in preventing allergic symptoms, allergen-specific immunotherapy can be tried. The goal of immunotherapy is to desensitize the pet to offending allergens. How immunotherapy blocks cutaneous inflammation is not totally understood. Changes in the immune system of a desensitized pet include lower concentrations of allergen-specific IgE, lower numbers of mast cells in the skin, and decreased release of histamine and other products from mast cells. Desensitization typically requires between 6 and 12 months—so immunotherapy helps prevent future allergic episodes and is not useful in dealing with acute flares of allergy-associated skin inflammation.

Immunotherapy injections (shots) are given **subcutaneously**. Reactions to immunotherapy are very uncommon in dogs and cats, so many veterinarians teach owners how to administer injections. The solution used for the injections contains very small amounts of the allergens identified by testing. Giving these allergen solutions for many months results in a gradual development of immunological tolerance. A specialist in veterinary allergy can help you develop a desensitization plan based on your pet's history and the results of allergy testing (with IDSTs or allergen-specific serum IgE assays).

If your pet initially responds to immunotherapy and later relapses, new allergies may have developed. So more than one testing and desensitization treatment may be needed. Once your pet's allergies are under control, you can reduce the frequency of immunotherapy injections to a maintenance schedule, with booster injections every 1 to 4 weeks for the rest of its life. Owners who discontinue immunotherapy injections in a pet that responded favorably typically see a return of clinical signs within a few months.

Not all animals with atopy will be successfully desensitized. Reasons may include failure to detect all allergens involved, poor control of coexisting problems such as ectoparasites, and decreased function of the animal's immune system. If your pet has atopy that was not helped by immunotherapy, reevaluation by your veterinarian for other possible allergens or contributory factors is indicated. It also is important to continue with efforts to minimize allergen exposure and to relieve clinical signs and decrease cutaneous inflammation.

Contact Allergies

In atopy, the allergic reaction occurs rapidly after exposure, so it is called an immediate (type I) **hypersensitivity** reaction (mast cell degranulation starts within minutes). By contrast, with **contact allergy**, the allergic reaction does not develop until 24 to 72 hours after allergen exposure and is therefore called a delayed (type IV) hypersensitivity reaction.

The best-known example of contact allergies in people is the occurrence of a rash with itching and blisters after exposure to poison ivy. Contact allergy and atopy are similar in that both require time for sensitization to develop before the animal becomes allergic to the substance. So if you notice a rash on your pet's skin after the first time you use a shampoo or dip, the rash is from an irritant reaction and not an allergic reaction.

If your pet has a contact allergy, you will notice skin problems mostly in thin-haired areas, such as between the toes or on the belly or scrotum. The lips or muzzle may be affected if the pet becomes allergic to a chew bone, rawhide toy, or food bowl. Other possible contact allergens include plants, carpet cleaners or deodorizers, detergents, wood decks, cedar or pine shavings, plastic or

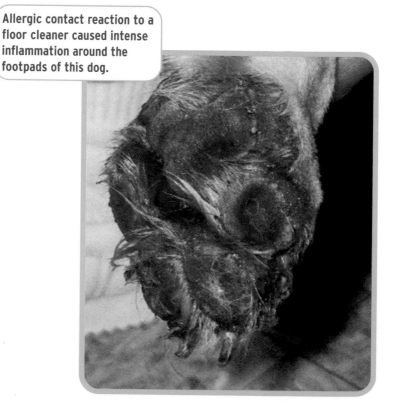

Allergic contact reaction to a floor cleaner caused intense inflammation around the footpads of this dog.

rubber in bowls or toys, wool, carpets, rugs, insecticides, fertilizers, topical medications, and shampoos. Initial signs may include redness of the skin, **papules** (pinpoint-size red bumps), oozing (of serum through the skin pores), small blisters (vesicles), crusts, **excoriations** (scratches), **lichenification** (skin thickening), and **hyperpigmentation** (darkening or blackening of the skin).

Diagnosing a Contact Allergy

Diagnosis of a contact allergy is made by ruling out other causes of skin inflammation including ectoparasites, other allergies, and bacterial or fungal infections of the skin. One way of doing this is patch testing: An allergen is applied to a small area of skin, which is covered with a patch; then the test site is observed for the next 72 hours to determine if a reaction develops. Another method of testing is "avoidance/provocation": The pet is removed from its normal environment until all skin lesions have resolved, and then possible allergens are brought back into the testing environment (reintroduced) to determine if symptoms recur. One potential allergen is reintroduced every 3 to 5 days.

Strategies for Managing a Contact Allergy

Avoiding the allergen is the best treatment. Using barriers such as socks or shirts will prevent exposure to allergens that are common in the environment. Bathing or rinsing with water can help to decrease the allergen "load" on the skin. Secondary skin infections should be treated with antibacterial or antifungal medications. Topical or systemic corticosteroids can be used to block the allergic reaction, but not on a long-term basis because of serious side effects. A drug called pentoxifylline also can be used to block delayed hypersensitivity reactions. This drug has fewer side effects than corticosteroids but must be given two or three times daily for maximum effectiveness.

Food Allergies

Food allergies may involve type I (immediate–similar to atopy) and/or type IV (delayed–similar to contact) hypersensitivity responses. As with all allergies, sensitization must occur before allergy develops. Clinical signs may then appear abruptly. The sensitization period may be 2 years or longer, so a pet that has eaten the same food with no problems for years may suddenly start to show intense itching from an allergy it has developed to that food. The allergen causing the food allergy usually is a meat protein but in some pets may be a carbohydrate or a contaminant present in the food, such as a mold or storage mite. Most pet foods contain similar ingredients, so food allergies usually are not related to a change in the brand of food. With certain diseases, the gastroin-

Food Ingredients Reported to Cause Allergies in Dogs and Cats

Dogs	Cats
Beef	Beef
Dairy	Dairy
Wheat	Fish
Chicken	Lamb
Egg	Wheat
Lamb	Chicken
Soy	Corn/corn gluten
Corn	Egg
Pork	
Rice	
Fish	

testinal tract becomes "leaky," allowing intact proteins (not properly digested) to be absorbed and then react with the pet's immune system. Examples of diseases that may predispose pets to food allergies are intestinal parasites (worms), viral infections (parvovirus, coronavirus, rotavirus, feline panleukopenia virus), inflammatory bowel disease, and IgA deficiency (hereditary defect in the production of antibodies normally present on mucosal cell surfaces).

Clinical Signs

Clinical signs due to food allergies in dogs include severe itching (pruritus), erythema (especially of the face, feet, ears, and perianal region), papules (pinpoint red bumps), hair loss (alopecia), recurrent infections (involving ears, feet, or skin), hives, and vomiting and/or diarrhea. Clinical signs of food allergies in cats include severe itching, especially on the head and neck, miliary dermatitis, hair loss, indolent ulcers, eosinophilic plaques, and

Clinical Signs of Food Allergies

Dogs	Cats
Generalized pruritus (itching)	Itching and scratching, especially of head and neck
Inflammation of ears, shaking head	Miliary dermatitis
Inflammation of anal sacs, "scooting"	Indolent ulcers
	Eosinophilic plaques
Recurrent skin infections	Eosinophilic granulomas
Recurrent ear infections	Overgrooming resulting in hair loss (bald belly and/or thighs)
Occasionally vomiting, diarrhea, and/or flatulence	

eosinophilic granulomas. These signs may appear within hours (with immediate hypersensitivity reactions) or develop over days (with delayed hypersensitivity reactions) following food consumption. Clinical signs of food allergies can last for days to weeks after an offending allergen is eaten by a sensitized pet.

Diagnosing Food Allergies

Unfortunately, no reliable laboratory tests for food allergies are available. Some laboratories offer serum IgE tests for food allergies, but these tests are not reliable in diagnosing specific food allergies. For one thing, not all food allergies involve IgE—some are delayed hypersensitivity reactions, which involve special white blood cells called T-lymphocytes. In addition, too many different types of allergens are present in a "food type" to allow testing for all of them—for example, "beef" in a pet food may include kidneys, tongue, heart, liver, and various beef "by-products," all of which contain antigens different from those in a sirloin steak. Another point is that changes in allergens themselves are caused by cooking and food processing and also by the digestive enzymes breaking down foods after they are eaten. Cross-reactivity between allergens from different sources is yet another problem. For example, 92% of people allergic to cow's milk are also allergic to goat's milk, 92% of people allergic to cantaloupe are allergic to bananas, and 10% of people allergic to cow's milk also are allergic to beef. Cross-reactivity between environmental allergens and foods also is possible—a lot of people who are allergic to birch pollen also are allergic to strawberries and other fruits. So for many reasons, serum tests and IDSTs should *not* be used for diagnosing food allergies.

Diagnosis of a food allergy must be based on "feeding trials." The diagnostic process has two stages: First is the restrictive feeding period, during which the pet is fed only a new diet (referred to as a **restrictive diet** or **elimina-**

tion diet) that does not contain allergens likely to be involved in the pet's suspected allergies. The second stage is performing "food challenges" to see whether the pet has a food allergy and to determine what food or foods are involved.

The diet used during a feeding trial often is referred to as a "hypoallergenic diet." This term is misleading because all diets contain some allergens, and therefore no diet is completely nonallergenic. Two general types of manufactured diets are available for use in feeding trials. The first type is "novel protein diets." As noted earlier, the allergens in most foods are proteins, and an animal cannot have an allergy to anything it has not already been exposed to (remember that a sensitization period is required to develop an allergy). So in these diets, the protein source is a new (novel) food that the pet has not ever eaten before. Examples of novel protein sources that may be suitable for use are lamb, pork, fish, rabbit, venison, kangaroo, duck, tofu, and pinto beans.

Food Allergies

Myth: My dog cannot be allergic to its food because it was fed the same food for years before the skin problem started.

Fact: A food allergy does not start until the immune system has been sensitized to the food. Sensitization does not occur until after multiple episodes of food proteins getting into the circulatory system. The average amount of time between when a food has been eaten and when allergies appear is 2 years. In dogs that have had intestinal parasites or other intestinal diseases, food allergies may develop more quickly, because such diseases may damage the intestine, allowing nondigested foods to enter the circulatory system and then sensitize the immune system.

Myth: My cat likes its food and never vomits or has diarrhea, so the food cannot be the cause of its skin disease.

Fact: Cats and dogs with food allergies rarely have gastrointestinal problems; food allergies in pets cause severe itching and skin lesions because the allergic reaction targets the skin.

Myth: We have tried many brands of food and have not seen any difference in our pet's skin disease, so food is not the problem.

Fact: A majority of pet foods have very similar ingredients, so changing from one brand to another probably will not make a difference in symptoms associated with food allergies.

Myth: My pet has been on a restrictive diet for almost 4 weeks with no improvement—it is time to try something else.

Fact: Improvements following diet change are very slow, because blood levels of histamine and other substances responsible for skin inflammation may still be high. Diet trials should be continued for 10 to 12 weeks and must be restarted if the pet consumes another food during the trial.

Examples of Commercial Novel Protein Diets

Product Line	Diets Available (Major Ingredients)
Eukanuba	F/P (herring meal, catfish, potato, beet pulp) K/O (kangaroo, oat flour, canola meal, beet pulp)
Hill's Prescription Diets	Canine D/D Rice and Duck (rice, duck) Canine D/D Rice and Egg (rice, egg) Canine D/D Rice and Salmon (rice, salmon) Canine D/D Rice and Whitefish (rice, whitefish) Feline D/D (lamb, rice)
Innovative Veterinary Diets (IVD) Limited Ingredient Diets	Canine Potato and Duck (potato, duck) Canine Potato and Rabbit (potato, rabbit) Canine Potato and Venison (potato, venison) Canine Potato and Whitefish (potato, whitefish) Feline Green Pea and Duck (green peas, duck) Feline Green Pea and Lamb (green peas, lamb) Feline Green Pea and Rabbit (green peas, rabbit) Feline Green Pea and Venison (green peas, venison)
Purina Veterinary Diet	LA Formula (salmon meal, rice, trout, canola meal, tallow, canola and fish oil)
Waltham	Selected Protein Catfish (catfish, rice)

The selection of a novel protein must be based on a review of the pet's dietary history. If it has been previously fed one of these foods, then that food is unsuitable for the feeding trial. Just because a pet has never eaten a food does not totally eliminate the possibility of an allergic reaction to it, because the pet may have eaten a cross-reacting food. For example, some pets allergic to beef also are allergic to venison, and some pets allergic to chicken also are allergic to duck. So more than one feeding trial may be needed.

Pure meat source diets are unsuitable for use because they are lacking in many important nutrients (such as some B vitamins) and have too much of others (protein and phosphorus). Thus, diets for feeding trials also must contain a carbohydrate source. Ingredients used for carbohydrate sources may include brown rice, potatoes, yams, barley, and oats/oatmeal. Ideally, the pet would not have previously consumed the carbohydrate source before the feeding trial. The incidence of food allergies to rice and potatoes is relatively low (less than 3% of food allergies), so these are used in most manufactured novel protein source diets. If your pet does not improve while being fed one type of carbohydrate, a second feeding trial using a different carbohydrate may be helpful.

Pets respond better to homemade elimination diets than to manufactured diets, so homemade diets are preferred when owners are willing to cook the special foods required. Large amounts can be prepared and then divided into meal portions and frozen.

The second general type of diet manufactured for use in feeding trials is the hydrolyzed protein diet. The basis for these diets is that allergens involved in type I hypersensitivity reactions must be large enough to interact with the IgE on a mast cell. If proteins are properly hydrolyzed (broken down using enzymes), the resultant protein fragments (peptides) are too small to cause a type I hypersensitivity reaction—although they may be involved in some type IV delayed hypersensitivity reac-

Homemade Diets for Food Allergy Testing

The ideal diet for food allergy testing is homemade using a protein the pet has not previously eaten plus a carbohydrate and/or vegetable (no corn). Start with 1 cup of cooked protein source + 3 cups of cooked carbohydrate (may substitute 1 cup of a vegetable) per 25 pounds of body weight, divided into 2 or 3 meals per day. Adjust amount fed to maintain normal weight.

Proteins	Carbohydrates
Duck	Barley
Fish	Brown rice
Lamb	Oatmeal (no milk) or oat groats
Pinto beans	Potatoes
Pork roast	Yams
Rabbit	
Venison	

tions. Hydrolyzed protein diets also must contain a carbohydrate to provide nutritional balance, and a few pets may be allergic to the carbohydrate portion of the diet.

Before choosing a diet for a restrictive feeding trial, review your pet's previous food exposures, and consult with a veterinarian experienced in managing animals with food allergies. Even those diets specially formulated for food-allergic pets contain some allergens, however, so they will cause allergy-related clinical signs in some animals. In these cases, more than one feeding trial may be needed to diagnose food allergies as the cause of the skin disease. Improvement following diet changes is gradual. Because of this, each restrictive feeding trial should be continued for a minimum of 12 weeks.

Examples of Hydrolyzed Protein Diets

Product Line	Diets Available (Major Ingredients)
Hill's Prescription Diets	Canine Z/D Ultra Allergen Free (starch, hydrolyzed chicken liver) Canine Z/D Low Allergen (potato, hydrolyzed chicken liver) Feline Z/D Low Allergen (rice, hydrolyzed chicken liver)
Purina Veterinary Diet	HA Formula (corn starch, modified soy protein)
Waltham	Royal Canin Canine Hypoallergenic HP 19 (rice, soy protein hydrolysate, chicken fat, beet pulp, fish oil) Royal Canin Feline Hypoallergenic HP 23 (rice, soy protein hydrolysate, chicken fat, beet pulp, fish oil)

During a restrictive feeding trial, do not give your pet any other foods or treats—no bones, rawhide chew toys, dog biscuits, or table foods, and no chewable medications (flavored vitamins and heartworm preventatives are not allowed). If the pet eats even one bite of a food that it is allergic to during the diet trial, another 12-week feeding period must be started.

Strategies for Managing a Food Allergy

If your pet's clinical signs decrease during the diet trial, it probably is allergic to an ingredient of its previous diet. But the improvement also could result from seasonal changes in environmental allergies or to other interventions (such as improved flea control, bathing, or treatment of a skin infection). Therefore, verification of a food allergy requires a "diet challenge." Begin by mixing small amounts (starting with 25%) of food from the previous diet with the food that was used during the feeding trial. If you see no change in your pet's clinical signs over the next week, gradually increase the amount of food from the old diet. If clinical signs do not reappear, the improvement was not due to a food allergy, and your pet may continue with its prior diet. If your pet starts to itch or show other signs of food allergies, return it to the diet used for the feeding trial. Then your options are either to feed the restrictive diet lifelong (paying attention to nutrient balancing if you are feeding a homemade diet), or to start doing individual food challenges.

Individual food challenges are accomplished by adding a single different ingredient from the prior diet to the pet's food every 2 weeks (such as cheese, beef, soy, chicken, wheat, or corn). Most pets are allergic to only one or two foods. So once a food allergy is confirmed, it usually is possible to identify a commercial pet food that does not include that ingredient. For example, if your pet turns out to be allergic to beef and milk proteins, you can feed a poultry-based commercial diet instead.

Parasite-Related Allergies

Dogs and cats may be affected by a large number of external and internal parasites. The response of an animal's immune system to parasites involves the same cell types (eosinophils) and antibodies (IgE class) as those involved in allergies. Therefore, it is not surprising that parasites almost always induce an allergic reaction in pets. IgE-mediated type I hypersensitivity reactions are most common, but other types of allergies, including delayed hypersensitivity reactions, may develop in some pets.

Fleas are the most common external parasite of companion animals and are a major cause of skin disease. In many areas of the world, flea allergy dermatitis is the most common disease affecting dogs and cats. Clinical signs of flea allergy dermatitis in dogs include pruritus (itching as indicated by scratching and chewing), papules (pinpoint red bumps), hair loss (alopecia), excoriations (scratches), lichenification (thickening of the skin), hyperpigmentation (darkening or blackening of the skin), and secondary skin infections. The base of the tail, dorsal rump, thighs, flanks, and belly are the most severely affected areas in most dogs. Clinical signs of flea allergy in cats may include "bald belly" (hair loss involving the underside of the abdomen and/or the thighs), miliary dermatitis, eosinophilic plaques, indolent ulcers, and pruritus involving the dorsal neck and/or rump.

Diagnosis of flea allergy dermatitis is based on finding fleas or "flea dirt" (flea feces), elevated serum IgE antibody to flea antigen, a positive result on intradermal skin testing for flea sensitivity, and/or a good response to flea control (symptoms resolve when fleas are eliminated). See Chapters 2 and 6 for information on flea control measures.

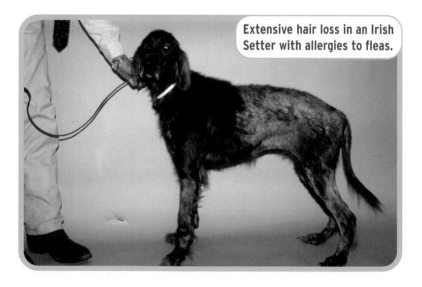

Extensive hair loss in an Irish Setter with allergies to fleas.

Mosquito bites produce a hypersensitivity (allergic) reaction in sensitized animals. Mosquitoes feed in areas with sparse hair; the most commonly affected areas in cats are the bridge of the nose, the outer ear pinnae (the "points"), and the footpads. Clinical signs include itching and swelling with papules (pinpoint red bumps), hair loss, and crusting. Diagnosis is based on a history of exposure to mosquitoes, biopsy specimens showing an eosinophilic dermatitis (in which the inflamed skin contains numerous eosinophils), and improvement when the cat is kept in a mosquito-free environment. Mosquitoes or other insect bites may result in an eosinophilic dermatitis affecting the nose and muzzle of dogs. Lesions in affected dogs may be very painful, with extensive swelling, papules, ulcers, blisters, and hemorrhagic (bloody) crusts. Treatment often requires corticosteroids to resolve inflammation plus antibiotics to treat secondary infections.

Allergic reactions to mosquito bites resulted in swelling, ulcers, and crusts on the nose and around the eyes of this dog.

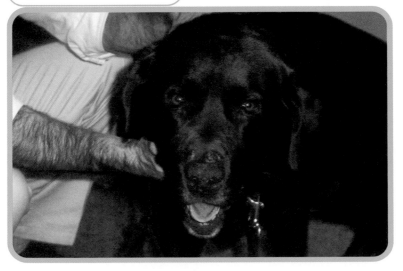

Other ectoparasites associated with hypersensitivity reactions in dogs and cats include mites (*Sarcoptes*, *Otodectes*) and ticks. These parasites are discussed in Chapter 6. Internal parasites are rarely proved to be the cause of allergic skin diseases in dogs and cats. Affected animals should be given anthelmintics (internal parasites are called helminths) and parasiticides to eliminate both internal and external parasites, respectively.

Miscellaneous Allergies

Organisms infecting the skin of cats and dogs can serve as allergens and produce additional cutaneous inflammation as a result of an allergic reaction to the bacterial or fungal allergen. *Staphylococcus* and *Malassezia* species are implicated in both type I (IgE-mediated) and type IV (delayed) hypersensitivity reactions in dogs. **Dermatophytes** are implicated primarily in delayed hypersensitivity reactions but also may result in other immune-mediated skin diseases including **pemphigus foliaceus** (Chapter 9). Diagnosis may be based on finding elevated levels of allergen-specific IgE, IDST results, or skin biopsy findings plus response to treatment (resolution of the allergy symptoms with elimination of the infection).

Drugs also can serve as allergens. A wide variety of clinical signs and lesions are possible, depending on the type of allergic reaction to the drug. As with all allergies, drug allergies require a period of sensitization—so a reaction occurring the first time a drug is given is a direct effect of the drug and not due to an allergy. Conversely, a pet that had no clinical signs the first time it was given a drug may have a life-threatening reaction the second time it receives the medication. Drug reactions vary, ranging from life-threatening **anaphylaxis** to pruritus, **angioedema**, hives, blistering lesions, areas of erythema (skin redness), and in some of the worst cases, widespread sloughing (separation and peeling) of the skin. Diagnosis is based on a history of prior exposure to the drug (or a closely related drug), typical skin biopsy findings, and improvement following withdrawal of the drug. A diagnosis can be confirmed by reexposing the pet to the drug, with recurrence of clinical signs, but such "rechallenge" is rarely done because the resulting reaction could be fatal.

Summary

A primary function of the immune system is to protect the body from potential sources of disease. In some animals, however, the immune system overreacts to certain antigens (allergens), resulting in an allergic reaction. Allergic reactions cause discomfort, itching, and inflammation of the skin. The inflamed skin is highly susceptible to both bacterial and yeast skin infections. Secondary infections worsen the inflammation in the skin and are additional sources of antigens that may produce new

Hives in a dog with an allergic reaction to penicillin.

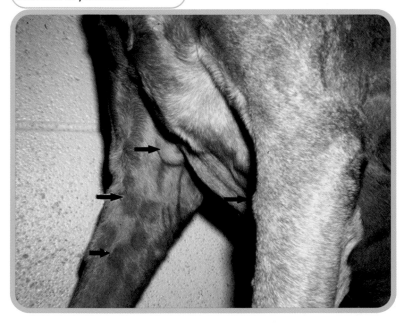

allergies. Medications given to treat infections may result in additional allergic reactions to the drugs themselves. Sorting out allergies is a complex challenge that often requires the involvement of a veterinarian specializing in allergies and both patience and cooperation of the owner of the affected pet.

BACTERIAL INFECTIONS

The term **pyoderma** refers to infections of the skin that produce pus. The most common cause of pyoderma in dogs and cats is the bacterium *Staphylococcus intermedius* (*S. intermedius*). Normal skin and hairs hold small numbers of bacteria; these are part of the normal flora of the skin and hair coat. The numbers of bacteria on normal skin are low because the **stratum corneum** (the outermost, horny layer of the skin) is hard, dry, and constantly shedding. Bacteria rapidly multiply when skin becomes damaged, moist, or inflamed. Certain bacteria, such as *S. intermedius*, produce toxins that cause further damage to the skin, allowing more bacterial growth. Bacteria normally are kept from penetrating past the horny layer of skin by the **immune system.** If the pet's immune system is weakened by other infections, diseases, drugs, or genetic problems, its skin will be more vulnerable to deeper infections, which can spread to the tissues beneath the skin. Cuts, puncture wounds, and damaged **hair follicles** allow bacteria into deeper tissues, slipping by the defense systems of the skin—the dry horny layer and skin immune system.

Skin infections generally develop after the skin's defense system is weakened somehow, so the presence of pyoderma is a clue to an underlying problem. Unless the problem is identified and corrected, the infection is likely to return when treatment for pyoderma is stopped. So treatment of a bacterial skin infection in your pet is much more complicated than simply using an **antimicrobial** on the skin surface or oral antibiotics—any underlying condition must be addressed as well, to allow your pet's skin to get healthy again.

Underlying Causes of Pyoderma in Pets

Factors That Compromise the Cutaneous Barrier

Inflammation: allergies, parasites, immune-mediated diseases

Self-trauma: obsessive-compulsive disorders, itching disorders

External trauma: scrapes, irritants, hair mats, weed seeds

Seborrhea: defects in keratin formation or excessive oils produced by sebaceous glands

Neoplasia: cancer cell infiltration of skin

Moisture: damp environment or frequent swimming

Other infections: dermatophytosis (ringworm), yeast

Factors That Weaken the Immune Defense System

Metabolic diseases: diabetes mellitus, liver disease

Hormonal (endocrine) imbalances: hypothyroidism, Cushing's disease, sex hormone imbalances, other endocrine disorders

Drugs: corticosteroids, chemotherapy agents, general anesthetics

Radiation: ultraviolet light exposure, radiation therapy

Nutritional deficiencies: protein, zinc, vitamin A, and essential fatty acids are vital for normal skin health and integrity

Hereditary immunodeficiencies: defects in production of anti-bodies, or in the ability of white blood cells to destroy bacteria

Stress: rapid growth, environmental conditions (too hot, too cold, overcrowding), surgery

Factors That Bypass the Cutaneous Barrier

Foreign bodies: splinters, grass awns, thorns

Ingrown hairs, ruptured hair follicles: keratin acts like a foreign body

Lacerations (cuts) and bite wounds

Hot Spots (Acute Moist Dermatitis)

Acute moist dermatitis is the term used by many veterinarians to describe the quickly developing skin lesions that are commonly called "hot spots." Another term used to describe this problem is **pyotraumatic dermatitis**. The lesion is seen as a rapidly enlarging area of moist, reddened skin with hair loss. The hair loss is caused by the pet's intense biting or scratching at the area. Hot spots are common in dogs, especially in thick-coated, long-haired 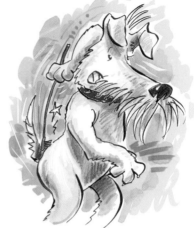 breeds; they are rare in cats. They occur most frequently in warm, humid weather and may be found on the face, back, tail base, or side of the thigh. Bacteria multiply in the discharge (**exudate**) on the skin surface, and the discharge then becomes pus-like (**purulent**).

Lesion of acute moist dermatitis (hot spot) on the thigh of a German Shepherd dog.

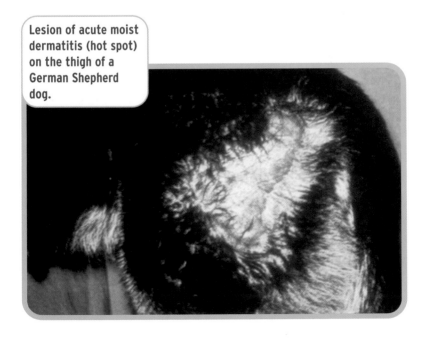

Underlying causes for acute moist dermatitis include:

- **Fleas, ticks, mites, lice, and other ectoparasites (non-internal parasites)**
- **Hair mats**
- **Foreign bodies, such as grass or weed seeds**
- **Anal sac disease**
- **Ear disease**
- **Allergies**

Diagnostic steps usually include taking **impression smears** to determine the number and type of bacteria in the lesion, examining **skin scrapings** to look for mites, flea combing to inspect for fleas, and reviewing the pet's health history to decide whether the pet may have another disease predisposing it to the development of hot spots.

The first step in treatment is to clip and clean the area. Your veterinarian may need to sedate your pet, because the affected area often is painful. A mild **antiseptic** solution, such as chlorhexidine, is used to remove purulent discharge and crusts. A mild **astringent** such as 5% aluminum acetate used on the lesion twice daily will help dry it. An **analgesic** or **corticosteroid** may be used directly on the area to decrease the pain and **inflammation**. Antiseptic or antibiotic sprays keep bacteria from multiplying on the lesion. Sprays generally are better than creams and ointments because the creams and ointments are **occlusive**–they tend to trap moisture on the skin, rather than helping it to dry. An **Elizabethan collar** may help keep the pet from continuing to chew the lesion. Feet may need to be hobbled or bandaged to keep the pet from scratching the lesions. Occasionally, the veterinarian will recommend giving oral corticosteroids for a few days to decrease the inflammation in the skin. If the lesions seem to be spreading, oral antibiotics are given for a minimum of 2 weeks. Additional treatment steps should address any problems that helped the lesion to develop in the first place (for example, these steps may include flea control, good grooming, and eliminating any mites).

Where We Stand

The initial cause of hot spots is a localized irritation that causes the dog to repeatedly bite at or scratch the irritated skin. Damage to the skin from the self-trauma results in oozing of serum (the liquid part of blood) and can lead to secondary bacterial infections.

The most important steps in stopping lesions from getting worse are to (1) stop the self-trauma and (2) help the lesion to dry. Oral antibiotics are needed only if the lesions are spreading. A sign of a spreading lesion is the appearance of raised, red, or pus-filled bumps in the skin surrounding the main lesion. Do not use ointments on these lesions because they trap moisture, rather than promoting drying.

A search should be made for factors that cause the pet to start chewing or scratching the area. Correction of underlying factors is essential in keeping new lesions from forming.

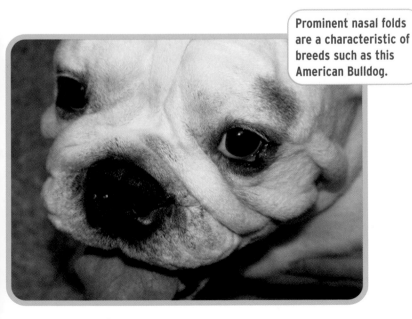

Prominent nasal folds are a characteristic of breeds such as this American Bulldog.

Skin Fold Pyoderma

The body shape of many dogs results in areas of skin that rub together or create folds. These warm, dark areas trap moisture, resulting in **maceration** (deterioration from too much moisture) of the skin and rapid growth of bacteria or yeast in the area. In addition to natural skin secretions, saliva collects in lip folds, tears collect in nasal folds, and licking adds moisture to skin folds around the tail and vulva. The growth of bacteria in the affected skin often produces an offensive odor. The areas may become painful.

Diagnosis is easily made by seeing purulent discharge in a body fold or friction area. Your veterinarian will use **cytology** (cell studies) to see whether bacteria or yeast is

Breed Predispositions to Skin Fold Pyoderma (Intertrigo)

Lip Folds
Saint Bernard
Cocker Spaniel
Springer Spaniel

Nasal Folds
Pekingese
Pug
Bulldogs
Boston Terrier
Boxer

Tail Fold
Bulldogs
Boston Terrier
Pug

Body Folds
Bulldogs
Chinese Shar Pei
Basset Hound (legs)
Dachshunds (legs)

Vulvar Folds
Obese dogs
Dogs spayed before
puberty (?)

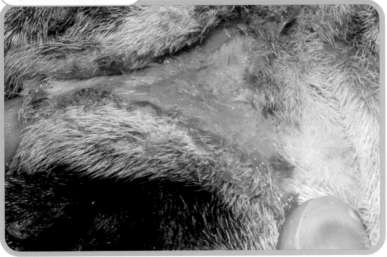

present. For cytologic study, a sample of the discharge is collected for staining and microscopic examination of cells in the discharge. Female dogs with infections in the folds around the vulva also should have a urine sample collected for culture because the infection can sometimes involve the bladder.

The first treatment goal is to clean and dry the lesions. If the area is hairy, clipping will make it easier to keep the area clean. Cleansing with a mild antiseptic shampoo containing chlorhexidine helps to remove crusts and discharge. Medicated wipes containing acetic acid and boric acid or miconazole and chlorhexidine may be used to clean the fold areas once or twice daily. Mupirocin cream also may be used daily to help control bacterial growth in the folds. Weight reduction may help if obesity is causing deeper skin folds. In chronic cases, skin folds can be surgically removed, or the tail may be amputated to eliminate tail folds or rubbing.

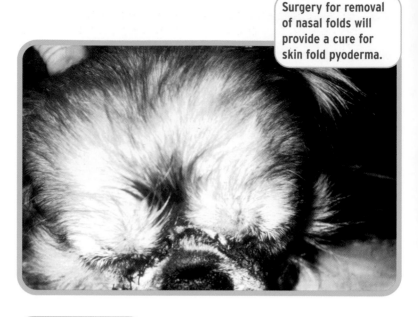

Surgery for removal of nasal folds will provide a cure for skin fold pyoderma.

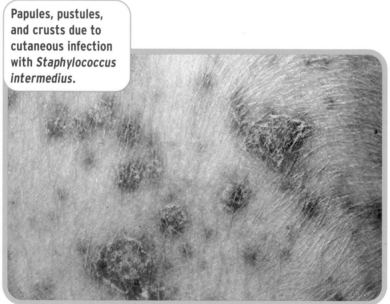

Papules, pustules, and crusts due to cutaneous infection with *Staphylococcus intermedius*.

Staphylococcal Pyoderma

The most common skin infection in dogs is staphylococcal pyoderma. These infections can cause a variety of skin problems, including:

■ **Reddened and raised papules, whitish pustules, and/or crusts**

- **"Bull's eye"** lesions with excess pigmentation in the center, surrounded by red, inflamed skin, and circular areas of scaling (epidermal collarettes)
- **"Moth-eaten"** appearance to the hair coat
- **"Blood blister"-like** lesions
- Thin hair coat with scaling
- Tufts of hair that appear to stick out more than surrounding hairs
- Increased shedding
- Offensive odor (especially when skin is wet)
- Variable pruritus (itching).

Similar-appearing diseases to look for include **demodicosis** (Chapter 3), **dermatophytosis** (Chapter 8), and **pemphigus foliaceus** (Chapter 9). Tests used to look for the causes of one of these diseases are skin scrapings (for *Demodex* mites), fungal cultures (for dermatophytes),

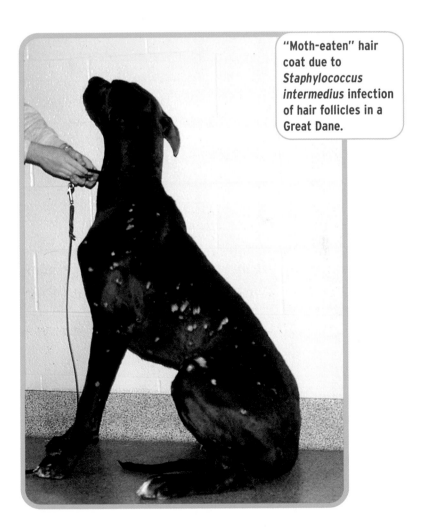

"Moth-eaten" hair coat due to *Staphylococcus intermedius* infection of hair follicles in a Great Dane.

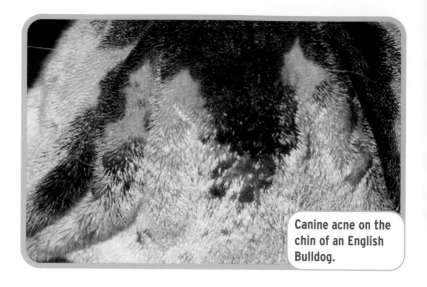

Canine acne on the chin of an English Bulldog.

skin cytology (for bacterial cocci and white blood cells without any **acantholytic keratinocytes**), and, on occasion, skin **biopsy** (for pemphigus foliaceus). Treatment trials also may be helpful—for instance, if the lesions heal with antibiotic therapy, the disease staphylococcal pyoderma was most likely the culprit. However, confirming the presence of staphylococcal pyoderma is only the first step in the pet's evaluation—next, have your veterinarian examine the pet for underlying conditions that may have made a bacterial infection more likely to develop.

Mild cases of staphylococcal pyoderma may respond to the use of **topical** (skin surface) antiseptics (for example, bathing every 2 or 3 days with a medicated shampoo containing chlorhexidine, benzoyl peroxide, or ethyl lactate) or topical antibiotics (such as mupirocin cream or benzoyl peroxide gel applied daily). However, most cases will require the use of **systemic** (given internally, usually by mouth) antibiotics to treat the infection. It is important that antibiotics be given at the correct dose and frequency, and for enough time to completely eliminate infections. Higher doses and longer treatment periods are needed to treat skin infections than with infections of other tissues. The skin receives only approximately 4% of cardiac output (blood flow), and the concentration of antibiotics in the skin averages less than 33% of the concentration in blood. The surface of the skin renews itself every 21 days, so treatment usually is for 3 weeks for simple skin infections and 6 to 12 weeks for deeper skin infections.

Proper dosages for antibiotics are based on the pet's weight. Always give the full dose, as often as directed by your veterinarian. Underdosing makes the antibiotic less effective and may even help bacteria become resistant to the antibiotic. If you are unable to give your pet the antibiotic as directed, request a different antibiotic from your vet. Several antibiotics are available that allow once-a-day dosing; these may be more expensive, but their convenience may make the additional cost well worthwhile. It is simplest to give pills by hiding them in a treat—try putting the pill in the middle of a marshmallow, meatball, or chunk of canned food, or wrapping it in cheese or a piece of soft bread. Coating the pill with peanut butter often works for pets that spit out pills, as the stickiness of peanut butter makes it harder to spit out! If your pet is on a special diet, ask your veterinarian what kinds of food or treats can be used to help give pills. Some pharmacies can compound medicines—that is, crush them and mix them with a tasty liquid or paste—for pets that are not cooperative in taking pills.

Because the main bacterium causing skin infections in dogs, *S. intermedius*, responds predictably to antibiotics, veterinarians usually prescribe an antibiotic known to work against all staphylococci. Some commonly used antibiotics for treating staphylococcal infections include:

cephalexin
cefadroxil
cefpodoxime proxetil
clavulanate plus
  amoxicillin
clindamycin
enrofloxacin
erythromycin
marbofloxin
orbifloxacin
ormetoprim/
  sulfadimethoxine
tetracycline
trimethoprim/sulfadiazine
trimethoprim/sulfamethoxazole

Antibiotic Dosing Frequency

Prescribed Frequency	Prescription Abbreviations	When to Administer to Your Pet
Once a day day	s.i.d, q.d., OR q24h	At the same time each
Twice daily	b.i.d. OR q12h	1. First thing in the morning 2. In the evening, about 12 hours after first dose
Three times daily	t.i.d. OR q8h	1. First thing in the morning 2. Mid-afternoon or when you get home from work or school 3. Just before bedtime

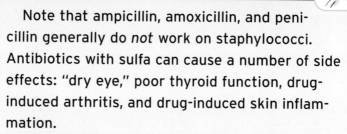

Where We Stand

Note that ampicillin, amoxicillin, and penicillin generally do *not* work on staphylococci. Antibiotics with sulfa can cause a number of side effects: "dry eye," poor thyroid function, drug-induced arthritis, and drug-induced skin inflammation.

Therefore, I do *not* recommend using these antibiotics for routine treatment of staphylococcal pyoderma.

A common mistake in the treatment of staphylococcal pyoderma is stopping oral antibiotics too soon. It is wise to continue giving the antibiotics a minimum of 1 full week after the infection is gone—and for infections that have recurred in the past, it is best to continue giving the antibiotics for a full 2 weeks after all lesions have disappeared. Longer treatment is needed to eliminate bacteria from deep within the hair follicles and skin. If treatment is stopped too soon, bacteria will return and may be harder to kill (the organisms may have developed **resistance** to the antibiotic used previously). Have your pet reexamined by your veterinarian *before* stopping antibiotics; the vet will be able to tell whether the skin infection has been eliminated.

Topical medications can be helpful for supplemental treatment of staphylococcal pyoderma. The easiest way to apply topical medications to multiple skin lesions is through use of an antimicrobial shampoo. Bathing with medicated shampoos reduces the amount of bacteria on the skin surface, removes discharges that aid bacterial growth, and helps relieve skin irritation, making the pet more comfortable. In order for the shampoo to penetrate into the skin and kill the bacteria, it should be left on for 10 minutes before rinsing. Shampoo ingredients with antimicrobial action include benzoyl peroxide, chlorhexidine, ethyl lactate, triclosan, acetic acid, and povidone-iodine (Chapter 2). The recommended frequency of bathing is every 2 to 4 days when infections are present, and every 1 to 2 weeks after that to help prevent return of infections. Medicated lotions, sprays, or wipes containing chlorhexidine or acetic acid plus boric acid will provide longer-lasting activity than shampoos and are particularly helpful in the treatment of infections affecting only one area of the body (such as the feet, chin, tail, head, or underside of the abdomen). Benzoyl peroxide gel and mupirocin cream also are useful in treating specific areas of infection (feet, chin, legs).

Once the pyoderma has been eliminated, it is important to control factors that contributed to the initial infection. Pets with **immunodeficiencies** may be helped by immunostimulant therapy. Immunostimulants are agents that activate the immune system. Three immunostimulant options for dogs with reoccurring staphylococcal pyoderma are:

- **Staphage Lysate (SPL, Delmont Laboratories, Inc.)**
- **Immunoregalin (Immunovet)**
- **Alpha-2 interferon (Roferon-A, Roche Pharmaceuticals)**

Staphage Lysate is a solution containing killed staphylococcal bacteria and tiny organisms called bacteriophages; it is given by injection into the skin twice weekly for several weeks and then once weekly for maintenance. Immunoregalin is a solution containing killed *Propionibacterium acnes* bacteria; it is given by injection into a vein every 2 weeks for two or three treatments. Alpha-2 interferon may be given orally (one to three times daily) or by injection into the skin (twice weekly). The goal of immunostimulation is to help the pet's immune system kill bacteria; it may require several weeks or months to achieve this result. Because response is slow and difficult to measure, immunostimulants usually are used only for pets that have had multiple infections, especially if the infections did not resolve or become less frequent after treatment of known underlying diseases.

Most cases of staphylococcal pyoderma in dogs and cats are due to *S. intermedius*, a normal inhabitant of the skin and hairs. This bacterium is not contagious to healthy people. Occasionally, however, dogs and cats become infected with *Staphylococcus aureus*, which also can cause skin disease in people. If a person in the family has a skin infection, any skin lesions of dogs and cats in the household should be cultured to find out if the pet is infected with *S. aureus*. **Culture and susceptibility testing** for antibiotic effectiveness also should be performed if the pet's skin infection has not started to heal after

2 weeks of antibiotic therapy or if multiple species of bacteria are found on skin cytology examination.

Miscellaneous Bacterial Infections

There are several other conditions in which bacteria contribute to skin disease. The names used for these conditions refer to the body location, breed, or age associated with the disease.

Chin Pyoderma (Acne)

Acne in dogs is most common in young (3- to 12-months-old), short-coated, large-breed dogs (such as Doberman Pinschers, Great Danes, English Bulldogs, and Labrador Retrievers). In this condition, blackheads, papules, and pustules develop on the chin and muzzle; these lesions often rupture and discharge blood or pus. Conditions with a similar appearance include demodicosis, contact dermatitis, juvenile pyoderma (puppy strangles), and dermatophytosis. Common diagnostic tests include examination of skin scrapings to rule out *Demodex*, fungal cultures to rule out **ringworm** fungus, and cytology to determine the numbers and types of organisms present in the lesions. Skin biopsy and bacterial cultures are helpful to evaluate severe cases. Mild cases are treated by gently cleansing affected areas with a benzoyl peroxide shampoo, followed by application of either a benzoyl peroxide gel (this will bleach fabrics that come in contact with the treated skin) or mupirocin cream. The gel or cream is reapplied once daily until lesions heal, and then once or twice a week as needed to keep them from returning. More severe cases require treatment with oral antibiotics; these should be continued for at least 2 weeks after the lesions disappear (typically for a total of 6 weeks). Canine acne rarely reoccurs in dogs older than 1 year of age, although a few dogs will continue to need preventive treatment (bathing the chin with benzoyl peroxide shampoo or applying mupirocin cream weekly) for several months.

Acne in cats may occur at any age and often waxes and wanes in severity. Many cases of feline acne do not involve a bacterial infection but result when hair follicles become plugged by excess **keratin** (a protein that normally is present in skin, hair, and nails), causing **comedones** (blackheads) to form. Comedones are found most often on the chin and occasionally on the lips. The keratin plugs may look like flea dirt, but they do not contain blood and do not produce a red color when moistened. Pus-filled and raised skin lesions and small nodules may develop if the lesions become infected with bacteria or yeast. Conditions that may have a similar appearance include demodicosis, dermatophytosis, and **eosinophilic granulomas** of the chin. Diagnostic tests include examination of skin scrapings, fungal cultures, skin cytology, and skin biopsy. No treatment is necessary if the lesions are not infected and do not bother the cat. Infected lesions are treated with warm compresses to help loosen the comedones, followed by gentle bathing with a benzoyl peroxide or ethyl lactate shampoo. Human acne treatment pads containing benzoyl peroxide, salicylic acid, or retinoic acid may be used every 1 or 2 days. Daily applica-

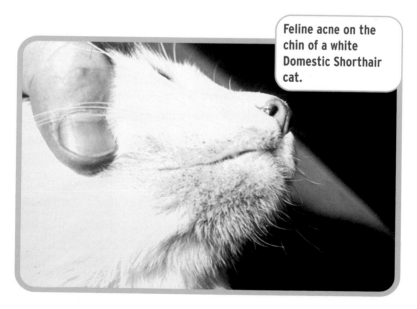

Feline acne on the chin of a white Domestic Shorthair cat.

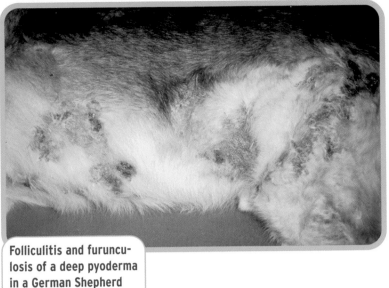

Folliculitis and furunculosis of a deep pyoderma in a German Shepherd dog.

tions of mupirocin cream are helpful in the treatment of bacterial or yeast infections. Oral antibiotics usually are prescribed for cats with draining tracts (openings within infected tissue leading to the skin surface) or when topical treatment has not resolved the infection.

German Shepherd Dog Pyoderma

German shepherd dogs are prone to a number of deep skin infections. The underlying reason for these infections is rarely found. These problems often are difficult to treat, and relapses are common.

Staphylococcal infections in German Shepherd dogs often are located deep in hair follicles and cause the follicle to rupture. After rupture, intense inflammation develops around the remainder of the follicle, forming a draining tract with a pus-like discharge. These lesions may look like puncture wounds but are a result of ruptured hair follicles, not trauma. The terms veterinarians use for these lesions are **folliculitis** and **furunculosis**. Lesions are most common on the rump, back, abdomen, and thighs. Affected dogs usually are middle-aged German Shepherd dogs or German Shepherd mixes. Other conditions that should be checked for include demodicosis, fungal infections, **immunodeficiency**, **hypothyroidism**, food allergy, **atopy,** and flea-bite dermatitis. Bacterial culture and antibiotic effectiveness testing are advised, because long-term treatment with oral antibiotics will be needed (12 weeks or longer). Shaving affected areas and daily whirlpool therapy are recommended to speed recovery.

Focal metatarsal fistulation is a disease affecting middle-aged to older German Shepherd dogs. Males are affected more often than females. This disease is believed to be an **immune-mediated disease** that causes **fistulas** (abnormal passages through tissue) to form between the metatarsal area and the skin surface. Lesions develop on the rear of the lower hind leg, often on both legs. Early lesions may appear as swellings that later rupture and develop deep into draining tracts. Bacteria often become involved. Other diagnoses that should be tested for include foreign bodies, trauma, fungal infections, and tumors. Skin biopsy usually is performed to confirm the

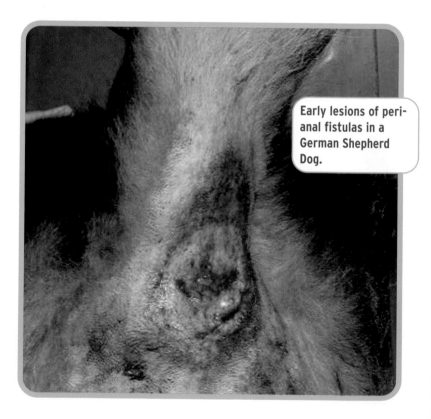

Early lesions of peri-anal fistulas in a German Shepherd Dog.

diagnosis. Long-term antibiotic and topical therapy (warm compresses or medicated whirlpool treatments) will help, but relapses are common. Some dogs respond well to vitamin E supplements, topical or oral corticosteroids, or a combination of tetracycline and niacinamide. A veterinary dermatologist should be consulted for the management of focal metatarsal fistulas.

Perianal fistula disease is most common in German Shepherd dogs and German Shepherd crosses. Lesions are located in the skin surrounding the anus. Early lesions appear as areas of raised red skin or **cysts**. These lesions rupture, forming draining tracts. The condition usually is painful; the dog may lick the perianal region, object to having its tail raised, and cry when defecating. Some affected dogs have underlying food allergies, but in most cases no underlying disease can be found. This disease may represent another immune-mediated disease in which bacterial infection occurs only after the development of the fistulas. Treatment options include surgery, immunosuppressive drugs (such as corticosteroids, azathioprine, cyclosporine, or tacrolimus), dietary management, and systemic antibiotics. Because this disease is difficult to manage, consulting a veterinary dermatologist is recommended.

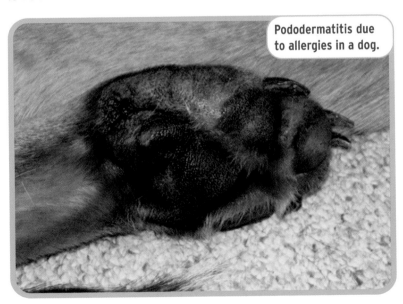

Pododermatitis due to allergies in a dog.

Interdigital Pyoderma (Pododermatitis)

Dogs' feet—their paws—are prone to bacterial infections caused by a variety of factors. These include:

- **Allergies (environmental, food)**
- **Embedded hairs**
- **Foreign bodies (grass and plant awns, splinters, thorns, glass fragments, sharp gravel)**
- **Irritants (chemicals, fertilizers, weed killers)**
- **Parasites (*Demodex, Pelodera*, hookworms, ticks)**
- **Ruptured cysts**
- **Trauma (such as from contact with rough surfaces or burns)**

One or more paws may be affected. Common findings include **erythema** (redness), swelling, and various skin lesions—**papules**, **pustules**, hemorrhagic **bullae** (blood-filled blisters), **nodules**, draining tracts, and **ulcers**. Dogs commonly lick at the lesions. Licking may make the condition worse by embedding hairs or rupturing follicles and cysts. Some affected dogs are lame, and most show signs of pain when their paws are touched. Possible diseases to test for include demodicosis, fungal infections, immune-mediated skin diseases, sterile **pyogranulomas**, and tumors. Examination of skin scrapings, cytologic study of any discharge, cultures, and skin biopsy are helpful in making a diagnosis. Treatment includes giving oral antibiotics for a minimum of 2 weeks after lesions resolve (often for 12 weeks or longer) and daily foot soaks in an antiseptic solution (chlorhexidine, aluminum acetate, acetic acid, boric acid, or magnesium sulfate). Topical mupirocin cream also may be useful in treating these infections. Surgical removal of infected tissue may be needed in severe or chronic cases. Consult a veterinary dermatologist to help manage recurring pododermatitis.

Deep Pyoderma

Deep pyoderma is defined as a skin infection involving the **dermis** (second layer of skin) and deeper skin structures. It develops when bacteria penetrate through the

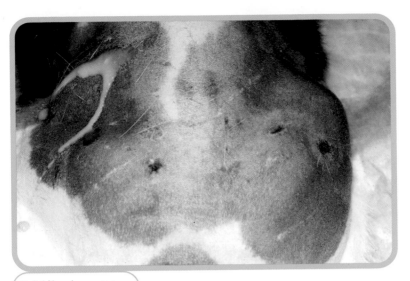

Cat-bite abscesses on the back of a Domestic Shorthair cat (the cat's back has been shaved).

top layers of the skin or through the walls of hair follicles. German Shepherd dog folliculitis and furunculosis and interdigital pyoderma are examples of deep pyoderma (see earlier sections of this chapter). Deep pyoderma may develop in any breed of dog and may affect any body region. Lesions may affect one specific area, a few specific areas, or the whole body. Red, raised, and pus-filled lesions, crusts, and draining tracts are common. The pet may be inactive and feverish. Other diseases that may have a similar appearance include demodicosis, fungal infections, immune-mediated skin diseases, and skin tumors. Skin scrapings, cultures (bacterial and fungal), cytology, and skin biopsy are helpful in making the correct diagnosis. Treatment includes finding and treating any underlying diseases and giving oral antibiotics for a minimum of 2 weeks after lesions resolve (typically for a total of 8 to 12 weeks). Daily whirlpool baths using an antiseptic solution (chlorhexidine, aluminum acetate, or potassium peroxymonosulfate) will help the lesions heal. If a whirlpool is not available, the dog should be bathed with a medicated shampoo every 2 or 3 days until the lesions heal.

Subcutaneous Abscess

Subcutaneous abscesses develop when bacteria multiply in lipid-rich (fatty) tissues beneath the skin (subcutaneously). The most common cause of subcutaneous abscesses is a fight injury, in which bacteria carried on teeth or on claws infect a wound. Other penetrating wounds, foreign bodies, and infections around teeth also may result in subcutaneous abscesses. The abscesses appear as painful swellings that may rupture and drain pus. Careful inspection of the swelling may reveal the site of the puncture wound. Subcutaneous abscesses are most common in cats and typically are found around the tail base or on the shoulders, neck, face, or legs (depending on whether the cat was facing its opponent or running away). The most common bacterium present in subcutaneous abscesses is *Pasteurella multocida*. Staphylococci, streptococci, and anaerobic bacteria also may be involved. Your veterinarian will surgically drain and clean the wound with an antiseptic solution. In addition, oral antibiotics are given for 1 to 2 weeks. Cat bites also may spread viral infections; therefore, cats that have been involved in fights should be tested for **feline immunodeficiency virus** (FIV) and **feline leukemia virus** (FeLV) infections. Neutering male cats may make them less likely to fight.

Juvenile Pyoderma (Puppy Strangles)

Juvenile pyoderma usually affects puppies between 3 weeks and 6 months of age. It is thought to be an immune-mediated disease, not a primary bacterial skin disease. Certain breeds are more prone to develop this disease than others, suggesting that genetics may play a role. Dachshunds, Golden Retrievers, Labrador Retrievers, Beagles, and Pointers have the highest incidence of this

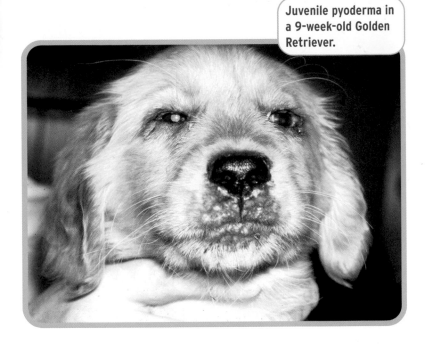

disease. Lesions may start in the ears, on the muzzle, or around the eyes. Affected skin is swollen and red, with raised and pus-filled (purulent) lesions, purulent discharge, and crusts. The ears often have a purulent discharge, and the ear flaps may show swelling and hair loss. The submandibular lymph nodes, located under the jaw, are greatly enlarged and sometimes rupture, draining a purulent fluid. Affected puppies often are inactive, feverish, and reluctant to eat. Other diseases that may have a similar appearance include canine acne, **otitis externa** (ear infection), demodicosis, allergies, fungal infections, deep pyoderma related to immunodeficiency, and lymphosarcoma (cancer affecting the skin or lymph nodes). Skin scrapings, impression smears for cytologic study, lymph node aspirates, bacterial and fungal cultures, and skin biopsy can be helpful in ruling out other causes and confirming the diagnosis of juvenile pyoderma.

Treatment includes daily antiseptic soaks to remove discharge and crusts, oral antibiotics to prevent secondary skin infections, and corticosteroids to decrease the inflammation. Most puppies show rapid improvement

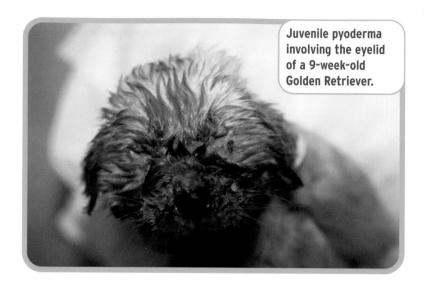

Juvenile pyoderma involving the eyelid of a 9-week-old Golden Retriever.

during treatment and live normal lives after recovery. With severe cases, the dog may have permanent scars and hair loss in affected areas.

Summary

Bacterial skin infections are common in dogs and, with the exception of cat-bite abscesses, rare in cats. Bacterial infections may involve only the surface of the skin or may extend into the subcutaneous tissues, beneath the skin. Bacterial skin infections may look like demodicosis, dermatophytosis, pemphigus foliaceus, and many other diseases. In addition, bacterial skin infections usually are caused by another underlying disease process (such as allergies, parasites, hormonal diseases, immunosuppressive diseases, and others). For these reasons, a series of diagnostic tests may be needed to rule out other diseases. Treatment of bacterial skin infections frequently involves a combination of topical medications and oral antibiotics. It is important to continue treatment for a minimum of 1 to 2 weeks after all skin lesions have disappeared, to be certain the infection has been eliminated from deeper areas of the skin. Consultation with a veterinary dermatologist is recommended for advice in managing reoccurring infections.

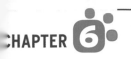
PARASITIC SKIN DISEASES

Ectoparasites are organisms that live on or within the skin of an animal host and feed and get nutrients from the host. Problems linked to ectoparasites range from mild irritations to severe allergic reactions to parasite bites and serious illness from diseases transmitted by the parasite. Many ectoparasite infestations are contagious to other animals and also may affect people; however, some ectoparasites (for example, lice) infest only certain animal species, and a few (such as certain *Demodex* mites) can't be transmitted at all. Some ectoparasites (fleas, lice, ticks) are easily seen on the pet's skin and hair coat, whereas others (like mites) may be found only by using a microscope to examine samples from the pet's skin or ears.

There are many antiparasitic agents that work against ectoparasites. Some are given orally, and others are delivered via collars, shampoos, sprays, dips, powders, or spot applications. Correct dosing and application of **parasiticides** are essential for them to work well and safely; thus, many products are available only when prescribed by a veterinarian who has examined the pet.

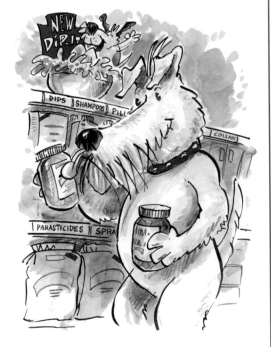

Fleas

Adult fleas are small, wingless, blood-sucking insects with strong hind legs that allow them to jump onto their hosts. There are over 2500 species of fleas worldwide. The most common flea affecting dogs and cats is *Ctenocephalides felis*. Flea infestations are contagious, and fleas can live on cats, dogs, mice, rats, rabbits, ferrets, birds, and people. Fleas feed on their hosts by piercing the skin and sucking the blood.

Life Cycle

Fleas have a complex life cycle with a complete metamorphosis (change in life forms): egg→larva→pupa→adult flea. The adult flea lives on its host. Female fleas start laying eggs 24 to 36 hours after a blood meal and produce 20 to 40 eggs each day. Eggs are oval in shape, white, and 0.5 mm long. The eggs are not "sticky," so they fall off the host into the environment. Under ideal conditions (64º to 80º F and 75% relative humidity or higher), eggs hatch into larvae in 4 to 6 days. After hatching, the larvae migrate into cracks in wood floors, deep into carpets, or under leaves or organic

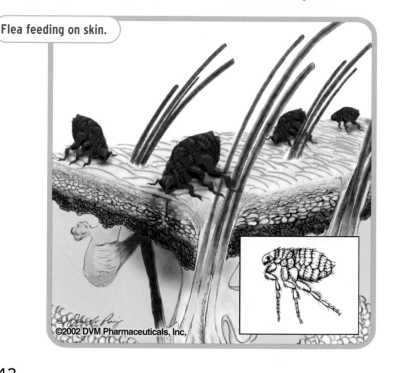

Flea feeding on skin.

©2002 DVM Pharmaceuticals, Inc.

debris if outdoors. Larvae feed on organic material (such as feces from adult fleas) and molt twice before spinning a cocoon; inside the cocoon, the larva develops into a pupa. The emergence of the adult flea from the cocoon is triggered by increases in temperature, vibration, or physical pressure—conditions caused by a potential host walking nearby. The length of this life cycle varies but ranges between 12 and 174 days, largely depending on temperature. Dryness (less than 33% relative humidity), low temperatures (below 8° C), and high temperatures (above 35° C) are lethal to flea larvae in a short time. Newly emerged fleas must find a host within a couple of days or they will die. The life span of fleas living on a host can be 100 days or longer. A single fertilized female flea and her offspring may produce over 20,000 adult fleas within 60 days. Because most of a flea's life cycle is spent in pre-adult stages, there may be 100 pre-adult fleas in the environment for every adult flea on a pet.

Clinical Signs

Symptoms of a flea infestation vary depending on the number of fleas and whether the pet is allergic to fleas. A single flea may cause intense biting and scratching in a flea-allergic pet, resulting in excoriations (scratch marks), crusting, and loss of hair (alopecia). In dogs, fleas usually are most numerous on the rump, base of the tail, hind

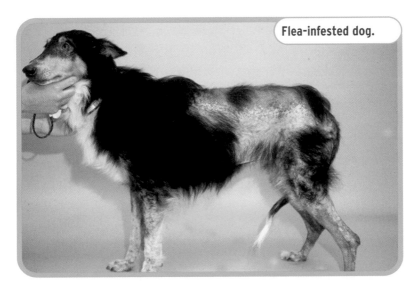

Flea-infested dog.

limbs (inner thighs and back of legs), and abdomen. Adult fleas avoid light and will scurry to hide when you try to find them by parting the pet's hair.

Perhaps because cats are very efficient groomers and will catch and swallow fleas that they can reach on their backs and abdomens, fleas in cats often group around the cat's head and neck. Flea bites produce pinpoint red spots (papules) that become crusted. Cats with flea allergies often have numerous crusted papules along their backs and around their necks. These lesions feel like millet seeds on the cat's skin, so the condition is called **miliary** ("millet-like") **dermatitis**. Some cats with flea allergies develop ulcers on their upper lips (indolent ulcers); others develop red plaques and skin ulcers that contain large numbers of cells called eosinophils (eosinophilic plaques). Because cats have a barbed tongue, cats that groom excessively to rid themselves of fleas often pull out large amounts of hair; this may result in a "bald belly" or other areas of alopecia.

Each flea feeds on approximately 0.014 mL of blood per day. Heavy infestations can cause anemia or even death from loss of blood. Fleas can serve as intermediate hosts that transmit tapeworms (*Dipylidium caninum*) and the nematode (worm) *Acanthocheilonema* (*Dipetalonema*) *reconditum*. Fleas also can be carriers of rickettsiae, *Bartonella*, and other disease-causing microorganisms.

Diagnosis

Fleas are large enough to be seen crawling or jumping on pets. Combing the pet with a fine-toothed flea comb often will catch fleas or pick up "flea dirt." Flea dirt (flea feces) is seen as comma-shaped particles, which consist primarily of dried blood. Flea dirt can be distinguished from environmental dirt by placing it on a moistened cotton ball or paper towel and observing a halo of red "bleeding" out of flea fecal particles. Flea allergies can be confirmed by intradermal skin testing (with injection of antigens just below the top horny layer) or by finding high titers (levels) of flea antigen-specific serum IgE anti-bodies.

Treatment

Control of fleas is best achieved with a program of total pest management. This involves the simultaneous use of **adulticides** to kill adult fleas and **insect development inhibitors** (IDIs) to keep pre-adult fleas from becoming adults, plus steps to remove and kill fleas in the pet's environment. Your veterinarian should be consulted to prescribe a control program appropriate for your individual household. Important things to consider in choosing one of the many available pesticides and IDIs include:

- **Types of pets in the household**
- **Ages and breeds**
- **Length of hair coats**
- **Overall health (any ill or debilitated pets?)**
- **Environment (inside or outside, carpets or hardwood floors, bedding, kennels)**
- **Frequency of bathing or swimming**
- **Other activities**

All of these factors may affect how well the product will work. Be sure that the flea control products you've chosen will not poison fish, birds, or exotic pets in the household.

Thorough cleaning of the environment is important in controlling fleas. Vacuuming carpets with a powerful machine equipped with a "beater bar" can remove many flea eggs, flea feces, larvae, and new-hatched fleas (the vibrations of the beater bar stimulate fleas to emerge from their pupas). Upholstered furniture also should be thoroughly cleaned and vacuumed often. Launder pet bedding weekly. If the pet travels in family vehicles, vacuum and clean the vehicles weekly. Outdoors, keep the pet away from areas under bushes, trees, decks, and porches. Rake and remove organic debris (leaves or mulch) from areas where the pet spends most of its time.

The best approach to flea control is prevention—once a flea population becomes established, there are often 100 developing fleas in the environment for every adult flea

Integrated Pest Management for Control of Fleas: Sample Regimen

Complete pest management involves the simultaneous use of adulticides and insect development inhibitors, plus environmental control steps.

Adulticides on Pets

- **Apply fipronil or imidacloprid or selamectin monthly.**
- **Treat all dogs and cats in the household or in contact with a flea-infested pet.**

Insect Development Inhibitors for Pets

- **Use lufenuron OR methoprene OR pyriproxyfen.**
- **Treat all dogs and cats in the household or in contact with a flea-infested pet.**

Environmental Control Measures

- **Vacuum and mop twice weekly.**
- **Wash pet bedding and disinfect kennels weekly.**
- **Use methoprene OR pyriproxyfen sprays or foggers monthly.**
- **If needed: Apply chlorpyrifos or diazinon sprays or powders to yard monthly.**
- **If needed: Use pyrethrin foggers or sprays in house monthly.**

seen on the pet. IDIs help to keep fleas from developing in the environment. Lufenuron is an IDI that keeps flea chitin (their protective covering) from forming. It is given orally to dogs and cats once monthly (found in the products Program and Sentinel, made by Novartis Animal Health). Lufenuron is stored in fat just underneath the skin and, when ingested by a flea feeding on the pet, prevents the eggs laid by the flea from hatching; larvae feeding on the flea's feces also are prevented from molting (so they can't progress to the pupa stage). Methoprene is a type of IDI that mimics juvenile growth hormones of insects—it keeps fleas from maturing into adults. Methoprene may be applied to the pet in "spot-on" ("onespot") formulations (Frontline Plus, made by Merial Animal Health), flea collars (Ovitrol, VetKem, and others), sprays (Ovitrol, VetKem, and others), or directly to the environment as a surface spray (Precor). Pyriproxyfen (Nylar and others) is another IDI that mimics juvenile growth hormones; it's available in collars, shampoos, and sprays for use on pets and in the environment.

Dozens of adulticide products (see the table on Antiparasitic Agents and Pest Control Management for Dogs and Cats in Chapter 2) are available to kill adult fleas on pets and in the environment. Examples include:

borax
botanicals (*d*-limonene, pyrethrins, rotenone)
pyrethroids (allethrin, cypermethrin, permethrin)
carbaryl
imidacloprid (Advantage)
nitenpyram (Capstar)
lindane
organophosphates (dichlorvos, phosmet, chlorpyrifos, diazinon, cythioate)
selamectin (Revolution)
fipronil (Frontline)

Many of these products are toxic to certain species—for example, fipronil is toxic to rabbits, organophosphates and pyrethroids can be toxic to cats, and most are toxic to fish. Be sure to use all products according to label directions, and select an adulticide only after consulting with a veterinarian familiar with the pet and its environment.

Mange and Other Mite Infestations

Mange is the term used for skin diseases caused by mites. Cats and dogs are affected by several species of mites. Many of these mites are tiny and can be seen only under a microscope. Different mites vary in their life cycles, signs and symptoms linked to their presence, measures needed for control, and ability to spread to other animals. So it's important for you to consult your veterinarian to identify the specific type of mange affecting your pet; the vet will then prescribe appropriate treatments.

Canine Demodicosis (Red Mange)

Mange resulting from large numbers of *Demodex canis* mites has been called "red mange" (skin of affected dogs is reddish in color as a result of intense inflammation), "follicular mange" (these mites live in hair follicles), and "demodectic mange." Small numbers of mites may be found in normal dogs and are transmitted to puppies from their mothers. In normal healthy dogs, the number of mites is low because the immune system blocks most mite reproduction. If a dog's immune system is weakened by stress, disease, drugs, or a genetic deficiency, the mites may multiply rapidly, leading to clinical signs of disease.

Life Cycle

Demodex canis mites can be transmitted to dogs only during their first few days of life. These mites are not transmissible between adult dogs or to other animals or people. *Demodex* mites are elongated with short stubby legs and spend their entire life living in the hair follicles and skin of their host. Eggs are fusiform ("teardrop"-shaped) and hatch into small, six-legged larvae. The larvae molt into eight-legged nymphs, which in turn mature into eight-legged adults. These four life stages can be easily identified by microscopic examination of skin scrapings taken from dogs with active infections. Adult mites average 40 micrometers in width and 250 to 300 micrometers in length. Short-tailed and long-bodied variants of *Demodex* mites have been found in some dogs.

Clinical Signs

Disease caused by the presence of too many *Demodex* mites can be **localized** to one area of the body or **generalized** over large areas. Localized demodicosis usually develops in dogs younger than 1 year of age (often near the time of puberty). The affected area of skin becomes scaly, with a focal patch of hair loss. The patches of hair loss are seen most commonly on the face, around the eyes, or on the muzzle. The front legs also may be affected. These lesions are not painful to the dog and will resolve within 4 to 8 weeks without any specific treatment. It is believed that the stresses caused by growth weaken the dog's immune system enough to allow the mites to overmultiply for a few weeks, after which the immune system recovers and keeps mites in check.

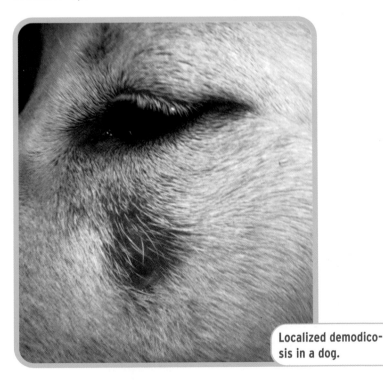

Localized demodicosis in a dog.

Generalized demodicosis affects more than one body region. It is either "juvenile-onset," starting in dogs younger than 1 year of age, or "adult-onset," developing in older dogs. Juvenile-onset generalized demodicosis is most common in purebred dogs and is thought to be caused by a genetic defect in the immune system, resulting in a failure in the control of mite reproduction. Adult-onset generalized demodicosis often is due to drugs (corticosteroids or chemotherapy drugs) or diseases—such as cancer, endocrine disease, and metabolic disease—that suppress the dog's immune system. Patches of hair loss develop and spread. The affected areas of skin become red and scaly, with bumps and crusts. Secondary bacterial infections develop in the skin and can become severe enough to kill the dog if not treated. Lesions can develop anywhere on the body and often involve the feet, which become swollen and painful. Some dogs become itchy, especially if the skin has secondary bacterial infections. Fever and enlarged lymph nodes are other possible findings; the dog also may become inactive.

Diagnosis

There are many possible causes of hair loss and scaling in dogs. Conditions with signs similar to those of demodi-

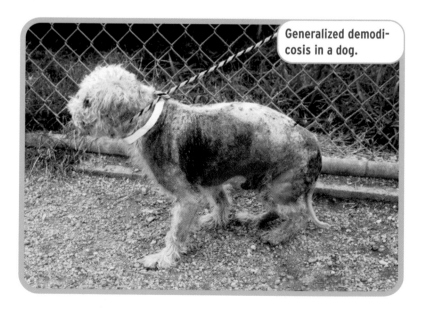

Generalized demodicosis in a dog.

cosis include dermatophytosis (ringworm infections), staphylococcal folliculitis (bacterial infections of hair follicles), and follicular dysplasias (hereditary diseases affecting hair follicles). Fortunately, demodicosis usually is easily diagnosed by microscopic examination of skin scrapings taken from an affected area of skin. The veterinarian will do counts of the numbers of each life stage present in the skin scraping (eggs, larvae, nymphs, adults) and note whether the mites are alive or dead. These mite counts are valuable in monitoring the response to treatments—if these are successful, the numbers of immature mites and eggs will decrease and a majority of mites will be dead; eventually, mites will no longer be found. Occasionally, in chronically affected skin, so much scarring is present that mites will be difficult to find; in those cases, skin biopsy may be needed for diagnosis. Biopsy also may be needed to diagnose demodicosis in Chinese Shar-Pei dogs because of their thick, mucin-filled skin, which makes it difficult to find mites on scrapings. After a diagnosis of demodicosis, your veterinarian will look for any co-existing diseases that may be suppressing the dog's immune system. Common screening tests include fecal examinations to detect other parasites, blood chemistry panels and urinalysis to look for metabolic diseases, cultures if secondary infections are present, and in some cases endocrine testing, x-ray studies (radiography), or ultrasound examinations to screen for cancer or other diseases.

Treatment

Localized demodicosis should resolve without any specific mite treatment, so try to keep the dog as healthy as possible: Avoid stressful situations (such as traveling, boarding, or nonrequired surgeries), feed high-quality dog food, and deworm as recommended by your vet. Prevent secondary infections by using a benzoyl peroxide shampoo, lotion, or gel. Specific mite treatment generally is not needed and is not recommended in pets intended for breeding—it is important to find out if the dog's immune system will be able to control the mites on its own. If it can't, the dog should not be used for breeding, because the immunodeficiency that allows demodicosis to develop may be passed on genetically to the puppies. Affected dogs should be rechecked by the veterinarian every 2 to 4 weeks. If repeated skin scrapings show increasing numbers of mites, specific anti-mite therapy may be needed, and the dog should be neutered following treatment.

Generalized demodicosis can be difficult and expensive to treat. Many dogs with juvenile-onset demodicosis will be cured following 2 to 6 months of anti-mite therapy. A few dogs with juvenile-onset demodicosis and many dogs with adult-onset demodicosis require lifelong anti-mite treatment to prevent flare-ups of the disease. As with localized demodicosis, it is important to have a veterinarian check the dog for any underlying diseases and treat those appropriately. Drugs that suppress the immune system (such as corticosteroids) should be stopped and avoided for the remainder of the dog's life. Weekly bathing with benzoyl peroxide shampoos will help prevent secondary skin infections and also help in flushing mites out of hair follicles. Severely affected dogs will benefit from several medicated whirlpool treatments. Several drugs are effective in killing *Demodex* mites. These include amitraz (Mitaban), ivermectin, milbemycin, and other avermectins. These drugs are not safe for all dogs, and some breeds of dogs are highly prone to adverse reactions. So treatment with any of these agents should *always* be closely supervised by a veterinarian experienced in managing generalized demodicosis. Follow-up appointments to evaluate the pet's response to treatment will be needed every 2 to 4 weeks until all mites are eliminated, and for several months afterward to watch for relapses.

Feline Demodicosis

Two different species of *Demodex* mites can cause disease in cats. The first is *Demodex cati*, an elongate slender mite that inhabits the hair follicles and has a life cycle similar to that of *D. canis* in dogs. The second is *D. gatoi*, a shorter mite with a rounded abdomen. *D. gatoi* lives within the surface layers of the skin (in the stratum corneum).

Life Cycle

Mites causing feline demodicosis do not affect other animals or people; the life cycles are completed on their host. *D. gatoi* can be spread to other cats by direct contact; *Demodex cati* is similar to *D. canis*, with transmission taking place only between queens (mother cats) and their kittens during the first few days of life. Immunosuppression from an underlying condition is present in a majority of cats that demonstrate clinical signs linked to large numbers of *D. cati* mites. Examples of underlying conditions include:

- **Diabetes**
- **Hyperadrenocorticism**
- **Cancers**
- **Feline leukemia virus infection**
- **Feline immunodeficiency virus infection**
- **Prior use of corticosteroids or other immunosuppressive drugs**

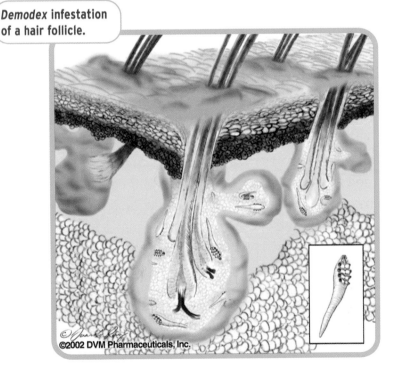

Demodex infestation of a hair follicle.

©2002 DVM Pharmaceuticals, Inc.

Clinical Signs

Localized demodicosis in cats may appear as patchy areas of hair loss on the eyelids, around the eyes, or on the muzzle, and mites occasionally live in the ear canals. Less commonly, lesions may develop on the neck, legs, chest, sides, or trunk and become widespread generalized demodicosis. Skin in affected areas may become reddened, scaly, crusty, and thicker than normal. Some cats become very itchy. Cats affected with *D. gatoi* infestation may overgroom, resulting in a widespread loss of hair from the rear legs, belly, and other regions.

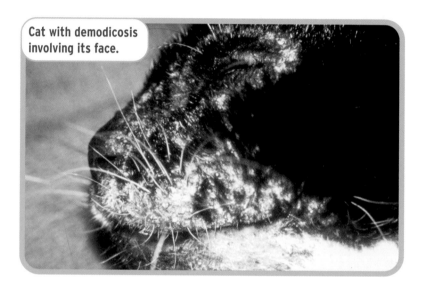

Cat with demodicosis involving its face.

Diagnosis

Demodex mites are tiny and can be seen only under a microscope. They sometimes can be found on examination of feces, because mites swallowed by cats during grooming remain intact as they pass through the digestive tract. Your veterinarian will obtain skin scrapings and swabs of the ears to find the mites. Cats affected with *D. cati* infestation should be checked for underlying immunosuppressive diseases such as diabetes and infections with feline leukemia virus or feline immunodeficiency virus. Because *D. gatoi* infestations are contagious, skin scrapings should be obtained in all cats that come in contact with an affected cat, to detect carriers of these mites.

Treatment

Demodex mites in cats often can be eliminated through the use of weekly lime-sulfur dips. These dips smell terrible but are very safe for use in cats. Dips should be continued for 1 month after skin scrapings from all affected sites are negative for mites. Other treatments that are sometimes used include amitraz dips and giving high doses of ivermectin daily or weekly. These alternative treatments are not approved for cats and should only be used with the advice of a veterinary dermatologist familiar with their use in the treatment of feline demodicosis.

Canine Scabies (Sarcoptic Mange)

Scabies in dogs, also known as **sarcoptic mange**, is caused by a microscopic mite, *Sarcoptes scabiei* var. *canis*. These mites burrow into the superficial layers of skin (stratum corneum) and cause intense itching in most affected pets. Many pets develop an allergic reaction to the mites, which worsens the skin inflammation and itching.

Life Cycle

Sarcoptes mites live approximately 3 weeks. Most of this time is spent on (or in) the skin of the host animal. Females lay eggs in tunnels within the stratum corneum of the skin; the eggs hatch into larvae, which leave the tunnels and form molting pockets in the stratum corneum. Larvae molt into nymphs, which mature into adults that mate on the skin surface. The fertilized female mite then burrows, forming new tunnels in the skin. Mites can survive only a day or two in the environment. Although the mites prefer *Canidae* (the dog family), they also can affect other mammals including people. Foxes and hedgehogs are believed to serve as reservoirs of these mites. Dogs coming in contact with foxes (increasingly common even in urban areas) or running through trails where foxes have recently run can become infected with *Sarcoptes*. Dogs also may become infected through contact with other dogs in boarding kennels, grooming facilities, dog parks, or dog shows.

Clinical Signs

The mites prefer thinly haired skin and are most numerous in the skin of the ears, elbows, legs, and belly. The skin becomes red, thickened, and crusty. Thick yellow crusts are sometimes found along ear edges and on the elbows. Most affected dogs are extremely itchy. Simply rubbing the dog's ears may cause the dog to scratch with the rear legs. Some affected dogs are itchy with little hair loss or crusting. In other dogs, widespread hair loss, scaling, and crusting develop. Skin lesions are most severe in immunosuppressed dogs (those that have received high doses of corticosteroids or that have underlying diseases suppressing the immune system).

Diagnosis

Definite diagnosis requires the finding of a *Sarcoptes* mite or egg by microscopic examination of skin scrapings taken from lesions on the dog. False-negative results are common, because mites can be very difficult to find—an affected dog may only have a dozen mites on its entire body, so the chances of finding one are slim. Blood tests showing the presence of antibodies against *Sarcoptes* sup-

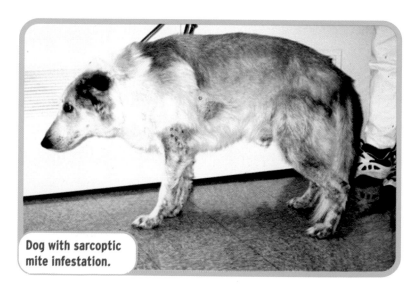

Dog with sarcoptic mite infestation.

port the diagnosis of scabies, although false positives are possible because of cross reactions with antibodies to other mites or from past infections. Dogs showing intense itching or other symptoms linked to sarcoptic mange should undergo a "treatment trial." If the symptoms resolve following treatment for sarcoptic mange, then it is likely that *Sarcoptes* mites were responsible for the symptoms.

Treatment

Several alternatives are available for the treatment of sarcoptic mange. Consult your veterinarian to select the most appropriate treatment. All dogs in contact with the affected dog also should receive treatment, even if they

Treatment Trials for *Sarcoptes scabiei* Infestation

All dogs with nonseasonal pruritus (itching) should undergo a treatment trial for *Sarcoptes scabiei* infestation. Each treatment trial must be limited to any ONE of the following:

- **Lime-sulfur dips every 5 to 7 days for six treatments**
- **Selamectin spot-on every 14 days for three treatments**
- **Fipronil spray every 14 days for three treatments**
- **Milbemycin orally every 7 days for six treatments**
- **Ivermectin orally or by injection every 7 days for four to six treatments (not in collies and other ivermectin-sensitive breeds or in dogs harboring heartworms)**
- **Phosmet dips every 7 days for four to six treatments**
- **Amitraz dips every 14 days for three treatments**

are free of symptoms, since they may be carriers of the mite and a source of reinfection later on. Infections in cats and other species usually are short-lived and rarely require treatment. If people in the family are affected, a physician should be consulted.

Lime-sulfur dips are highly effective in killing *Sarcoptes* mites and have the added benefit of soothing the skin and decreasing itching; they also help eliminate secondary bacterial or fungal skin infections. The dog is bathed to remove crusts, followed by soaking the entire body with a 2% solution of lime-sulfur. Dips are repeated weekly for a total of 6 weeks. The main disadvantage of lime-sulfur dips is the "rotten egg" smell of the wet solution. The dips also may stain white hairs on the dog a yellow color, although this color change is temporary. Bathtubs will need to be bleached to remove the yellow stain. Jewelry should not be worn by anyone applying the solution because it also can be discolored by contact with lime-sulfur solutions. Many veterinarians prefer to perform the dips in their clinic to make sure that the solution is properly applied and to minimize the owner's involvement with the unpleasant aspects of handling lime-sulfur.

Properties of Lime-Sulfur

- **Good safety profile (low risk of toxic effects)**
- **Antiparasitic (kills most mites and lice)**
- **Antifungal (kills most dermatophytes and yeasts)**
- **Antibacterial (kills most bacteria)**
- **Antipruritic (relieves itching)**
- **Antiseborrheic (keratolytic and keratoplastic, decreases scaling)**
- **Odiferous (smells like rotten eggs)**
- **Staining (yellow discoloration of hair, bathing tubs, jewelry)**

Several other dips also are effective at killing *Sarcoptes* mites. These include phosmet, malathion, mercaptomethyl phthalimide, lindane, and amitraz. These dips do not smell unpleasant or cause yellow staining, but they are much more toxic than lime-sulfur, although not more effective. So the risk of side effects far outweighs the benefit with these products.

Selamectin (Revolution) is highly effective in killing *Sarcoptes* mites. For the treatment of sarcoptic mange it is applied every 2 weeks for three applications. Monthly use will prevent reinfection with *Sarcoptes*, as well as heartworm infections, and will help control fleas and ticks. This product is recommended for routine use on hunting dogs and other dogs at high risk of reinfection from contact with foxes or free-roaming dogs.

Fipronil spray (Frontline Spray) applied to the entire body (for a total dose of 6 mL per kg of body weight) every 2 weeks for three treatments also will kill the mites. Monthly use will help prevent reinfection with *Sarcoptes*, fleas, and ticks. The spot-on formulations of fipronil (Top-Spot, Frontline Plus) are less effective against *Sarcoptes*, so it is important to use the spray formulation in treating sarcoptic mange.

Alternative miticides (anti-mite agents) that are effective but should be used only on the advice of a veterinarian familiar with their side effects and indications include ivermectin (given orally once weekly or by injection every 2 weeks) and milbemycin oxime (given once weekly). In some dogs, these medications can have serious side effects at the doses necessary to kill *Sarcoptes* mites. Ivermectin should not be used to treat *Sarcoptes* in collies and related breeds.

Dogs that are severely pruritic (those showing intense chewing and scratching) will benefit from short-term treatment with an oral corticosteroid (prednisone, prednisolone, or methylprednisolone). Steroid treatment should be stopped after about 2 weeks to evaluate the pet's response to the miticide. Antibiotics may be needed for the treatment of secondary skin infections. Although mites can survive only a short time off the host, washing or changing the pet's bedding also may be beneficial in preventing reinfection.

Feline Scabies (Notoedric Mange)

Feline scabies (notoedric mange) is caused by a mite, *Notoedres cati*, that is slightly smaller than the canine *Sarcoptes scabiei* mite. In comparison with disease due to *Sarcoptes* and *Demodex* mites, infestation with this mite is much less frequently diagnosed in the United States. The mite can infest dogs, rabbits, and people for short periods of time but can complete its life cycle only on cats.

Life Cycle

Similar to *Sarcoptes* in dogs, *N. cati* burrows in the superficial layers of skin. The mites most commonly affect the ears, head, face, and neck but can spread across the body. Eggs are laid in tunnels in the skin. Larvae hatch and move into molting pockets on the skin surface, where they molt into nymphs and later into adults. Mites are spread from one cat to another through direct contact.

Clinical Signs

Infested skin becomes thickened and crusty, with hair loss. Tunneling of the mites in the skin causes severe itching and scratching. Lesions may rapidly spread from the ear edges to involve the entire ear, head, face, and neck. In advanced cases, the cat also may have lesions on the legs and body. Over time the cat will become weak and ill and lose weight, and it may die if the infestation is not treated.

Diagnosis

Affected cats usually carry large numbers of mites, making it easy to find mites by using a microscope to examine skin scrapings. Other diseases that may look like feline scabies include ear mites, ringworm, *Demodex*

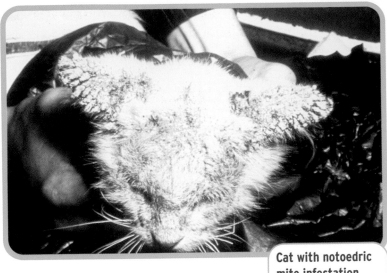

Cat with notoedric mite infestation.

infestation, allergies, and immune-mediated diseases. So it is important to confirm a diagnosis of notoedric mange by examining skin scrapings.

Treatment

All cats in contact with the affected cat, whether showing signs or not, should be treated with a miticide effective against *Notoedres*. The traditional treatment has been 2% lime-sulfur dips, repeated every 2 weeks for three treatments. The pros and cons of lime-sulfur dips are discussed under the treatment of canine scabies. An additional consideration with use of dips in cats is that many of them dislike getting wet–giving owners an additional reason to have their veterinarian perform the dips. Alternatives to lime-sulfur dips include topical selamectin (Revolution) and systemic ivermectin (given orally or by injection). Treatment selection and scheduling should be made by the pet's veterinarian.

Feline Fur Mites

Lynxacarus radosky is a hair-clasping mite that can be found on cats. It can be transmitted to other cats but does not affect dogs. It may cause a red, raised rash in people. This mite is relatively rare. It has been reported as a problem in parts of Florida, Texas, and Hawaii.

Life Cycle

Fur mites spend their entire life cycle on the pet. The mites attach themselves to hair shafts and feed at the base of the hair. The mites are spread by direct contact with an affected cat.

Clinical Signs

Fur mites generally cause little irritation or itching, although in some cats, miliary dermatitis with multiple crusted papules (red, raised bumps) will develop around the neck and along the back. Mites may be so numerous that the coat has a "salt and pepper" appearance from the hordes of mites clasping onto hairs. Hairs pull out easily, leaving a patchy alopecia. Severely affected cats have a dull and dirty-appearing hair coat with dandruff (scaling).

Diagnosis

The mites are small and are best identified by plucking hairs or trapping the mites with sticky acetate tape and examining the hairs or tape under a microscope. Other diseases that may have a similar appearance include pediculosis (lice infestation) and cheyletiellosis ("walking dandruff"). Fur mites are identified by their elongated body and legs that have suckers on them to help grasp hairs.

Treatment

Fur mites are killed by most flea control products and also by products used to treat other mite diseases. Lime-sulfur dips and systemic ivermectin (given orally or by injection) both are effective treatments.

Cheyletiellosis (Walking Dandruff)

Cheyletiella mites live in the fur of dogs, cats, and rabbits. They may be seen as tiny white specks scurrying around among the hairs—hence the nickname "walking

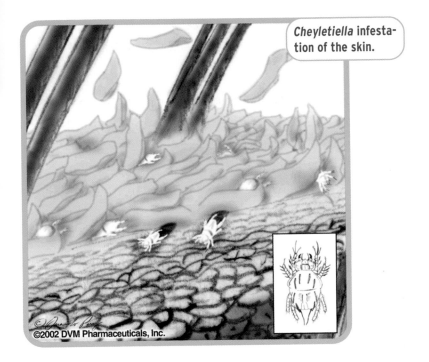

Cheyletiella infestation of the skin.

©2002 DVM Pharmaceuticals, Inc.

dandruff" for this condition. They may live on people briefly.

Life Cycle

Eggs are cemented onto hairs of the host. These hatch into larvae that feed on the host before molting into nymphs. Nymphs also feed on the host before molting into adults. The mites usually are spread to other hosts by direct contact. Adult female mites may survive up to 10 days in the environment. Adult mites form tunnels in epidermal debris and pierce the skin with their large mouthparts when feeding.

Clinical Signs

The most common sign of *Cheyletiella* infestations is excessive scaling (dandruff), especially over the back. In cats, miliary dermatitis with crusted papules may develop over the back and around the neck. Pruritus (itching) may or may not be present. Some pets show no clinical signs but serve as reservoirs for infecting others. Bites on people result in papules that become vesicles (fluid-filled

163

bumps) and pustules (pus-filled bumps), which rupture and become crusted.

Diagnosis

Your veterinarian will look for mites or mite eggs on acetate tape preparations or skin scrapings to confirm the diagnosis of cheyletiellosis. Some pets have only a few mites. Two methods are used to increase the chances of finding mites: (1) combing the whole body with a flea comb and (2) vacuuming the pet after placing a piece of filter paper in the vacuum nozzle to trap the mites. The samples collected are examined under a microscope. *Cheyletiella* mites have distinct large, pincher-shaped, piercing mouthparts.

Treatment

Cheyletiella mites are killed by most flea control products and also by products used to treat infestations by other mites. Lime-sulfur dips and systemic ivermectin (given orally or by injection) both are effective treatments. Be sure to tell your veterinarian about all of the pets in the household. All dogs, cats, and rabbits in contact with the affected pet should receive treatment. Keep in mind that pets vary in their ability to tolerate different medications. Ivermectin should not be used for treating cheyletiellosis in collies and related breeds of dogs. Permethrin is safe for dogs but toxic to cats and rabbits. Fipronil is safe for cats and dogs but highly toxic to rabbits. The environment should be thoroughly cleaned and treated with an insecticide—those effective against fleas also will kill *Cheyletiella* mites.

Trombiculiasis (Chiggers, Harvest Mites)

Adult harvest mites live in the environment and do not feed on dogs and cats. However, chiggers—harvest mite larvae—feed on birds and mammals. Pets acquire mites during the warmer months of the year through contact with infested vegetation.

Life Cycle

Adult harvest mites feed on decaying vegetation in the environment. Eggs are laid on the ground and hatch into six-legged red larvae that crawl up grasses and bushes to parasitize animals coming in contact with the vegetation. During feeding, chiggers form a temporary attachment of their mouthparts to the host's skin. After feeding on an animal, the larvae drop back on the ground and molt into nymphs and then adults.

Clinical Signs

Bites result in red, raised bumps, which often are very itchy. Lesions are found on the legs, feet, head, ears, and belly—areas in contact with the ground or with vegetation. Chiggers are most numerous during the late summer and autumn in the temperate zones of North America.

Diagnosis

Chiggers are tiny red-orange mites. They may appear to be tightly stuck to the skin during their feeding phase. When removed from the host for microscopic evaluation, they will be found to be six-legged mites. They can move rapidly when not attached to a host for feeding.

Treatment

Affected pets should be given one or two applications of a dip or spray generally effective against parasites. Pets should be kept away from areas known to harbor large numbers of mites. Use of environmental insecticides can be helpful in killing chiggers in yards.

Ear Mites (*Otodectes*)

Otodectes cynotis is a tiny white mite that lives on the surface of the skin and in the ear canals of dogs, cats, foxes, and ferrets. These mites feed primarily on discharges from the ear and are most numerous in the deep portion of the ear canal. Ear mites occasionally may be found on the head, back, and around the base of the tail. These mites spread quickly to dogs and cats in contact with an affected pet.

Life Cycle

All life stages are found on the host animal. Females lay eggs that hatch in approximately 4 days. Larvae feed on earwax and skin oils for approximately 1 week and then molt into protonymphs. After a few days the protonymph molts into an asexual deutonymph that mates with an adult male. After mating, the deutonymph develops into either a female or a male adult mite. If the deutonymph develops into a female, it will begin laying eggs. The total life cycle from egg to adult is completed in about 3 weeks.

Clinical Signs

Ear mites stimulate the ears to produce large amounts of a dark earwax that resembles coffee grounds. Ears that also become infected with yeast will have a moist, dark brown discharge. Secondary infections with bacteria may cause a pus-like discharge from the ears. A majority of pets infested with ear mites rub and scratch at their ears and also may show vigorous head shaking. Scratching and shaking of the head may rupture blood vessels in the ear flaps, resulting in the formation of an aural hematoma (blood-filled pocket on the inner surface of the ear flap). Mites living outside of the ears may cause red, raised lesions with itching and hair loss on the head, neck, rump, or tail. Miliary dermatitis develops in some cats with ear mite infestations. Some affected pets show few clinical signs but serve as carriers of the mites, which then infest other pets in the household.

Diagnosis

Your veterinarian will look for mites through a magnifying otoscope or use a cotton-tipped applicator stick (such as a Q-tip) to collect debris from the ear canal and examine it under a microscope. Discharge in the ears will also be examined for evidence of secondary infections (yeast or bacteria).

Treatment

The ear canals should be cleaned to remove built-up debris. Although this can be done at home, you should consult your veterinarian for instructions on ear cleaning techniques and cleaning solutions that are safe to use in pets. Use of the wrong products or improper cleaning technique can cause deafness. The affected pet and all dogs and cats in contact with it must receive appropriate treatment to avoid further spread of mites between animals. There are several options for treatment. Topical parasiticide solutions for the ears should be dropped in the ears at the dose and frequency, and for the length of time, prescribed by your veterinarian (treatment generally is continued for a minimum of 3 weeks). Selamectin (Revolution) applied topically at the base of the head twice, 1 month apart, is effective in killing mites in the ears and also on the body. When ear medications are used, a flea spray or spot-on treatment also should be used to kill any mites outside of the ears. Specific anti-yeast or antibacterial treatments may be needed for secondary ear infections; these should be used according to your veterinarian's recommendations.

Ticks

Ticks are long-lived arachnids with four pairs of legs and no antennae as adults. They directly weaken hosts by sucking blood and also can transmit a wide variety of diseases. Ticks have four major stages in their life cycle: egg, larva, nymph, and adult. Eggs are laid in the environment. The larvae, nymphs, and adults all are intermittent blood feeders. They remain on a host feeding for several days and then drop off. This periodic feeding pattern means that one tick may feed on several animals—this can result in the transmission of diseases between animals. "One-host" ticks feed on a single host species during all life stages (for example, a brown dog tick may feed on multiple dogs, but feeds only on dogs). "Two-host" ticks have one host species for the larva and nymph stages and a second for the adult stage. "Three-host" ticks have different host species for each life stage. The identification of a species of tick is made by examination of its size, shape, color, and any special markings.

Environmental control measures such as trimming grass and brush and applying pesticides to yards and kennels will help to minimize tick infestations. Avoid walking dogs in areas known to harbor ticks. Amitraz collars (Preventic) and permethrin sprays and spot-on treatments (Advantix, BioSpot, and others) are effective in preventing tick infestations in dogs; however, these products are highly toxic to cats. Fipronil (Frontline) spray and spot-on treatments are effective in preventing tick infestations in both cats and dogs. Selamectin (Revolution) is useful in the control of *Dermacentor variabilis* (American dog tick) but does not work well against other species of ticks. Several other dips and sprays labeled for use against ticks may be used to kill ticks already on a dog or cat—consult with your veterinarian and be careful that the product is approved for use in your pet's species (many dips safe for dogs, for example, are highly toxic to cats). Ticks already on a pet may be manually removed using tweezers (avoid rupturing the tick or leaving its mouthparts buried in the skin).

Rhipicephalus Ticks

Rhipicephalus sanguineus is commonly known as the brown dog tick. It feeds almost exclusively on dogs and can be found both outdoors and inside homes and kennels. Adults attach to the ears and between the toes. Larvae and nymphs often are found along the back of the dog. During feeding, female mites become engorged with blood, which swells their body to 1/2 inch long by 1/4 inch wide. The normal red-brown color changes to a gray-blue or olive color on the distended portion of the body. Females drop off the dog and lay eggs in cracks and crevices, under boards, and indoors under plaster or carpeting. Brown dog ticks sometimes are seen in homes crawling on carpeting, walls, or furniture. They are an intermediate host of *Babesia canis*, which causes piroplasmosis in dogs.

Dermacentor Ticks

Dermacentor variabilis is commonly known as the American dog tick. It is a three-host tick found outdoors. Larvae and nymphs feed on mice and other rodents; adults feed on many species but prefer dogs. Adults generally are brown but become slate-gray when engorged with blood. Diseases spread by this tick include Rocky Mountain spotted fever, tularemia, and tick paralysis. *Dermacentor andersoni* is the Rocky Mountain wood tick. It is found throughout the Rocky Mountains, where it is the principal vector for Rocky Mountain spotted fever. It also can produce tick paralysis. Larvae and nymphs generally are found on small wild rodents. Adults feed on larger mammals, including dogs and people.

Amblyomma Ticks

Amblyomma americanum is commonly known as the Lone Star tick because it has a single white spot on its back—as on the flag of Texas, the "Lone Star State." It is a three-host tick that feeds on many animals, including humans. It can transmit tularemia and Rocky Mountain spotted fever.

Amblyomma maculatum is the Gulf Coast tick. It is a three-host tick that feeds in the ears of cattle, horses, sheep, dogs, and people. It can cause tick paralysis.

Ixodes Ticks

Ixodes dammini is the common deer tick. It is a three-host tick that feeds on mice and voles as larvae and nymphs and on deer as adults. It also may feed on dogs and people and transmits *Borrelia burgdorferi*, the cause of Lyme disease in dogs and humans.

Otobius Ticks

Otobius megnini is commonly known as the spinous ear tick. This is a soft-bodied tick. The adults are not parasitic, but larvae and nymphs feed in the ear canals of cattle, sheep, goats, horses, and, rarely, dogs or cats. These ticks can produce severe inflammation within the ear canals. Infested animals show vigorous head shaking, ear scratching, pain, and a waxy discharge within the ear canal.

Diagnosis

The larvae and nymphs can be seen within the ears with use of an otoscope. Discharge from the ears should be examined for secondary bacterial or yeast infections.

Treatment

Ticks may be manually removed using forceps. Your veterinarian may need to sedate your pet for this procedure, because the affected ear often is very painful. The pet should be sprayed or dipped with a topical product labeled for use against ticks (make sure that the product is licensed for use in your pet's species). Any secondary ear infections should be treated as directed by your veterinarian. The environment should be treated with an insecticide labeled for use against ticks, to help prevent reinfestation.

Miscellaneous Ectoparasites

Pediculosis (Lice)

Lice are relatively rare parasites of cats and dogs in the United States. Lice are small, wingless insects that are highly host-specific, which this means they affect only one host species. Dogs and cats are never the source of human head lice infestations. There are two types of lice—biting lice (Mallophaga) and sucking lice (Anoplura). The most common biting louse of dogs is *Trichodectes canis*.

Heterodoxus spiniger is a biting louse of dogs found in warmer climates. *Felicola subrostratus* is the only biting louse that affects cats. *Linognathus setosus* is the only sucking louse of dogs. Cats are not affected by sucking lice.

Life Cycle

The entire life cycle is completed on the host. Eggs (nits) are cemented onto the hairs of the host. Eggs hatch into nymphs that are similar in shape to the adult but smaller. Lice can only survive a few days off a host; they usually are transmitted by direct contact or through grooming equipment.

Clinical Signs

Some pets show few symptoms of infestation; others are restless as a result of itching and have hair loss. Severely infested pets may have secondary seborrhea (dandruff), scruffy or matted hair coats, excoriations (scratches), and papules (red, raised bumps) or crusts. Miliary dermatitis may develop in affected cats. Heavy infestations may result in anemia from blood loss. Lice may serve as intermediate hosts for tapeworms.

Diagnosis

Lice are large enough to be seen as small specks moving in the pet's fur. Your veterinarian will pluck hairs or use sticky acetate tape to trap lice for examination under a microscope. Biting lice have a large, rounded head with large jaws (mandibles) fitted with teeth for chewing. Sucking lice have a more oval head with sucking mouthparts. Nits (eggs) can be found cemented to hair shafts.

Treatment

Hair mats should be removed and the entire body treated with 2% lime-sulfur or another insecticidal spray or dip. Fipronil (Frontline) and imidacloprid (Advantage) spot-on products applied twice 1 month apart also are effective in killing lice. Severely anemic pets may need a blood transfusion. All in-contact animals of the same species also should receive treatment. Pet bedding and grooming tools must be thoroughly cleaned and disinfected.

Cuterebra Larvae
Life Cycle

Adults of the genera *Cuterebra* are beelike insects that deposit eggs near the burrows of rodents and rabbits. Larvae hatch and move onto a passing mammal—usually a rabbit or rodent, but also perhaps a dog or cat that sticks its head into the burrow. The larva migrates through body openings such as the nose or mouth, under the eyelids, or through a wound. Larvae then migrate through the tissues just beneath the skin of the head, neck, or trunk. A nonpainful, 1-cm swelling develops around each larva. The swelling develops an opening (fistula) that serves as a breathing hole for the larva. When mature, the larva drops to the ground, pupates, and emerges as an adult fly.

Clinical Signs

The skin around the larva's breathing hole may be erythematous (red) and swollen. Lesions usually are solitary and located on the head, neck, or trunk. Rarely, larvae may migrate to sites such as the throat or nose, or even into the brain. Migration into the brain is fatal.

Diagnosis

The larvae are large enough (1 cm long) to be easily seen within their breathing holes. When removed, the larva can be identified by its stout black spines on a white, cream, brown, or black body.

Treatment

Your veterinarian will need to gently enlarge the breathing hole and remove the larva using forceps. This procedure requires care not to crush the larva, since doing so may produce anaphylaxis, a life-threatening allergic reaction. The wound heals slowly, and any infection present will need to be treated with appropriate topical or oral antibiotics.

Flies

Flies may be responsible for two types of lesions in cats and dogs—irritation from fly bites and infestations of fly larvae (myiasis).

Biting flies feed on ear tips, ear margins, the nose, eyelids, and other thinly haired or hairless areas. Irritation and resulting inflammation result in red raised bumps, bloody crusts, and hair loss. Dogs and cats may make the lesions worse by scratching at them. Treatment involves preventing fly bites and resolving any secondary infections. Topical antibiotic creams or ointments usually are enough to treat infections. The dog or cat should be kept indoors in a fly-free environment until the lesions are healed. Fly repellents can be applied to help prevent future bites. If possible, the source of the flies should be identified and treated with insecticides plus other fly control measures (such as frequent removal of animal wastes from yards and removal of decaying vegetation).

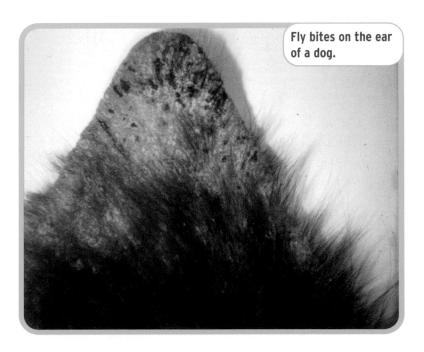

Fly bites on the ear of a dog.

Flies lay eggs on moist skin and in wounds. The eggs hatch into larvae (maggots), which produce enzymes that break down the surrounding tissues. Lesions expand into foul-smelling, saucer-shaped or irregularly shaped ulcers containing the maggots. This infestation is called **myiasis**. Lesions are most commonly found around the nose, eyes, anus, or vulva, or in wounds.

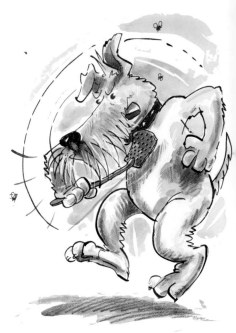

Diagnosis is based on finding the maggots. Lesions are gently cleaned and thoroughly flushed with warm water or saline. Pyrethrin sprays can be used to kill any remaining larvae. The pet should be given oral antibiotics and the wound cared for daily until it is healed. The pet should be kept in a fly-free area until all wounds have healed. The cause of any contributing factors such as diarrhea or urine scalding should be identified and corrected.

Mosquitoes

Adult mosquitoes are small, slender, winged insects with long legs. Adult females are blood suckers and can produce skin irritation and allergic reactions, and also can transmit diseases such as heartworm and West Nile virus infection.

Life Cycle

Adult females lay eggs on the surface of water. Eggs hatch into larvae known as "wigglers." Wigglers molt three or four times and enter the pupal stage, when they are known as "tumblers." Adult mosquitoes emerge from the pupal case. Males feed on nectar and plant juices;

females require blood meals, which they obtain from animals (including dogs and cats).

Clinical Signs

Mosquitoes feeding on the skin cause irritation. In many cats and some dogs, allergic reactions to mosquito antigens develop. The skin of allergic pets becomes red and inflamed in areas bitten by the mosquito. The lesions may become hairless and crusted. Mosquito bites can cause eosinophilic plaques and granulomas over the nose, around the eyes, and on the face of cats. Mosquito bites can cause eosinophilic folliculitis and furunculosis on the muzzle of dogs.

Diagnosis

Mosquito-bite hypersensitivity is likely in a cat or dog, with crusted hairless or hemorrhagic lesions involving the nose, muzzle, periocular (around the eyes) skin, or face in an pet with exposure to mosquitoes. The lesions often arise rapidly and resolve when the pet is protected from mosquitoes. Skin cytology and skin biopsies show large numbers of eosinophils.

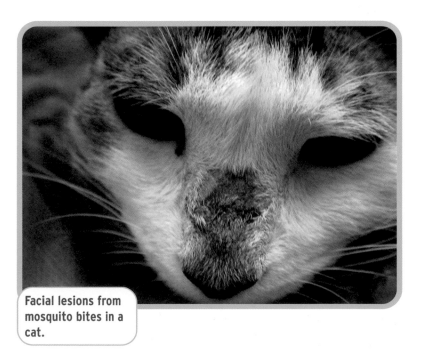

Facial lesions from mosquito bites in a cat.

Treatment

Corticosteroids are useful in relieving allergy-related skin inflammation. The pet should be kept in mosquito-free quarters during the mosquito season. When this is not possible, fly repellents offer some protection against mosquito bites. Sources of mosquitoes should be eliminated (clean bird baths regularly, eliminate standing pools of water, use a mosquito larvicide to treat water that cannot be drained).

Pelodera Infestation (Rhabditic Dermatitis)

Dogs are occasionally infested by larvae of *Pelodera strongyloides* (also called *Rhabditis strongyloides*), a free-living nematode found in damp soil, decaying organic debris, and straw bedding.

Life Cycle

Adult *Pelodera* nematodes are 1 to 2 mm long and live in damp organic material. Their larvae move around and can penetrate into the hair follicles or skin of animals, causing inflammation.

Clinical Signs

The larvae produce intense inflammation in the skin, resulting in itching, erythema (redness), hair loss, and formation of papules, crusts, and scales. Lesions are found on areas that have been in contact with infested ground or bedding—the feet, legs, front of the belly, perineum (area between the genitals and anus), and underside of the tail.

Diagnosis

Skin scrapings of affected areas will contain moving nematode larvae on microscopic examination. Biopsy specimens of affected areas will show nematode larvae within hair follicles.

Treatment

Bathe the dog in an antiseborrheic shampoo to remove crusts and scales, followed by application of a topical parasiticide (2% lime-sulfur or another scabicide). Kennels should be thoroughly cleaned. All bedding should be discarded, and the kennel sprayed with a long-lasting parasiticide. If pruritus is severe, short-term oral corticosteroids may be given to relieve the itching. If bacterial skin infections are present, these should be treated with oral antibiotics for 2 to 3 weeks.

Hookworms

Hookworms are intestinal parasites of dogs. Female hookworms can produce 16,000 or more eggs daily. The eggs are passed in feces and develop into infective larvae in the environment. Larvae enter hosts following ingestion or by penetration of the skin. Larval migration in the skin produces irritation and may cause an allergic reaction that increases skin inflammation. Affected skin becomes red, hairless, thickened, and itchy. Lesions involve areas in frequent contact with the ground such as the skin between the toes. The feet become swollen, hot, and painful (pododermatitis).

Diagnosis is based on ruling out other causes of foot inflammation (such as *Demodex* mites, chiggers, *Pelodera* larvae, bacterial or fungal infections, or other allergies). Hookworm eggs can be found on fecal examination.

Treatment involves regular deworming of all dogs and cats in the area. Regular removal of dog and cat feces and cleaning of kennels and runs also are important control steps. If secondary bacterial infections are present, they are treated with oral antibiotics. Soaking the feet in a solution of lime-sulfur, aluminum acetate, or magnesium sulfate (Epsom salts) is soothing and speeds healing.

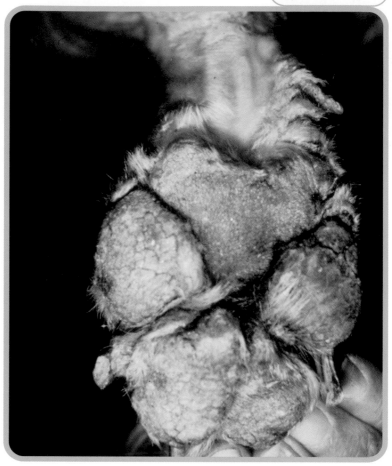

Dracunculiasis

Dracunculus is a nematode (worm) that parasitizes sub-cutaneous tissues. Immature stages of this worm develop inside microscopic aquatic crustaceans. Pets become infected by drinking water containing these crustaceans. The immature worms migrate through the body to the subcutaneous tissues, where they develop into adults within a nodule (swelling in the skin). A fistula (opening between the skin surface and the inside of the nodule) develops over the front end of the worm. When water contacts the opening to the fistula, female worms will come out part way to expel numerous infective larvae into the water. An old treatment was to wet the opening to lure the worm out and then wind the worm up on a stick to pull it out of the body (a process taking several days to slowly pull the worm out without breaking it). Modern treatment is to surgically remove the nodules and keep the pet away from contaminated water.

Spiders

Spiders are not parasitic on animals, but their bites can be painful and in some cases deadly. Brown recluse spider bites cause a painful, fluid-filled blister to form at the bite site. Within a couple of days the skin begins to die and **slough** (shed off). The sloughing may continue for several days. Your veterinarian may recommend surgical removal of the dying tissue to speed healing and to prevent secondary bacterial skin infections from developing. Bites of black widow spiders can produce weakness, incoordination, excessive drooling, and in severe cases, difficulty breathing, muscle spasms, seizures, and death. Pets bitten by a black widow spider should be taken to a veterinary clinic for supportive treatment.

Inflammation from a spider bite on a dog's abdomen.

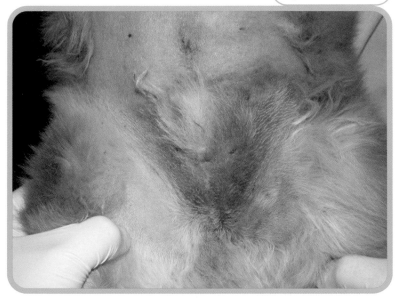

Summary

Skin is exposed to attack by many kinds of parasites. Knowledge of the life cycle of each parasite will help you in developing strategies to minimize your pet's exposure to that parasite and also adds understanding about why certain treatment approaches work best. When the parasite spends all of its life cycle on the pet, treatments are applied to the pet itself. Environmental control measures are important with parasites that spend most of their life cycle in the environment, rather than on the pet. The many available insecticides and pesticides can be toxic and differ in their effects when used in different animal species, so it is important to work closely with a veterinarian who is familiar with all of the pets in your household to develop safe and effective treatment plans for parasite-related skin diseases.

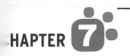

HORMONE-RELATED SKIN DISEASES

Endocrine-related skin diseases are common in dogs and occasionally are seen in cats. The hallmark of these disorders is a bilaterally symmetrical **alopecia**—hair loss that occurs on both sides of the body in a "mirror-image" pattern. A majority of endocrine skin diseases occur in combination with disorders of other body systems as a result of abnormalities in **hormone** secretion.

The endocrine system is composed of **glands** and other tissues that produce hormones. Hormones are chemicals that regulate the functioning of specific body organs and tissues. Endocrine glands release hormones directly into the bloodstream. Hormones are carried in the blood to tissues that have receptors for a specific hormone. The interaction of a hormone with its receptor causes the "target tissue" (with the receptors) to perform a specific function.

Hormone secretion is regulated by feedback mechanisms—changes in hormone levels act as signals to increase or decrease hormone production. This feedback allows precise control of hormone concentrations in the blood and regulation of target tissue activity. Many hormones affect the skin and its associated structures, such as **hair follicles** and **sebaceous** (oil) glands. These same hormones also affect many other body tissues, so a majority of endocrine diseases that affect the skin also produce changes in other body tissues. The most common **cutaneous** (skin) clinical finding in endocrine-related disease is bilaterally symmetrical alopecia. The endocrine problem results in hair loss because hair growth is regulated by hormone receptors within hair follicles.

Adrenal Disorders

The **adrenal glands** are located near the kidneys. The outer layer of the adrenal gland is called the adrenal cortex and produces **cortisol** and sex hormones—estrogens, progesterones, testosterone, and other androgens. The activity of the adrenal cortex normally is controlled by adrenocorticotropic hormone (ACTH) secreted by the anterior pituitary gland. This hormone stimulates the secretion of cortisol from the adrenal glands. ACTH production, in turn, is controlled by corticotropin-releasing hormone (CRH) produced by the hypothalamus. A decrease in cortisol in the blood results in an increase in CRH production, leading to an increase in ACTH production. An increase in cortisol concentration above its optimal range tells the hypothalamus and the pituitary gland to stop secreting CRH and ACTH. Under normal circumstances, this feedback between hypothalamic production of CRH, pituitary gland production of ACTH, and adrenal gland production of cortisol works to keep the concentration of cortisol in the blood within a narrow range. However, cancer cells in tumors of either the pituitary gland or the adrenal gland continuously secrete their own ACTH or cortisol, respectively, and do not respond to negative feedback signals; this results in overproduction of cortisol.

Hyperadrenocorticism (Cushing's Disease)

Causes

Cushing's disease (**hyperadrenocorticism**) is a **metabolic disease** caused by excessive amounts of **corticosteroid** hormones. There are three common forms of Cushing's disease:

Pituitary-dependent hyperadrenocorticism (PDH) is caused by a tumor of the anterior pituitary gland that produces too much ACTH. High levels of ACTH result in enlargement (**hyperplasia**) of the adrenal cortex and production of too much cortisol.

Adrenal-dependent hyperadrenocorticism occurs when an adrenal tumor produces too much cortisol.

Iatrogenic Cushing's disease is caused by giving large amounts of corticosteroids, either through pills taken by mouth or by injections. The corticosteroids usually are given to treat another problem such as destructive inflammation, immune-mediated diseases, or certain cancers.

Clinical Signs and Symptoms

High levels of corticosteroids affect most organs and tissues of the body, producing the **clinical signs** characteristic of Cushing's disease. Hair growth is inhibited, resulting in thinning of the hair coat as old hairs fall out and lack of hair regrowth when the coat is shaved. Empty hair follicles become plugged with **keratin** (a type of protein), forming **comedones** (blackheads). Sebaceous (oil) and **apocrine** (sweat) **glands** do not function well and decrease in size, and the decrease in the production of **sebum** (an oily substance) and apocrine secretions (a thick, milky sweat) results in dull, dry hairs and dry, scaly skin. The skin becomes thinner and is easily bruised. The risk of bacterial skin infections greatly increases, and the skin does not heal well after injury. The skin of cats with hyperadrenocorticism becomes fragile and tears easily. High levels of corticosteroids sometimes cause formation of calcium deposits in the **dermis** (deep layer of the skin)—a condition called **calcinosis cutis**. The most commonly affected areas are the top of the neck and the back and the **inguinal** (groin) region.

Clinical Signs and Symptoms of Cushing's Disease in Dogs

- Increased thirst (polydipsia) and urination (polyuria)

- Increased appetite (polyphagia) and weight gain (obesity)

- Abdominal enlargement (enlarged liver and increased intra-abdominal fat)

- Muscle weakness (decreased exercise tolerance)

- Panting

- Thin skin that bruises easily

- Alopecia (hair loss, usually bilateral, starting on trunk) and comedones (blackheads)

- Reoccurring skin infections

- Calcinosis cutis (skin calcification)

- Hyperpigmentation (skin darkening)

- Infertility—*in males*: testicular atrophy (shrinkage); *in females*: prolonged anestrus (lack of "heat" cycles)

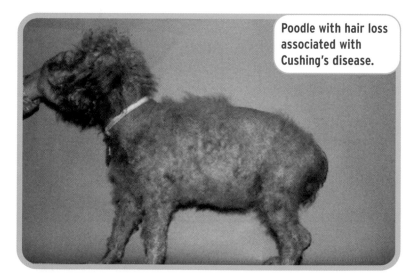

Poodle with hair loss associated with Cushing's disease.

Corticosteroids stimulate the appetite, resulting in **polyphagia** (overeating), weight gain, and elevated blood glucose levels. Many cats and some dogs with Cushing's disease

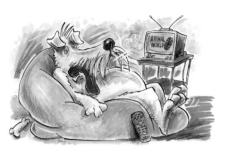

become diabetic and require insulin injections for control of blood glucose concentration. Corticosteroids cause muscle wasting; **atrophy** (shrinkage) of the facial muscles may occur, and movement may become stiff. Muscle weakness contributes to the development of an **abdomen** that sags. The liver enlarges from deposits of **glycogen** (a form of carbohydrate the body uses to store food) and fat within the liver cells (**steroid hepatopathy**). This also contributes to a larger abdomen. Excess corticosteroids make it hard for the kidneys to concentrate urine. For that reason, urine production increases (**polyuria**) and the pet becomes excessively thirsty (**polydipsia**). Bladder infections are also common because of the **immunosuppressive** effects of corticosteroids. High levels of corticosteroids cause osteoporosis, a weakening of the bones. Increased panting is common, and pets with Cushing's

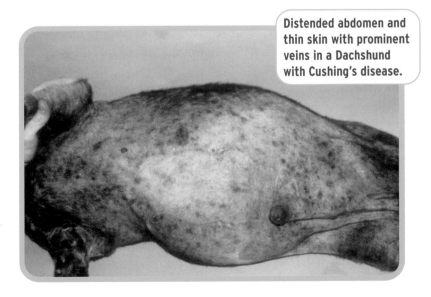

Distended abdomen and thin skin with prominent veins in a Dachshund with Cushing's disease.

disease are more likely to have thromboembolism (blood clots in the lungs). Increased levels of corticosteroids also result in hypertension (high blood pressure) and may cause affected pets to be more likely to develop congestive heart failure.

Cushing's disease is fairly common in dogs but is rare in cats. Iatrogenic Cushing's disease (which results from corticosteroid treatment) can occur at any age and in any breed. Pituitary-dependent hyperadrenocorticism (caused by pituitary gland tumors) is the most common naturally occurring (noniatrogenic) form of Cushing's disease. Boston Terriers, Boxers, Dachshunds, and Miniature Poodles are breeds with an increased risk of developing PDH. Adrenal-dependent hyperadrenocorticism (due to adrenal gland tumors) causes about 20% of the cases of naturally occurring Cushing's disease.

Diagnosis

Diagnosing Cushing's disease and figuring out which of the three forms is present often require a series of tests. A history of previous corticosteroid administration is the best way to diagnose iatrogenic Cushing's disease. Pets vary in how prone they are to developing this form of Cushing's disease. If symptoms appear, it is wise to consider using alternative medications to control the underlying disease before the pet develops serious complications related to Cushing's disease.

If Cushing's disease is suspected, the veterinarian examining the pet will usually recommend submitting blood samples for a **complete blood cell count** (CBC) and **biochemical profile**. In addition, urine samples will be evaluated by **urinalysis** and bacterial culture. High levels of corticosteroids cause increases in the total **white blood cell** count, with increased numbers of **neutrophils** and **monocytes** and decreased numbers of **lymphocytes** and **eosinophils**. Red blood cell and **platelet** counts may be increased slightly. The blood glucose (blood sugar) concentration usually is increased slightly, along with increases in liver enzymes (particularly serum alkaline phosphatase) and cholesterol. The urine concentration usually is decreased (this is referred to as having a low specific gravity), because cortisol interferes with the ability of the kidneys to concentrate urine. Urine may contain increased levels of protein as a result of kidney damage or urinary tract infections. Bacterial infections of the urinary tract are common because of the immunosuppressive effect of cortisol, which makes it hard for the body to fight infection. If blood pressure is measured, it usually is higher than normal.

Abdominal **ultrasonography** (ultrasound examination, sonogram) is useful in evaluating a pet suspected of having Cushing's disease. The liver is evaluated for the "hypoechoic" pattern of steroid hepatopathy (liver disease caused by steroids). **Fine-needle aspiration** (see Chapter 3) of the liver can be performed under the guidance of the ultrasound operator. **Cytology** (analysis of the cells under a microscope) of the aspirated specimen will confirm whether the liver has steroid hepatopathy. The adrenal glands are examined for enlargement. If both adrenal glands are enlarged, pituitary-dependent hyperadrenocorticism is the likely diagnosis, whereas enlargement of one gland is suggestive of an adrenal tumor. **Computed tomography (CT) scans** or **magnetic resonance imaging (MRI)** may be used to evaluate the pituitary and adrenal glands for tumors.

The next phase in evaluating a pet suspected of having Cushing's disease is testing adrenal gland function. Three different tests are used: the ACTH stimulation test, the dexamethasone suppression test, and measurement of ACTH blood levels. The ACTH stimulation test assesses the ability of the adrenal glands to produce the cortisol needed by the body. The other two tests are used to help distinguish between adrenal and pituitary tumors.

Adrenal Function Tests

Name of Test	Procedure	Interpretation
ACTH stimulation test	Blood sample taken before and 1-2 hours after administration of ACTH	Increased levels on the second sample indicative of Cushing's disease. (*Exception*: Will be low if the hyperadrenocorticism is a result of corticosteroid treatment.)
Dexamethasone suppression test (low dose and high dose)	Blood taken before, then 4 and 8 hours after administration of dexamethasone	Normal dogs have decreased cortisol levels in the 4- and 8-hour samples. Dogs with PDH may have decreased cortisol levels at 4 hours in the low-dose test and at both 4 and 8 hours in the high-dose test. Dogs with adrenal tumors have normal to increased cortisol levels in all samples.
Endogenous ACTH level determination	Blood taken in special tubes	High levels of ACTH are suggestive of PDH. Low levels of ACTH are suggestive of an adrenal tumor or iatrogenic Cushing's disease.

ACTH, Adrenocorticotropic hormone; *PDH*, pituitary-dependent hyperadrenocorticism.

An ACTH stimulation test will determine whether the adrenal glands are capable of overproducing cortisol. A high dose of synthetic ACTH is given. In pets with enlarged adrenal glands (hyperplasia with pituitary-dependent hyperadrenocorticism or an adrenal tumor), the measured cortisol levels will be much higher than normal. This finding points to a diagnosis of noniatrogenic Cushing's disease.

Dexamethasone suppression tests are done to help distinguish between a pituitary tumor and an adrenal tumor. These tests will determine whether the pituitary and adrenal glands respond normally to increased levels of circulating corticosteroids by slowing or stopping production of cortisol (negative feedback). Dexamethasone, an injectable corticosteroid drug, will cause a drop in cortisol levels in normal cats and dogs. Dogs with pituitary-dependent hyperadrenocorticism will show a drop in cortisol levels, but with a faster-than-normal rebound of cortisol after a low dose of dexamethasone. Both cats and dogs with this form of hyperadrenocorticism will show a drop in cortisol that lasts over 8 hours after a high dose. "Functional" (hormone-producing) adrenal tumors are not affected by dexamethasone suppression, and cortisol levels remain high.

Measuring blood levels of ACTH also is helpful in distinguishing between a pituitary tumor and an adrenal tumor. If a pet has a pituitary tumor, it will have high levels of ACTH. An adrenal tumor will cause low levels of ACTH, because the high levels of cortisol produced by the adrenal tumor cells inhibit pituitary secretion of ACTH. Only a few laboratories perform measurement of ACTH, and special handling of the blood is required, so this test is not used as frequently as the other tests are.

Treatment

When the cause of Cushing's disease has been diagnosed, your veterinarian will consider several options for treatment. If the pet has the iatrogenic form of the disease, it should be slowly "weaned" off corticosteroid drugs. Gradual decrease in dosage of these drugs is necessary because rapid withdrawal may cause an **Addisonian crisis**–sudden cardiovascular collapse with extremely low blood pressure, shock, and death. When a pet has been receiving high doses of oral or injectable corticosteroids, an unwanted effect of these medications on the pituitary gland and the adrenal gland is to stop production of ACTH and cortisol, respectively. With time, the glands even begin to atrophy (shrink). When the pet stops receiving oral or injectable corticosteroids, the atrophied adrenal glands are incapable of producing sufficient cortisol to sustain life. Cortisol has many essential roles in normal functioning of the circulatory system, gastrointestinal tract, and other organs. When a pet doesn't have enough cortisol, it may experience an Addisonian crisis. To prevent this, pets with iatrogenic Cushing's disease should be slowly weaned off exogenous corticosteroids (those not produced by the body itself); the dose administered is decreased by approximately 25% per week (for example, first week 75%, second week 56%, third week 42%, and so on). Slow "tapering" of the corticosteroid dosage provides time for the pituitary gland to resume production of ACTH, resulting in regrowth of the adrenal cortex's cells, which then resume production of cortisol. At the same time the pet is weaned off corticosteroids, alternative strategies should be developed to treat the condition for which the corticosteroids were originally prescribed (for example, immunotherapy and antihistamines to treat **atopy**, diet changes to treat food allergies, nonsteroidal anti-inflammatory drugs to treat arthritis, and cyclosporine to treat **immune-mediated diseases**).

Medical therapy is recommended for most dogs with pituitary hyperadrenocorticism. Occasionally, **radiation therapy** is recommended to treat a large pituitary tumor; however, in most cases, treatment is directed at decreasing the production of cortisol by the adrenal glands.

Options for Treatment of Canine Cushing's Disease

Treatment	Advantages	Disadvantages
Wean off corticosteroid drugs	Necessary for resolution of iatrogenic Cushing's disease	Must wean slowly; must look for alternative drugs to treat any underlying diseases
Radiation therapy	For treatment of pituitary tumors	No immediate effect on excessive cortisol production; must be performed at a specialized facility
Mitotane (Lysodren) (*o,p′*-DDD)	Proven effective in destruction of cortisol-secreting cells of the adrenal cortex	Requires frequent follow-up blood tests and careful monitoring to prevent fatal overdosing; is given daily at first, then twice weekly for maintenance
Ketoconazole	Blocks the pro-duction of cortisol; can be used to stabilize dogs before surgery; most side effects are reversible	May cause liver damage in some dogs; may cause anorexia and vomiting; must be given twice daily; expensive; does not work in all dogs
Trilostane	Blocks the production of cortisol	Must be given daily; death has been reported in some dogs with heart disease; unavail-able in the United States
L-Deprenyl (Anipryl)	Also improves cognitive function; few side effects	Must be given once or twice daily; effective in only 10-30% of dogs with PDH
Adrenalectomy [surgical removal of adrenal gland(s)]	Curative for dogs with non-malignant adrenal tumors	High risk of surgical complications; careful monitoring required for several days following surgery

Mitotane (Lysodren), also known as *o,p'*-DDD, is the drug most often used to treat pituitary-dependent hyper-adrenocorticism. Mitotane is given by mouth and destroys cells of the adrenal cortex. Destruction of the adrenocortical cells results in a decrease in the amount of corticosteroids circulating in the blood system. Treatment with mitotane begins with an "induction phase" in which the medication is given daily for 7 to 10 days. At the end of this induction, an ACTH stimulation test is performed. During the induction phase, you should monitor your pet closely for a decrease in appetite, a decrease in drinking, weakness, or depression. If any of these signs are observed, the medication is stopped, and your veterinarian will repeat an ACTH stimulation test to determine how low the cortisol levels have dropped. The goal of the induction phase of mitotane therapy is to decrease cortisol production to the low-normal range in both the first and the second blood samples taken during an ACTH stimulation test. If cortisol levels are too high, mitotane will be administered daily for several more days, and then cortisol levels will be rechecked with the ACTH stimulation test. If cortisol levels are too low or the pet is showing signs of an Addisonian crisis, mitotane will be stopped and oral corticosteroids will be administered. When cortisol levels are in the ideal range, maintenance treatment with mitotane is given to maintain control of Cushing's disease. Dogs receiving maintenance treatment usually are given mitotane twice weekly (for example, on Monday and Thursday). Recheck evaluations will be performed every few months. These evaluations should include repeating blood work (biochemical profile, ACTH stimulation test) and checking urine for infections (urinalysis and cultures). Overdosing with mitotane is dangerous because it may result in an Addisonian crisis or death. Underdosing with mitotane results in worsening of Cushing's disease. For these reasons, dogs that are receiving treatment for Cushing's disease require close monitoring and frequent blood tests to ensure proper regulation of their medications. Mitotane is ineffective for treating Cushing's disease in cats.

Ketoconazole is a drug most commonly used for treating fungal infections. It also slows the activity of two enzymes involved in making cortisol. Fairly high blood levels of ketoconazole must be maintained for best results in slowing cortisol production. That's why ketoconazole must be given twice a day, every day, when it is used to treat Cushing's disease. Side effects of ketoconazole can include **anorexia** (loss of appetite), lethargy, lightening of the hair color, and liver damage. Dogs receiving ketoconazole should have frequent blood tests to monitor liver function and ACTH stimulation tests to make sure cortisol production is suppressed. Ketoconazole is not effective for treating Cushing's disease in cats.

Trilostane is another drug that inhibits enzymes involved in cortisol production. It is used in Europe for treating Cushing's disease in people and dogs. It must be given every day for optimal effectiveness. Death has been reported in a few dogs with heart disease, so it should not be used in pets with heart problems. Trilostane is not currently available for use in the United States.

L-Deprenyl (Anipryl, from Pfizer Animal Health) is another drug sometimes used in treating Cushing's disease in dogs. It inhibits enzymes in the brain involved in the metabolism of **dopamine**. One function of dopamine in the brain is to inhibit the secretion of ACTH by the pituitary gland. Another function is to support cognition (thought processes)—in fact, L-deprenyl has been found to improve memory, especially in older dogs with signs of senility. Unfortunately, only 10% to 30% of dogs with pituitary Cushing's disease treated with L-deprenyl show reduction in clinical signs of the disorder. So although L-deprenyl is safe and has a side benefit of improving memory in senile dogs, it usually is reserved for use in dogs with early or mild signs of Cushing's disease.

The preferred treatment for adrenal tumors in dogs is surgical removal. Dogs with Cushing's disease have many problems (for example, high blood pressure, high risk of blood clots, and slow healing) that make them high-risk patients for anesthesia and surgery, so it may be beneficial to stabilize their condition by treating them with ketoconazole for several weeks before surgery. Close monitoring of the pet is important after surgery. Supplemental corticosteroids usually are given for several weeks during recovery to help the pet cope with the stresses associated with surgery.

Cats with Cushing's disease rarely respond to medical therapy. For that reason, removal of one or both adrenal glands is the treatment of choice. If an adrenal tumor is present, removal of the affected adrenal gland will cure the disease. With the pituitary form of hyperadrenocorticism, removal of one gland may decrease cortisol levels, but it seldom resolves the problem. Removal of both adrenal glands will cause an Addisonian crisis unless supplemental corticosteroid drugs and a synthetic form of aldosterone are administered. Cats are rarely diagnosed with Cushing's disease until late in the clinical course. Affected cats frequently have complications such as diabetes and fragile skin, so they are much less likely to recover.

Thyroid Disorders

The thyroid gland is located in the lower neck next to the trachea (windpipe). It produces two hormones: **thyroxine,** also known as tetraiodothyronine (T_4), and triiodothyronine (T_3). Thyroid hormones have important roles in regulating **metabolism**: They stimulate protein synthesis (production) and increase tissue oxygen consumption. Thyroid hormones are important in the differentiation of skin (specialization of skin cells), maintenance of normal cutaneous (skin) function, and the initiation of hair growth. Two of the most common endocrine diseases of dogs and cats involve the thyroid gland. **Hypothyroidism** (low production of thyroid) often develops in dogs as a result of atrophy (shrinkage) or destruction of the thyroid gland. **Hyperthyroidism** (excess production of thyroid) often develops in older cats as a result of nodular hyperplasia (enlargement of gland) or **neoplasia** (tumor) of the thyroid gland.

The secretion of thyroid hormones is regulated by a series of interactions among the hypothalamus, pituitary gland, and thyroid gland. The hypothalamus produces thyrotropin-releasing hormone (TRH), which stimulates the anterior pituitary gland to produce thyrotropin, also called thyroid-stimulating hormone (TSH). Thyrotropin stimulates the synthesis and release of T_4 and T_3 from the thyroid gland. Increases in thyroid hormone concentrations (T_4 and T_3) have a negative feedback effect on the hypothalamus and pituitary gland to inhibit the production of TRH and TSH.

The most common hormone in circulation is a protein-bound form of T_4. Smaller amounts of protein-bound T_3 and of free (not bound to proteins) T_4 and free T_3 also are in circulation. Free T_4 and free T_3 are the active forms of the thyroid hormones that enter cells and bind to receptors to influence gene activity and protein synthesis. Free T_3 is three to five times more potent than free T_4.

Hypothyroidism
Causes

Hypothyroidism may result from abnormal function (dysfunction) of any part of the hypothalamic-pituitary-thyroid axis. The two most common causes of hypothyroidism are lymphocytic **thyroiditis** (inflammation of the thyroid gland) and **idiopathic** (of unknown cause) thyroid atrophy. Less often, thyroid dysfunction is caused by a nonfunctional tumor of the thyroid gland or pituitary gland. Congenital hypothyroidism (existing from birth) may result from a pituitary **cyst**, iodine deficiency, or inherited defects in the enzymes required for synthesis of thyroid hormones. Iatrogenic (treatment-related) hypothyroidism may result from surgical removal of the thyroid gland, destruction of the thyroid gland by radiation or radioiodine, or drugs inhibiting the secretion of thyroid hormones (for example, sulfonamide antibiotics, some anticonvulsants, and certain heart medications).

Lymphocytic thyroiditis is an immune-mediated disease in which lymphocytes (a type of white blood cells) and **plasma cells** infiltrate the thyroid gland and over time

Possible Causes of Hypothyroidism in Dogs

Primary Hypothyroidism
Lymphocytic thyroiditis

Idiopathic atrophy

Nonfunctional* thyroid tumor

Surgical removal of thyroid gland

Antithyroid drugs

Congenital

    Inborn malformation of thyroid glands

    Inborn defects in thyroid hormone synthesis

Iodine deficiency

Secondary Hypothyroidism
Pituitary malformation or cyst

Nonfunctional† pituitary tumor

Other causes of pituitary dysfunction

Tertiary Hypothyroidism
Destruction or malformation of hypothalamus

*Does not secrete thyroid hormone.
†Does not secrete pituitary hormone (TSH).

destroy thyroid hormone-producing cells. Lymphocytic thyroiditis is hereditary in Beagles and Borzois. It is suspected of being hereditary in many other breeds, including:

Akita	Golden Retriever
Basenji	Great Dane
Border Collie	Irish Setter
Boxer	Maltese
Chesapeake Bay Retriever	Old English Sheepdog
Cocker Spaniel	Rhodesian Ridgeback
Dalmatian	Shetland Sheepdog
Doberman Pinscher	Siberian Husky
English Setter	

Most dogs with lymphocytic thyroiditis have circulating **autoantibodies** directed against **thyroglobulin**—antithyroglobulin antibodies (ATA). However, clinical signs of hypothyroidism do not develop in all dogs with ATA.

In idiopathic thyroid gland atrophy, the hormone-producing follicular cells of the thyroid gland degenerate and are replaced with fatty tissue. The cause of this degeneration is not known.

The reported prevalence of hypothyroidism in dogs is from 0.2% to 0.8%. The mean age at diagnosis is 7 years (range, 0.5 to 15 years). The disease occurs earlier in large and giant breeds and in predisposed breeds. It is not related to the pet's gender or to whether it has been neutered. The two breeds with the highest risk of hypothyroidism are Doberman Pinschers and Golden Retrievers, although any breed may be affected.

Clinical Signs and Symptoms

Because thyroid hormones affect the function of numerous organs, hypothyroid pets may show many different clinical signs and symptoms. Changes to the skin and hair coat occur in 60% to 80% of hypothyroid dogs. Thyroxine is required for hair growth to start—so hypothyroid dogs will show a lack of hair regrowth after shaving. Over time, bilaterally symmetrical alopecia (hair loss in a mirror-image pattern on both sides of the body) develops as a result of the failure to grow new hairs to replace those lost normally. Sebaceous (oil) and apocrine (sweat) gland activity also decreases. The skin may become dry and scaly. The hair coat often becomes faded and dull. Hairs are easily epilated (pulled out). Hair follicles may become plugged with keratin, forming comedones (blackheads). Bacterial and fungal (**yeast**) skin infections are more likely, and so is adult-onset **demodicosis**. The skin may be easily bruised. Another problem seen with hypothyroidism is **ceruminous** (waxy) **otitis externa**, an outer ear inflammation associated with more frequent

Clinical Signs and Symptoms of Hypothyroidism in Dogs

- **Alopecia (usually bilateral, starting on trunk)**
- **Seborrhea (greasy or dry and scaly)**
- **"Rat tail"**
- **Dry, dull hair coat**
- **Reoccurring skin infections**
- **Hyperpigmentation (skin darkening)**
- **Ear inflammation with waxy discharge**
- **Myxedema (thickened skin with exaggerated skin folds)**
- **Lethargy, decreased activity**
- **Weight gain**
- **Heat-seeking behavior**
- **Facial nerve paralysis**
- **Weakness, circling, incoordination**
- **Lipid deposits or ulcers of the cornea**
- **Slow heart rate**
- **Infertility (failure of heat cycle)**
- **Gynecomastia (mammary gland enlargement)**

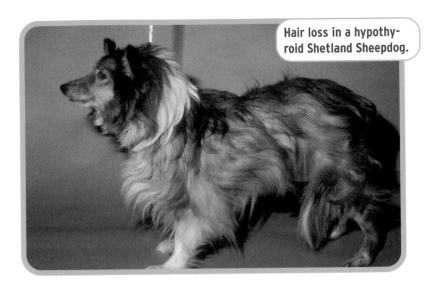

Hair loss in a hypothyroid Shetland Sheepdog.

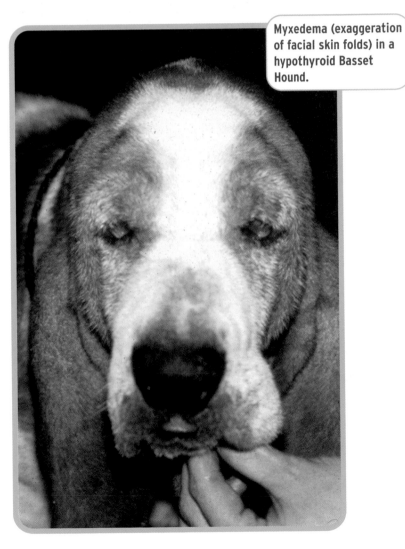

Myxedema (exaggeration of facial skin folds) in a hypothyroid Basset Hound.

bacterial and **Malassezia** (yeast) ear infections. In some dogs, the amount of **mucin** in the skin increases. Presence of this excess mucin results in an exaggeration of normal facial folds and swelling of the eyelids, cheeks, and forehead; these changes create a "tragic" facial expression in the affected dog.

The clinical signs of hypothyroidism can be vague and barely noticeable at first. Obesity develops in approximately 40% of hypothyroid dogs as a result of decreased metabolic rate, lethargy, and unwillingness to exercise. Affected dogs may seem mentally "dull" and typically show a preference for the warmest places in the home, such as near heat registers or a fireplace (heat-seeking behavior). The heart rate slows, and changes may be seen on electrocardiograms (ECGs). Eye abnormalities may include lipid deposits in the **cornea** or corneal ulcers. Reproductive system abnormalities include failure of the "heat" cycle (prolonged **anestrus**), lack of **libido** (sex drive), testicular atrophy, and infertility. A variety of nervous system dysfunctions have been reported to be associated with hypothyroidism. Examples are:

Paralysis of the nerves controlling the muscles of the face

Vestibular disease (resulting in balance problems)

Paralysis of the larynx

Myasthenia gravis (a disease affecting the junctions of the nerves with muscles)

Seizures

Disorientation

Circling

Profound mental dullness

Stupor

Coma

Hypothyroidism that is congenital (present at birth) results in mental retardation and dwarfism. Affected dogs have abnormally large heads, broad skulls, short thick necks, short limbs, large tongues, and delayed eruption of teeth. Similar signs are seen in kittens with congenital hypothyroidism.

Diagnosis

Pets with hypothyroidism often have a mild **anemia** (low numbers of red blood cells) and increased concentrations of serum cholesterol and triglycerides. These changes are present in many diseases, so they are of limited value in making a diagnosis of hypothyroidism. Numerous tests are available to measure the concentrations of the various thyroid hormones, as well as to measure ATA, anti-T_4, and anti-T_3 autoantibodies. Test results can be confusing, however, because thyroid hormone levels vary a lot in normal dogs. Your veterinarian will use a series of tests to confirm the diagnosis.

The most readily available test for evaluating thyroid status is measurement of total T_4 concentrations in the blood. Finding normal concentrations rules out a diagnosis of hypothyroidism. Unfortunately, finding low levels of total T_4 does not prove that a dog is hypothyroid. Time of day, season, breed, age, ambient temperature, other diseases, drugs, and many other factors can affect total T_4 concentrations. Greyhounds and Scottish Deerhounds have lower total T_4 concentrations than those typically found in other breeds. Hour-to-hour fluctuations in thyroid hormone secretion may result in total T_4 concentrations below the normal range in as many as 20% of samples from normal dogs. So veterinarians often recommend additional testing when a test shows decreased total T_4.

Tests to measure total T_3 concentrations are readily available; however, they are of minimal help in diagnosing hypothyroidism. Total T_3 concentrations are affected by the same factors affecting total T_4 levels and tend to have even greater hour-to-hour fluctuations.

Free T_4 is the only form of T_4 that can enter cells. It is not affected by as many factors as total T_4, so the free T_4 level gives a more accurate picture of thyroid function. Measurement of free T_4 by the equilibrium dialysis method is the most accurate single hormone measurement for diagnosing hypothyroidism in dogs. Because free T_4 measurement is more expensive than total T_4 measurement, many veterinarians request a free T_4 measurement only if the total T_4 is low.

Free T_3 assays are available, but the circulating levels of free T_3 are low even in normal dogs. So the diagnostic accuracy of this test is no better than that of a free T_4 test performed by itself.

Canine TSH assays are used to help diagnose hypothyroidism. When thyroid hormone concentrations are low in a normal animal, the pituitary gland secretes TSH to stimulate the thyroid glands to produce more T_4 and T_3. When the thyroid gland can't produce T_4 and T_3, the pituitary gland responds by producing even more TSH. In people, measurement of TSH is considered the most accurate single test for diagnosing hypothyroidism. The diagnostic accuracy is not as high in dogs—for unknown reasons, up to one third of hypothyroid dogs have TSH concentrations within the normal range. Approximately 10% of dogs with normal thyroid function have increased levels of TSH; this increase may reflect the time of day when the sample was collected, a very early stage of hypothyroidism, the effects of certain drugs (for example, sulfonamides), or a nonthyroid-related illness. Finding increased levels of TSH in a dog with low total or free T_4 helps in confirming the diagnosis of hypothyroidism. If the TSH assay is less expensive than a free T_4 assay, your veterinarian may use it instead as the second test. So the diagnostic steps are as follows: (1) observe clinical signs consistent with hypothyroidism; (2) verify that the dog does not have other illnesses and has not been given sulfonamides or other drugs that interfere with thyroid hormone secretion; (3) submit blood for measurement of total T_4; (4) if total T_4 is low, submit blood for measurement of free T_4 or TSH; (5) if free T_4 is low or TSH is elevated, the diagnosis of hypothyroidism is confirmed and treatment should be started.

The most accurate method for diagnosing hypothyroidism is to perform a TSH response test. With this test, a baseline blood sample is taken for total T_4 measurement. The dog is then given TSH intravenously, and a second blood sample is taken 4 to 6 hours later. Dogs with hypothyroidism do not show an increase in thyroid hormone concentrations in the second blood sample. Unfortunately, the cost of TSH has made this test too expensive to be practical.

Treatment trials in which a pet suspected of being hypothyroid is given thyroid hormone replacement therapy and observed for a favorable response are not recommended, because giving thyroid hormone to a pet with a normal thyroid gland results in atrophy of the thyroid gland. In addition, giving excess thyroid hormones to pets with other diseases may make their condition worse.

A diagnosis of thyroiditis can be made by measuring ATA or anti-T_3 and anti-T_4 antibodies. Presence of these antibodies is an indicator of lymphocytic thyroiditis but does not confirm the diagnosis of hypothyroidism. Lymphocytic thyroiditis may be present for many years before the ability of the thyroid gland to secrete adequate amounts of T_4 and T_3 is impaired. Some dogs have transient increases in ATA after vaccinations. Measurement of ATA, anti-T_3, and anti-T_4 antibodies has been recommended before breeding in dogs that have a high breed-related risk of developing hypothyroidism. Eliminating ATA-positive dogs from breeding pools should decrease the prevalence of hereditary forms of lymphocytic thyroiditis and thereby decrease the prevalence of hypothyroidism in those breeds. The Orthopedic Foundation for Animals (OFA) maintains a Thyroid Registry to help breeders interested in identifying breeding stock free of hereditary lymphocytic thyroiditis. Further information can be obtained from the OFA website (http://www.offa.org/thyinfo.html). The OFA recommends evaluating dogs for hypothyroidism and thyroiditis at 1, 2, 3, 4, 6, and 8 years of age.

Treatment

Hypothyroidism is treated with thyroid hormone replacement therapy. The preferred drug for treatment is synthetic sodium levothyroxine (a form of T_4). Intestinal absorption of this supplement varies and ranges from 10% to 50% in dogs. Because of this wide range, the optimal dose and frequency of supplementation will require individual adjustments based on testing after the drug is given. Different brands vary widely in their absorption, so once a brand is selected, only that brand should be used. Despite their higher cost, name brands of levothyroxine are preferred because of their more reliable absorption by dogs. Changes in diet also may affect absorption of the drug given by mouth because of changes in the binding of levothyroxine to undigested proteins in the intestinal tract. Be sure to have your pet's thyroid hormone concentrations re-tested after any change in the brand of levothyroxine being given or in the brand or type of food being fed.

Treatment should be started with twice-daily doses of levothyroxine. T_4 concentrations should be evaluated in 6 to 8 weeks. A blood sample is taken between 4 and 6 hours after the morning dose of levothyroxine. The serum T_4 concentration should be in the high-normal range. If the T_4 concentration is too low, the dose should be increased. Conversely, if it is too high, the dose should be decreased. Clinical signs and symptoms of levothyroxine overdosage may include panting, nervousness, increased thirst, increased urination, and weight loss. If any of these signs occurs, the dose being given is probably too high, and your veterinarian should be consulted for advice on dosage adjustment. T_4 levels should be rechecked 6 to 8 weeks after each change in dosage. Many dogs require dosage adjustments during the first few months of supplementation as a result of changes in their metabolism. When serum T_4 levels have stabilized, monitoring can be decreased to once or twice a year.

Improved "attitude" and energy level usually are seen within a couple of weeks after the start of T_4 supplementation. Hair loss at first may seem worse, because the pet sheds the old hairs before new hairs start growing. The skin and hair coat should return to normal after several months of treatment. Nerve function usually improves gradually over a period of 8 to 12 weeks. Weight loss may be noticeable within 2 months, although often the pet's food intake must be restricted for good control of obesity.

Hyperthyroidism
Causes

Hyperthyroidism (thyrotoxicosis) results from excessive production of T_4 and T_3 from an abnormally functioning thyroid gland. It is one of the most common endocrine disorders affecting older cats. Hyperthyroid cats have an enlargement of one or both lobes of their thyroid gland. (This resembles the thyroid disease known as toxic nodular goiter in people.) Factors that may possibly be associated with the development of hyperthyroidism in cats are:

- **Siamese and Himalayan breeds (higher incidence in these breeds)**
- **Diet of predominantly canned cat foods**
- **Diet of fish-flavored or liver-and-giblet-flavored foods**
- **Use of litter boxes**
- **Genistein and daidzein—goitrogenic (goiter-producing) soy isoflavones in commercial cat foods**

Clinical Signs and Symptoms

Almost any organ system can be affected by hyperthyroidism. Ninety-five percent of affected cats are older than 10 years of age; the average age at onset is 12 to 13 years. Weight loss is the most common sign (seen in more than 80% of hyperthyroid cats). The weight loss is caused by an increased metabolic rate and occurs despite an increase in food consumption (polyphagia). Many hyperthyroid cats are hyperactive, pant excessively, and have rapid heart rates (tachycardia). Most hyperthyroid cats show increased thirst and urination, occasional vomiting and diarrhea, and an increase in stool volume. Muscle weakness may result in decreased ability to jump and in fatigue after running. In some hyperthyroid cats, congestive heart failure and dyspnea (difficulty breathing) may develop.

Clinical Signs and Symptoms of Hyperthyroidism in Cats

- **Notably increased appetite (polyphagia)**
- **Weight loss**
- **Increased thirst (polydipsia) and urination (polyuria)**
- **Increased stool volume and frequency**
- **Vomiting**
- **Panting, dyspnea (difficult breathing)**
- **Hyperactive, but fatigues easily**
- **Heat intolerance (seeks cool places)**
- **Overgrooming (with hair loss)**
- **Matted, unkempt appearance to hair coat**
- **Rapid heart rate**
- **Long, deformed claws**

Skin and hair coat changes often are present in hyperthyroid cats. Some overgroom, perhaps because of their elevated body temperature—the spreading of saliva on hairs during grooming helps the cat cool itself. The overgrooming leads to alopecia (hair loss), because many hairs are pulled out by the barbs on the cat's tongue during grooming. Long-haired cats are the most likely to overgroom. Some short-haired cats decrease their grooming, so their hair coats become matted and unkempt in appearance. The claws often grow faster and become long and brittle.

Diagnosis

The physical examination of cats with hyperthyroidism usually identifies an enlarged thyroid gland (a goiter that can be felt). The diagnosis of hyperthyroidism is confirmed by finding elevated levels of total T_4. Approximately 10% of hyperthyroid cats have total T_4 values within the normal range; these cats should be tested to see if their free T_4 values are elevated. If both total and free T_4 levels are within the normal ranges but the cat has symptoms of hyperthyroidism, it should be evaluated by a specialist in feline internal medicine (a diplomate of the American College of Veterinary Internal Medicine). Thyroid **radionu-clide** uptake and **nuclear imaging** studies (**nuclear scans**) can be used to identify hyperfunctioning thyroid tissue.

Treatment

Treatment of hyperthyroidism is aimed at reducing the damaging effects of increased thyroid hormone concentrations, blocking the production of thyroid hormones, or removing or destroying abnormally functioning thyroid tissue. Medical treatments may be used to block the pro-

Treatment of Hyperthyroidism in Cats

Treatment	Advantages	Disadvantages
Oral antithyroid drugs (methimazole, carbimazole, others)	Usually effective; side effects usually reversible; do not require special facilities or surgery	Must be given daily; some cats are difficult to medicate, side effects of medication (appetite loss, vomiting, bone marrow suppression, itching)
Surgery	May provide a permanent cure; relatively inexpensive	Risks associated with anesthesia and surgery; occasional postoperative complications
Radioactive iodine	Usually effective; one dose may provide permanent cure	Requires hospitalization in a specialized facility until cat is no longer radioactive

duction of thyroid hormones and to protect the heart from the damaging effects of high levels of these hormones. Drugs used to block the production of thyroid hormones include methimazole and carbimazole. For short-term use (for example, before surgery), calcium ipodate or potassium iodate can be used to block the synthesis of thyroid hormones. Propranolol and atenolol are drugs that are used to slow rapid heart rates and stabilize cardiac function.

The thyroid gland can be removed surgically as a cure for hyperthyroidism. Medical therapy often is used for several weeks before surgery to stabilize the cat and improve its likelihood of surviving the surgery. A possible complication of surgical thyroidectomy is unintended removal of the parathyroid glands, which are necessary to maintain proper levels of blood calcium. Cats are monitored closely for several days after surgery to be certain they do not suffer from low blood calcium levels or other complications.

Radioactive iodine treatment is the safest, simplest, and most effective treatment for feline hyperthyroidism. To minimize human exposure to radioactive compounds, this treatment can be administered only at specially licensed facilities. After treatment, the cat must be kept within the licensed facility until it is no longer radioactive. This typically requires hospitalization at the facility for 2 to 3 weeks.

Sex Hormone Disorders

Sex hormones are produced by the ovaries and testicles of females and males, respectively, and also by the adrenal cortex in both genders. The adrenal cortex is the only site for sex hormone production in neutered pets.

Estrogens have variable effects on hair growth, sebum production, and skin thickness. The variability may result from regional differences in estrogen receptors on hair follicles. Androgens stimulate epidermal mitosis (skin cell division) and dermal mucin production, resulting in a thickening of skin. Androgens also stimulate sebaceous (oil) gland activity and hair growth. Progesterone suppresses sebaceous gland activity, decreases hair growth, and causes thinning of skin.

Numerous dermatological (skin and hair) syndromes in pets may involve sex hormones. Several of these are discussed in the following sections.

Hyperestrogenism

The most common cause of hyperestrogenism in dogs is a Sertoli cell tumor. Sertoli cells are found in the testicles of male dogs, where they help spermatozoa to mature and also produce estrogens. Cryptorchid males (those with "undescended" testicles that have failed to move down to the scrotum) are at increased risk of developing Sertoli cell tumors. Breeds at risk for Sertoli cell tumors include Boxers, Shetland Sheepdogs, Weimaraners, Cairn Terriers, Pekingese, and Collies. These breeds also have a high incidence of cryptorchidism. The high levels of estrogen produced by a Sertoli cell tumor often cause feminization–replacement of typically "masculine" features by "feminine" ones–and alopecia. The hair loss often begins around the dog's neck and in the **perineum** (area between anus and genitals), with gradual thinning of hair over the trunk. Hairs in affected areas epilate (pull out) easily. The skin may be thinner than normal. The prepuce may have a linear area of erythema (reddening) or hyperpigmentation (skin darkening). Signs of feminization include nipple enlargement (**gynecomastia**), a pendulous (droopy) prepuce, decreased libido, decreased sperm production, and attraction of other male dogs. High levels of estrogen sometimes cause bone marrow suppression, resulting in anemia, neutropenia (low level of certain white blood cells), and thrombocytopenia (decreased number of blood **platelets**). Bone marrow suppression can be irreversible and fatal. A tentative diagnosis of hyperestrogenism may be made on the basis of clinical signs of feminization and alopecia in a cryptorchid dog. Sertoli cell tumors also may develop in noncryptorchid males. In those cases, the testicle with the tumor usually is enlarged, while the nonaffected testicle is shrunken. Diagnosis is confirmed by castrating the dog and submitting the testicles for laboratory examination to identify the Sertoli cell tumor. Castration usually is curative, with hair regrowth within 3 months. Sertoli cell tumors rarely spread to other parts of the body; however, if hair regrowth does not occur, the tumor may have spread to nearby lymph nodes before surgery.

Hyperestrogenism in female dogs is very rare. It is associated with cystic ovaries or ovarian tumors that produce excessive amounts of estrogen. Clinical signs include a history of irregular or prolonged estrous cycles (heats), symmetrical alopecia that begins in the perineum, gynecomastia (enlargement of the nipples), enlargement of the vulva, hyperpigmentation, and in some cases, a greasy **seborrhea** (oily skin) and ceruminous (waxy) otitis externa. Diagnosis may be made by using an ultrasound examination (ultrasonography, sonogram) to identify

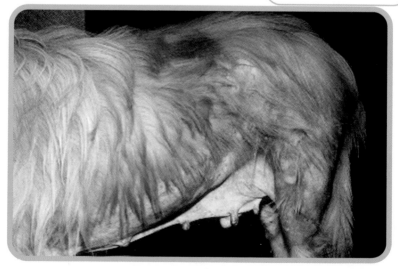

Feminization and alopecia in a Collie with a Sertoli cell tumor.

ovarian cysts or tumors. The recommended treatment is spaying. Hair regrowth usually occurs within 3 to 6 months after surgery.

Hyperandrogenism in Male Dogs

Hyperandrogenism (excessive production of male hormones) is a rare disorder that affects intact (non-neutered) male dogs. It can cause a greasy seborrhea (**seborrhea oleosa**) and hyperplasia (enlargement) of the tail gland and circumanal (around the anus) glands. Hyperplasia of the tail gland results in hair loss and crusting in an oval area along the top of the tail. Hyperplasia of the circumanal glands results in a donut-like enlargement of the tissue surrounding the anus. Dogs with hyperandrogenism usually are aggressive and show strong libido (sex drive). The testicles of affected dogs may contain androgen-secreting tumors known as inter-

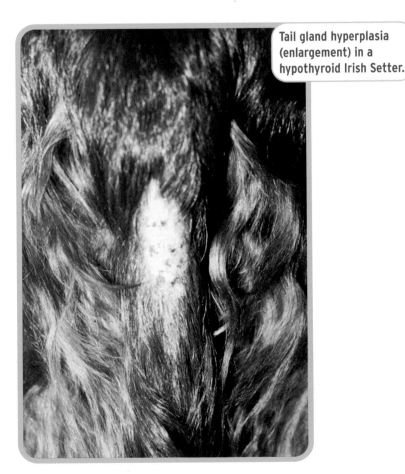

Tail gland hyperplasia (enlargement) in a hypothyroid Irish Setter.

stitial cell tumors. Castration is the recommended treatment for affected dogs. Problem behaviors may require months to change, and some dogs may need behavioral modification therapy (special training). Frequent bathing with **antiseborrheic** shampoos will improve the condition of the skin and hair coat. The enlarged tail glands may shrink over a period of several months.

Sex Hormone-Responsive Skin Diseases

Numerous skin disease syndromes involving hair loss have been described that respond to manipulations of sex hormones in dogs. The exact cause-and-effect relationship between the alopecia and sex hormones has not been established for most of these syndromes.

Estrogen-Responsive Dermatosis

Estrogen-responsive dermatosis (noninflammatory skin disease) occurs primarily in female Dachshunds and Boxers that were spayed at a young age. Affected dogs have thin skin and a sparse hair coat. Hair loss begins in the perineum (between anus and genitals) and progresses to involve the abdomen, thighs, neck, and head. The nipples and vulva are infantile. The diagnosis is based on ruling out other causes of hair loss and observing hair regrowth after treatment with estrogens (female hormones). Unfortunately, treatment with estrogens may have serious side effects, including irreversible bone marrow suppression. Some pets with skin problems that suggest an estrogen-responsive dermatosis will regrow hair after treatment with **melatonin** (as discussed later in the chapter). I advise against using estrogen supplements for a cosmetic disease, but I do prescribe melatonin.

Testosterone-Responsive Dermatosis

Testosterone-responsive dermatosis is a very rare condition that occurs in older neutered male dogs; Afghan Hounds may be have a greater-than-normal risk of developing this condition. The hair coat becomes dull and dry, and the color looks "faded." The skin may be abnormally thin. Hair loss begins with gradual thinning on the trunk. Diagnosis is based on ruling out other causes of hair loss. Options for treatment include observation (no treatment), methyltestosterone, and mibolerone (Check Drops). Methyltestosterone use must be monitored carefully, because this agent can cause liver disease in dogs and also has the potential for human abuse as an anabolic steroid.

Castration-Responsive Dermatosis

In Keeshonds, Alaskan Malamutes, Chow Chows, Samoyeds, Pomeranians, and Miniature Poodles that have not been neutered, a bilaterally symmetrical alopecia may develop that is reversible after castration (the hair regrows). Hair loss in these pets begins around the neck, flanks, belly, and **perineum**. Guard hairs are lost first, giving the coat a woolly, "puppy coat–like" appearance. Affected dogs are normal except for the hair loss. Diagnosis is based on ruling out other causes of hair loss and observing hair regrowth after castration. Many veterinarians believe that castration-responsive dermatosis is the same syndrome as alopecia X (discussed later in the chapter).

Feline Endocrine Alopecia

In middle-aged, neutered cats, a symmetrical alopecia occasionally develops beginning in the genital area and perineum, with diffuse (widespread) thinning of the hair that progresses to involve the belly, thighs, and tail. The back typically retains a normal coat. Hairs in the affected areas usually epilate (pull out) easily. The exact cause of this condition is unknown. It originally was thought to be caused by either a deficiency in sex hormones or hypothyroidism (underproduction of thyroid hormone); however, no consistent hormonal deficiency has been identified. Most cats with this pattern of hair loss are actually "secret groomers" that pull hairs out. A skin **biopsy** can be performed to determine whether hairs are actively growing (they will be if the cat is a secret groomer) or are all in the telogen (resting) phase. When overgrooming is ruled out, the cat should be evaluated for other causes of hair loss. These include **demodicosis** (parasitic infection), **dermatophytosis** (ringworm), Cushing's disease, hypothyroidism, and **paraneoplastic** alopecia (hair loss as a side effect of cancer). If no cause for the hair loss is identified, treatment options include observation (no treatment), a thyroid supplementation trial (being cautious to avoid overdosing), and sex hormone supplements (combinations of estrogens, androgens, testosterone, progesterone, and megestrol acetate). With sex hormone therapy, caution is advised because of the potentially serious side effects associated with the use of these supplements.

Possible Side Effects of Sex Hormone Treatments

Hormone	Possible Side Effects
Estrogen	Feminization, gynecomastia, infertility, bone marrow suppression
Androgens (testosterone, methyltestosterone)	Liver damage, behavioral changes (aggression), infertility, potential for abuse by people (anabolic steroids)
Progesterones (progesterone, megestrol acetate)	Increased blood glucose, diabetes, acromegaly, behavioral changes, mammary enlargement or cancer, pyometra (infection of uterus), infertility

Miscellaneous Disorders

Miscellaneous endocrine diseases include those that respond to other hormones including growth hormone and **melatonin**. A direct cause-and-effect relationship has not been established for most of these conditions. Management of the skin and hair problems may include manipulating hormone levels to stimulate hair growth. A good response to hormone therapies, however, does not necessarily prove that the pet was deficient in the hormones being used in the treatment.

Where We Stand

Treatments that may be harmful to the pet should be avoided, especially if the condition being treated is purely a cosmetic problem. Bald pets are happier and healthier than ones made sick by treatment with a hazardous drug.

Pituitary Dwarfism

Pituitary dwarfism is a hereditary disorder affecting mostly German Shepherd dogs, Carnelian Bear dogs, and crosses of these breeds. Affected dogs may appear normal at birth, but their growth rate slows by 2 to 3 months of age. The hair coat of pituitary dwarfs remains "puppy-like," with a soft, woolly texture. Hairs are easily epilated (pulled out), and hair loss develops beginning around the neck and on the sides. The head and legs remain haired. The hairless skin becomes hyperpigmented (darkened). Permanent teeth may fail to come in, and the testicles or nipples and vulva may remain infantile (they fail to mature). Superficial skin infections and a secondary **seb-orrhea** (oily, scaly skin) are more common among dogs with pituitary dwarfism. Some affected dogs also are hypothyroid. Diagnosis is most often based on the breed, history, and clinical signs. Management consists of controlling secondary skin infections and seborrhea, plus thyroid hormone replacement therapy if the dog also is hypothyroid. Growth hormone is difficult to obtain for use in dogs and can result in side effects including diabetes and **acromegaly**.

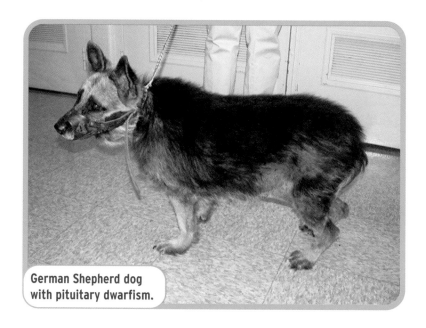

German Shepherd dog with pituitary dwarfism.

Growth Hormone-Responsive Alopecia

A syndrome referred to as "hyposomatotropism in the mature dog," "adult-onset growth hormone deficiency," and "pseudo-Cushing's disease" was described in the early 1990s. Affected dogs usually were young males between 1 and 2 years of age. Commonly affected breeds included the Chow Chow, Keeshond, Pomeranian, Samoyed, Miniature Poodle, and American Water Spaniel. Clinical signs included a loss of primary hairs (guard hairs) that began around the neck and thighs and progressed to involve most of the body, except for the head and legs. The loss of primary hairs left the softer, woolly secondary hairs, resulting in a "puppy coat" appearance. With time, the secondary hairs also were lost, and the skin became hairless, thin, and hyperpigmented. Growth hormone levels were low in these dogs (when measured by a laboratory that discontinued offering the assay in the early 1990s). Many affected dogs had hair regrowth after treatment with growth hormone supplements.

Despite these findings, the precise role and importance of growth hormone in hair growth in adult dogs still have not been clearly defined. The same breeds of dogs reported to have "growth hormone-responsive alopecia" also have been suggested to have adrenal sex hormone abnormalities or "alopecia X." Currently, a majority of veterinary dermatologists believe that the growth hormone abnormalities described in the 1990s were actually caused by another, still poorly understood endocrine or hair follicle disease (that is, alopecia X). Growth hormone assays are not readily available for testing in dogs; this has prevented further investigations related to the role, if any, of growth hormone in skin diseases of dogs that result in alopecia.

"Alopecia X"

Alopecia X is a syndrome that has been given *many* names—adrenal sex hormone imbalance, hyposomatotropism, growth hormone-responsive dermatosis, pseudo-Cushing's disease, and others. Numerous theories about the cause of this disorder have been proposed; however, none have been proved. Affected dogs are normal, with the exception of their skin and hair coat. Hair loss begins around the neck, rear and inner thighs, and tail. Primary (guard) hairs are lost first, leaving the soft, woolly secondary hairs. This results in a puppy-like appearance to the hair coat. Gradually the secondary hairs also are lost, and the exposed skin becomes hyperpigmented (darkened). The head and legs usually retain a normal-appearing hair coat. Most affected dogs are of breeds that normally have plush coats (for example, the Chow Chow, Pomeranian, Keeshond, Samoyed, Malamute, Husky, and Poodles). The age when the disease appears varies (range from 9 months to 11 years); however, most cases are young adults. Neutered dogs may be more likely to develop the condition. Diagnosis is based on history, physical examination findings, and ruling out other diseases causing hair loss.

Other Names for "Alopecia X"

- **Adult-onset growth hormone deficiency**
- **Adrenal sex hormone imbalance**
- **Biopsy-responsive alopecia (hair regrows at biopsy sites)**
- **"Black skin disease"**
- **Castration-responsive alopecia**
- **"Coat funk"**
- **Congenital adrenal hyperplasia-like syndrome**
- **Growth hormone-responsive dermatosis**
- **Hyposomatotropism**
- **Pseudo-Cushing's disease**

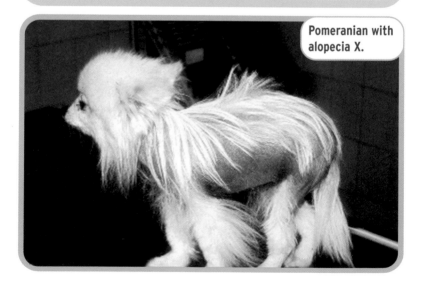

Pomeranian with alopecia X.

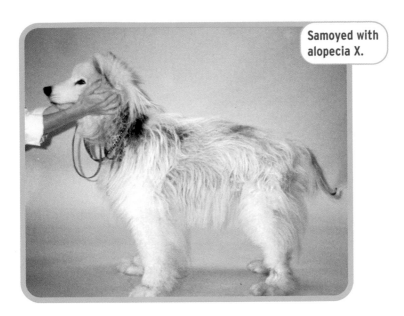

Samoyed with alopecia X.

A variety of treatments have been reported to help stimulate hair growth in affected dogs. All pets with this condition should be neutered. Approximately 25% of pets with alopecia X have hair regrowth within 3 months after neutering. Melatonin often is the first drug prescribed for treatment in neutered dogs. It is effective in approximately one third of the cases and has a low incidence of side effects. Ketoconazole (an antifungal drug) inhibits adrenal gland production of several sex hormones and cortisol; it has been successfully used in the treatment of alopecia X. Side effects of ketoconazole include anorexia (loss of appetite), liver disease, lightening of the hair color, and interference with the metabolism of other drugs. Trilostane, another drug that inhibits the synthesis of steroid hormones, is being investigated for use in the treatment of alopecia X. Early reports have shown that 80% of pets respond to this treatment. Trilostane currently is unavailable in the United States, and its safety profile is not completely known (there have been a few reports of death when the drug was given to dogs with heart disease). Mitotane also has been used for the treatment of alopecia X. However, mitotane is a potent drug that requires careful monitoring to prevent fatal overdoses. Many veterinarians question whether it is wise to use a potentially dangerous drug for treating a cosmetic disease.

Estrogen, testosterone, and growth hormone all have been reported to be effective in stimulating hair regrowth in some dogs. Each of these hormonal agents has potentially serious side effects, however, so they are rarely recommended for use in dogs. If hair loss does not resolve with neutering or melatonin therapy, an attractive T-shirt or sweater is the safest means of providing a covering for the dog's bald spots. Affected dogs should not be used for breeding, because hair loss in alopecia X appears to be inherited.

Treatment Options for Dogs with Alopecia X

Treatment	Advantages	Disadvantages
Observation or sweater	Safest, cheap	Does not stimulate hair growth
Neutering	Safe, protects against breeding (and passing on genes for the condition), protects against pyometra (infection of uterus) in females and both testicular and prostatic disease in males	Effective in only 25% of cases; effectiveness may be temporary; many affected dogs are already neutered
Melatonin	Safe, cheap	Effective in only 30-35% of cases; effectiveness may be temporary

Treatment Options for Dogs with Alopecia X—cont'd

Treatment	Advantages	Disadvantages
Ketoconazole	Also controls any secondary yeast infections	Expensive; must be given twice daily; side effects may include appetite loss, vomiting, liver damage; interferes with metabolism of other drugs
Trilostane	Reported to be effective in 80% of cases	Unavailable in United States; reports of death in dogs with heart disease
Mitotane (Lysodren) (*o,p'*-DDD)	Many veterinarians are familiar with its use in treating Cushing's disease	Expensive; requires frequent monitoring to prevent fatal overdose
Growth hormone	Effective in many dogs	Side effects may include increases in blood glucose, diabetes, and acromegaly; unavailable for use in dogs in United States
Estrogen	Some reports of effectiveness	See earlier table for side effects
Androgens	Some reports of effectiveness	See earlier table for side effects

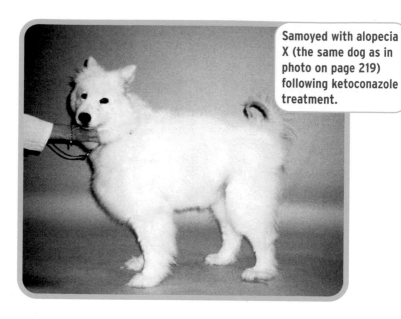

Canine Recurrent Flank Alopecia (Seasonal Flank Alopecia)

Canine recurrent flank alopecia, also known as seasonal flank alopecia, is a condition most commonly observed in Airedale Terriers, English Bulldogs, Boxers, and Schnauzers, although it also has been described in many other breeds. Alopecia and skin hyperpigmentation develop on both sides of the trunk. The hair loss occurs in cycles and in a pattern with well-defined borders, sometimes in the "saddle" region. Hair loss may begin in the fall, with regrowth in the spring, although seasonality varies from one dog to another. Approximately 80% of affected dogs have more than one episode of hair loss. Diagnosis is based on breed, clinical signs, and ruling out other causes of hair loss. Skin biopsy specimens show characteristic changes in hair follicles. Because hair loss in this type of alopecia fluctuates with the season and the disease is purely a cosmetic problem, many veterinarians feel that treatment is unnecessary.

Melatonin therapy may be useful in stimulating new hair growth. Melatonin is most effective when given soon after the start of the hair loss. In dogs with predictable cycles of canine recurrent flank alopecia, treatment with melatonin 1 to 2 months before the anticipated beginning of hair loss may prevent the next episode of hair loss.

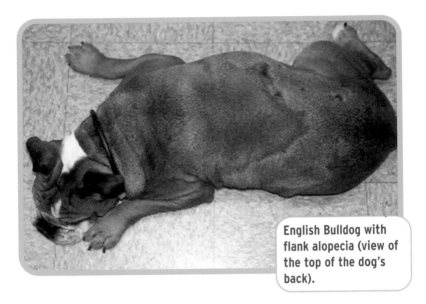

English Bulldog with flank alopecia (view of the top of the dog's back).

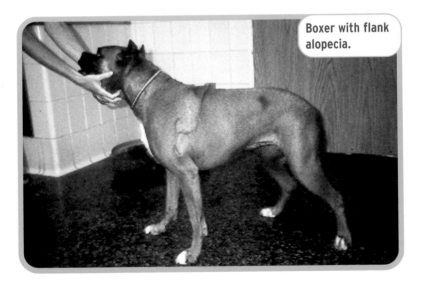

Boxer with flank alopecia.

Summary

Endocrine-related skin diseases are characterized by a slowly worsening, bilaterally symmetrical alopecia (hair loss in a mirror-image pattern on both sides of the body). Clinical clues that hair loss results from an endocrine disorder include hairs that are easily epilated (pulled out) and a dull, dry, faded appearance to the hair coat. Many endocrine diseases affecting the skin and hair coat also have effects on other organs. The early diagnosis and treatment of these disorders are important to prevent more serious systemic diseases. Other endocrine skin diseases are purely cosmetic disorders; for these problems, treatment with medications that have the potential of causing serious side effects probably should be avoided.

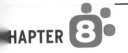
FUNGAL INFECTIONS

Fungal organisms are widespread in the environment. **Fungi** include **yeasts** and **molds.** Yeasts are single-celled organisms that reproduce by budding. Molds are multicellular and grow as fluffy colonies composed of multiple filamentous (strand-like) organisms. Fungal filaments also are referred to as **hyphae.** Some fungi are capable of existing in both yeast and mold forms; these are referred to as dimorphic ("two-form") fungi. Diseases produced by fungi are referred to as **mycoses.** More than 300 fungi have been found to cause disease in animals; however, only a few commonly produce skin disease in dogs and cats.

Dermatophytosis (Ringworm)

Dermatophytes are fungi that infect keratinized tissues. These tissues include hair, nails, and the horny layer of skin (**stratum corneum**). A term commonly used in describing dermatophyte infections (dermatophytoses) is **ringworm.** This name comes from the appearance of hair loss in a circular pattern. Why is the hair loss circular? When dermatophytes invade a growing hair, the fungal hyphae (filaments) within the hair shaft weaken it. Weakened hairs break off near the skin surface. The fungi then invade hairs adjacent to the one originally infected. This results in a progressive spreading of the infection in a widening circle—so the hairs break off in a spreading circular pattern.

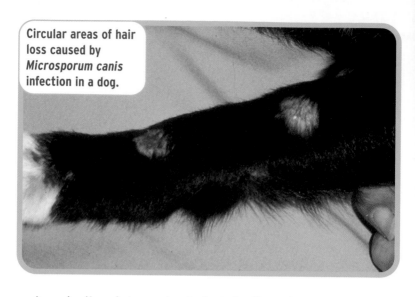

Circular areas of hair loss caused by *Microsporum canis* infection in a dog.

A majority of dermatophyte infections in cats and dogs are caused by three organisms: *Microsporum canis*, *Microsporum gypseum*, and *Trichophyton mentagrophytes*. It is important for your veterinarian to determine which one of these species is causing the ringworm in your pet, so that the source of the infection can be found. Knowing the source of the infection is important for identifying ways to protect pets from reinfection. *M. canis* usually is acquired from an infected cat. *M. gypseum* is found in the soil; dogs and cats usually acquire the organism when digging in contaminated soil. Rodents are the normal host for *T. mentagrophytes*; dogs and cats are infected by contact with an infected rodent or when digging or nosing around rodent burrows.

Clinical Signs and Symptoms

Hairs are the tissue most commonly affected by ringworm, and the most common **clinical sign** of infection is a circular patch of **alopecia** (hair loss) that expands around the infected area. However, many other signs can be associated with dermatophyte infections. **Papules** (red, raised bumps) and **pustules** (bumps that contain **pus**) may develop around the base of an infected hair. These lesions are produced by the pet's **immune system** responding to the infection. Papules are formed when the immune system causes an inflammatory reaction resulting in the accumulation of **white blood cells** and fluid around an infected **hair follicle**. Pustules are formed when increased numbers of white blood cells infiltrate the hair follicle.

Infected hair follicles sometimes rupture, resulting in an intense inflammatory reaction called **furunculosis**. Pus may drain from the sites of ruptured hair follicles. Sometimes a mass of inflammatory cells and scar tissue—

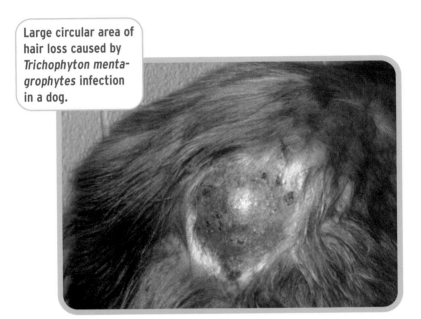

Large circular area of hair loss caused by *Trichophyton mentagrophytes* infection in a dog.

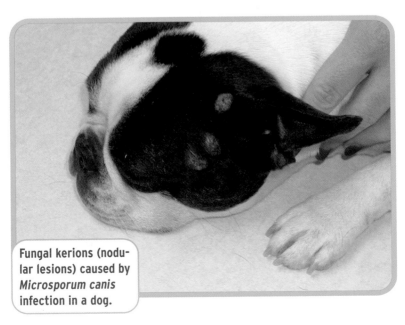

Fungal kerions (nodular lesions) caused by *Microsporum canis* infection in a dog.

a fungal kerion—forms around a fragment of an infected hair. These **lesions** sometimes rupture and drain pus.

In dogs that acquire *M. gypseum* from rooting in soil, or *T. mentagrophytes* from sticking their noses in a rodent burrow, a scaly rash on the nose frequently develops that slowly spreads up and over the face. The skin in hairless areas becomes hyperpigmented (dark-colored or black). Similar lesions may develop on the front legs of a dog that digs in infected soil or on the legs of young puppies that play in dirt.

In some cats with dermatophyte infections, multiple papules and crusts develop. This reaction pattern is called **miliary dermatitis**, because rubbing your hand over an affected cat's hair coat feels similar to rubbing a surface that has been sprinkled with millet seeds (*miliary* means "millet-like"). Other cats have a more typical pattern of multiple areas of alopecia (hair loss) with scaling.

Infections of the nails (**claws**) may result in the growth of deformed nails, often accompanied by pus around the base of the nail. Dermatophytosis of the chin looks very much like canine or feline **acne**. Some pets become pruritic (itchy), and ulcerated areas may result from intense scratching or chewing.

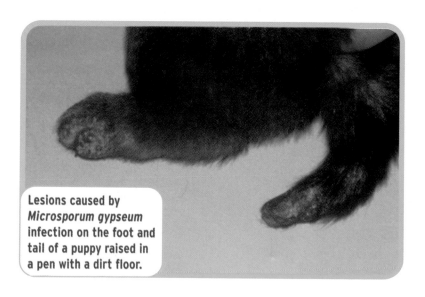

Lesions caused by *Microsporum gypseum* infection on the foot and tail of a puppy raised in a pen with a dirt floor.

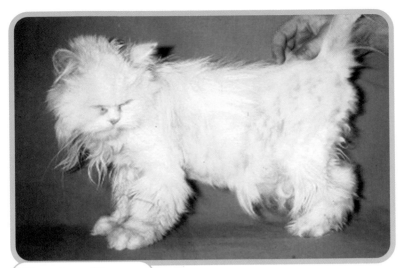

Miliary dermatitis lesions in a Persian cat infected with *Microsporum canis*.

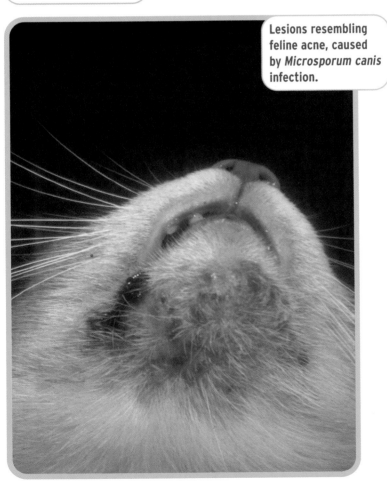

Lesions resembling feline acne, caused by *Microsporum canis* infection.

Dermatophytes are contagious to people. In approximately one third of households with an infected pet, one or more ringworm lesions also develop in a family member.

Diagnosis

It is impossible to diagnose ringworm by just looking at the lesions. The most common cause of circular patches of alopecia (hair loss) is a bacterial skin infection (staphylococcal **pyoderma**), not ringworm. The most common cause of miliary dermatitis in cats is fleas, not ringworm. The most common cause of alopecia on the face is *Demodex* (a parasitic mite), not ringworm. The most common cause of **cutaneous** nodules is a **tumor** (cancer), not ringworm. And the most common cause of nail deformities is an immune-mediated disease called **symmetric lupoid onychodystrophy**, not ringworm. Because of differences in treatment and prognosis (predicted outcome), your veterinarian will perform laboratory testing to confirm a diagnosis of ringworm and rule out other possible causes of skin disease.

Many cats harbor infections of *M. canis* without showing signs of hair loss or skin disease. These cats are termed asymptomatic **carriers** because they do not show outward evidence of being infected with ringworm; however, they can transmit the infection to other pets and people. The most reliable method of identifying asymptomatic carrier cats is to perform a toothbrush culture: First, the entire hair coat is brushed with a sterile toothbrush. Hairs infected with *M. canis* are more brittle than normal hairs; these break off and are collected by the toothbrush, along with any **spores** spread throughout the hair coat. The toothbrush bristles are then cultured on dermatophyte test medium. This often is called the McKenzie toothbrush screening procedure for dermatophytes, in honor of the first person who described the technique.

Treatment

In most pets, fungal infections activate the immune system. This results in the production of **antibodies** (proteins produced in response to a foreign substance) and in a cell-mediated response against the invading organism. Effector cells (the ones that do the work) in a cell-mediated response are called killer cells; these are **white blood cells** that engulf the organism or secrete enzymes and other chemicals, thereby destroying the invading organisms. The development of this immune response may take several weeks. Eventually the pet may be able

Where We Stand

Although ringworm infections in pets often are self-resolving, spores can remain infective in the environment for months to years. So it's important to be aggressive in treating dogs and cats infected with ringworm.

An aggressive treatment protocol will include (1) screening all in contact with pets for infections; (2) clipping infected pets in a closed room, destroying the clipped hairs, and disinfecting the entire room and all utensils used; (3) confining (isolating) all infected pets to one room that is cleaned daily and disinfected at least once per week; (4) dipping all infected pets with lime-sulfur (or enilconazole when available) once weekly; (5) treating all infected pets with a systemic antifungal medication; and (6) continuing the isolation, dips, and systemic medications until all lesions have healed and results of two consecutive fungal cultures are negative.

to "self-cure" and eliminate a ringworm infection. Most healthy dogs and short-haired cats eliminate localized ringworm infections within 3 months. Despite the possibility of a self-cure, treatment of ringworm is almost always recommended, to decrease the risk of spread of the infection to other pets or people.

Goals in treating ringworm include:

- **Maximizing the pet's ability to produce an effective immune response to the organism**
- **Reducing the spread of infective organisms**
- **Killing the organisms**

Several steps can be taken to maximize the pet's ability to produce an effective immune response to the organism. The most important thing is reviewing the drugs being administered to the pet and discontinuing any drugs that may suppress the immune system. These include **corticosteroids**, other anti-inflammatory drugs, and cancer chemotherapy. Consultation between an oncologist (cancer specialist) and a dermatologist (skin and hair specialist) is recommended if the pet has any type of cancer or a disease requiring immunosuppressive drugs. The nutritional status and overall health of the pet should be evaluated and appropriate steps taken to improve these areas as needed.

Several management strategies are helpful in minimizing the spread of infectious dermatophyte spores in the environment and to other pets and people. These include:

- **Isolation of infected pets**
- **Environmental decontamination**
- **Clipping to remove infected hairs**
- **Topical therapy**

M. canis infection is the most contagious dermatophytosis and is particularly contagious among cats. It is essential to test all cats within a household or cattery for ringworm and to isolate infected cats from noninfected ones. Cats that don't have visible lesions (diseased areas) should be tested for ringworm with the McKenzie toothbrush culture technique. Ideally, infected pets should be confined to a single room or individual cages—both to make environmental decontamination easier and to minimize the spread of infectious spores throughout the house, kennel, or cattery. Isolation is especially important for pets infected with *M. canis*; it also is helpful when the infections involve *M. gypseum* and *T. mentagrophytes*.

Environmental decontamination is extremely important in preventing the spread of dermatophyte infections and in preventing reoccurring infections. Dermatophyte spores on hairs shed by an infected pet retain their ability to infect other pets and people for as long as 18 months. Spores are resistant to most cleaning agents. Agents that may be effective in killing dermatophyte spores include:

- **Sodium hypochlorite (bleach, used in a 1:10 dilution in water)**
- **Formalin**
- **Chlorine dioxide (Oxygene, from Oxyfresh USA)**
- **Glutaraldehyde and quaternary ammonium chloride (GPC 8, from Solomon Industries)**
- **Potassium monoperoxysulfate (Trifectic, from EVSCO Pharmaceuticals, Vetoquinol USA, Inc., and Virkon, from S. Durvet)**
- **Enilconazole (Imaverol, from Janssen)**

Brushes, combs, and bedding used for an infected pet should be sterilized or discarded. Rugs and carpets should be disinfected with a steam cleaner with an antifungal disinfectant added to the water. Heating and cooling vents should be vacuumed and disinfected. Air filters should be changed weekly. Furnaces should be cleaned with commercial high-power suction equipment. The entire house should be cleaned thoroughly. Rooms housing infected pets should be mopped or vacuumed daily. Cages, bowls, and litter boxes should be disinfected daily. Crates, cages, pens, or vehicles that may be contaminated should be cleaned thoroughly and disinfected.

The major source of environmental contamination with dermatophyte spores is infected hairs. The most effective way of decreasing environmental contamination is to remove and destroy infected hairs. If an infected pet has only one or two localized areas of infection, scissors may be used to carefully trim away hairs that are within $2\frac{1}{2}$

inches of a lesion. If there are more than two lesions, or if the infected pet is a long-haired cat, the entire hair coat should be clipped. Clipping should be done carefully to avoid traumatizing the skin. Although clipping may spread the infection to other areas of the skin, removal of infected hairs is important, to decrease the probability of spreading ringworm to other pets or people. Extreme caution must be used to catch all of the shaved hair so that it can be destroyed. Clipping should be done in a closed room, without any fans or ventilation system running during the procedure. The entire room and all equipment used during clipping should be cleaned thoroughly and disinfected. The person clipping the pet(s) should wear protective clothing—ideally, a disposable gown and gloves that can be discarded after use.

Topical treatment is useful in further decreasing the contagiousness of an infected pet. Whole-body dips with lime-sulfur solution (2% LymDyp, from DVM Pharmaceuticals) are the preferred treatment. These dips should be repeated every 4 to 7 days for a minimum of 8 weeks. An alternative product for use in Canada and Europe is 0.2% enilconazole (Imaverol, from Janssen). Enilconazole also is applied as a whole-body dip every 4 to 7 days. Dips should be sponged over the pet until the entire hair coat is thoroughly saturated. Do not rinse the solution off the pet; it must dry on the hairs to provide maximal antifungal activity. Users should wear gloves and work in a well-ventilated area, because the odor, especially of lime-sulfur, can be very unpleasant. Lime-sulfur will stain the tub yellow and will also stain the hair coat of light-colored pets a yellowish color. Bleach can be used to remove stains from the tub. Prevent the pet from licking the dip solution, because ingesting the dips may cause vomiting or diarrhea. Keep puppies and kittens in a warm area until they are dry.

Antifungal creams and lotions are available for spot treatment of localized lesions. These should be applied twice daily to an area extending 2½ inches past the edges of lesions.

Topical Antifungal Agents

Lotions or Creams	Whole-Body Rinses	Shampoos
Amphotericin B lotion/cream (Fungazone)	Acetic acid (vinegar)	Chlorhexidine (ChlorhexiDerm, Hexadene, Nolvasan)
Chlorhexidine spray, cream (Nolvasan, ChlorhexiDerm)	Acetic acid + boric acid (Malacetic)	Chlorhexidine + sulfur (SebaHex)
Chlorhexidine + miconazole spray (Malaseb)	Chlorhexidine + miconazole (Malaseb Rinse Kit)	Ketoconazole (Nizoral)
Clotrimazole cream, lotion	Enilconazole (Imaverol)	Ketoconazole + chlorhexidine (Ketochlor)
Clotrimazole + gentamicin + betamethasone (Otomax)	Lime-sulfur (LymDyp)	Miconazole (Miconazole, Dermazole)
Miconazole cream, lotion, spray (Conofite)	Dilute sodium hypochlorite (diluted bleach)	Selenium sulfide (Head & Shoulders Intensive Treatment, Selsun Blue)
Nystatin cream, gel		
Nystatin + polymyxin B + neomycin + triamcinolone cream, ointment (Panolog, Animax)		Sulfur + benzoyl peroxide (SulfOxyDex)
Terbinafine cream (Lamisil)		
Thiabendazole + neomycin + dexamethasone (Tresaderm)		

Antifungal shampoos are of minimal benefit because they have little residual activity, and the process of lathering the pet may actually spread the infection. Normal **sebum** (body oil) provides some antifungal protection to the skin; bathing a pet removes these protective lipids.

Several topical agents have been shown to be ineffective in treating ringworm in dogs and cats. These include solutions of dilute chlorhexidine, iodine, and captan.

Systemic antifungal treatment generally is required to cure ringworm in long-haired cats and dogs, those with severe disease, and those not cured of infection after several weeks of topical therapy (with medication applied directly to skin or hair). I recommend systemic antifungal therapy for all cats with *M. canis* infections and also for all dogs with *T. mentagrophytes* infections. There are several options for systemic therapy.

Griseofulvin has the longest history of use in veterinary medicine. It is highly effective in treating ringworm infections. Griseofulvin must not be used in pregnant females or breeding males because it is a teratogen (it causes birth defects). The most common side effect of griseofulvin is bone marrow suppression (a reduction in the production of red blood cells, white blood cells, and **platelets**). Cats infected with **feline immunodeficiency virus** are particularly susceptible to bone marrow suppression. Cats should be tested for this virus and also **feline leukemia virus** before griseofulvin is prescribed; an alternative drug should be used if the pet is infected with either virus. Griseofulvin also may cause liver damage and should not be used in pets that have liver disease. Other reported side effects include nausea, vomiting, diarrhea, **pruritus** (itching), and **neurological signs** (incoordination, depression). Griseofulvin is deposited in newly formed **keratin,** so only newly growing hairs and skin are free from the fungus. Treatment should be continued until a series of three toothbrush cultures of samples taken at 1-week intervals all show negative results in tests for fungal growth. The average length of treatment

Systemic Medications Used in Treating Fungal Infections

Medication	Indications for Use	Cautions
Amphotericin B	Blastomycosis, cryptococcosis, coccidioidomycosis, histoplasmosis, sporotrichosis, (also aspergillosis); NOT effective against dermatophytes	Highly toxic to the kidneys; usually given with intravenous fluids; kidney function is monitored
Griseofulvin	Dermatophyte infections (ringworm); NOT effective against other fungal infections or against yeast	Side effects include bone marrow suppression (especially in cats infected with FIV), vomiting and diarrhea, liver disease; teratogenic (causes birth defects), not used in pregnant pets; blood counts and liver enzymes are monitored
Iodides (sodium iodide and potassium iodide)	Sporotrichosis (may be drug of choice for this disease)	Signs of iodide toxicity include sweating, rapid heart rate, dry scaly coat, diarrhea, drooling, increased thirst and urination; side effects are most common in cats

Systemic Medications Used in Treating Fungal Infections—cont'd

Medication	Indications for Use	Cautions
Itraconazole	Dermatophytoses, blastomycosis, cryptococcosis, histoplasmosis, sporotrichosis, coccidioidomycosis (not always effective), pythiosis (use in combination with terbinafine), *Malassezia* infections	May cause liver enzyme elevations, poor appetite, vomiting; liver enzymes are monitored; vasculitis, a rare side effect, may result in areas of skin necrosis and ulceration
Ketoconazole	Dermatophytes, blastomycosis (use in combination with amphotericin B), cryptococcosis, sporotrichosis, *Malassezia* infections	Must be given with food; may alter metabolism of other drugs; side effects include poor appetite, vomiting, liver damage, lightening of coat color, behavioral changes, itching, teratogenicity/infertility; liver enzymes are monitored
Lufenuron	Chitin inhibitor; effective in inhibiting flea development; minimal effect on dermatophytes	Do not depend on this drug to treat fungal infections in dogs and cats
Terbinafine	*Malassezia* infections, pythiosis, sporotrichosis, dermatophytoses	Expensive

for skin and hair infections is 12 weeks. Nail infections may require 6 to 12 months of griseofulvin treatment. Absorption of griseofulvin is enhanced when it is given with a fatty meal—so adding butter to the food given with the griseofulvin pill is often recommended.

Ketoconazole is an antifungal drug frequently used for treating ringworm infections in dogs. Ketoconazole is best absorbed when given with a meal. Absorption requires the presence of stomach acid—so antacids should NOT be given to pets being treated with ketoconazole. Side effects may include **anorexia** (appetite loss), vomiting, increased liver enzymes, lightening of the hair coat color, and decreased metabolism of other drugs. Side effects are observed in approximately 10% of treated dogs and 25% of treated cats. Because of a higher risk of side effects, this drug is rarely used in cats. Ketoconazole is embryotoxic (it can harm the growth or development of an embryo) and teratogenic (it causes birth defects) and should not be used in pregnant females or breeding males. It also may decrease the production of **cortisol** and sex hormones (resulting in infertility). Treatment with ketoconazole should be continued until three consecutive fungal cultures have shown negative results. The average duration of treatment for skin and hair dermatophyte infections is 10 to 12 weeks.

Itraconazole is commonly used for treating ringworm infections, especially in cats, because of its excellent effectiveness and low incidence of side effects. It is more expensive than griseofulvin or ketoconazole. Although it occasionally causes anorexia, vomiting, and increased liver enzymes, these side effects are rare. Another rare side effect in dogs is skin **necrosis** (death of skin cells) resulting from drug-induced damage to blood vessels (**vasculitis**). Itraconazole reaches high concentrations in keratinized tissues, so it remains very effective against fungal growth for days to weeks after it is given. Several protocols have been employed successfully to treat ring-worm infections of dogs and cats. Some protocols use "pulse dosing" in which itraconazole is given 2 days per week, or alternating 7 days on and 7 days off, or alternating 15 days on and 15 days off. Treatment should be continued until negative results on three consecutive fungal cultures have been obtained.

Terbinafine is another systemic antifungal drug that is useful in treating ringworm infections. It is well tolerated by dogs and cats but is expensive. As with the other systemic antifungal drugs, treatment with terbinafine should be continued until negative results on three consecutive fungal cultures have been obtained.

Lufenuron is a chitin inhibitor developed as a flea preventive (**chitin** is a protein that is part of the outer covering of insects). Chitin also is found in fungal cell walls. It has been proposed that monthly or biweekly administration of lufenuron may be an effective treatment for ringworm infections. Unfortunately, scientific studies in the United States have failed to demonstrate any effectiveness of lufenuron in preventing or hastening the cure of ringworm infections in cats. Lufenuron is a good flea preventive and is safe to use in pets with ringworm—but it won't cure the disease.

A commercial vaccine against *M. canis* was previously available for use in cats. Unfortunately, scientific studies failed to demonstrate a protective effect from the vaccine or to confirm a more rapid cure in vaccinated cats. The only benefit noted in vaccinated cats was a slight improvement in affected skin. Because of its low effectiveness, the use of *M. canis* vaccine is not recommended.

Prevention

The key to preventing *M. canis* infections is to protect pets from exposure to infected hairs. The most common source of infection is a carrier cat. When a pet or human is diagnosed with *M. canis* infection, all cats that have had contact with that person or pet should be screened for infection using the McKenzie toothbrush technique (the entire coat is brushed with a sterile toothbrush to collect organisms, and samples from the brush are cultured). Cats with a positive dermatophyte culture result should receive a systemic antifungal medication and topical antifungal rinses until three subsequent culture results are negative. Aggressive environmental treatment is necessary to remove infected hairs. In a cattery, all new cats and all cats returning from a cat show or breeding should be tested for infection using the McKenzie toothbrush technique and isolated until the results are known.

M. gypseum is a soil-borne dermatophyte. Prevention of infection requires restricting access to areas where the organism is found. Dogs and cats should be discouraged from digging in soil rich in organic material. If kenneled dogs become infected with *M. gypseum*, dirt runs should be covered with a stone and gravel base or a concrete surface that can be disinfected regularly.

T. mentagrophytes usually is acquired from rodents or their burrows. Improved rodent control and preventing access to rodent burrows will help minimize the incidence of infection with this organism. Pet rodents in the house should be tested for ringworm and treated if infected.

Yeast Infection (*Malassezia* Infection)

Malassezia is a yeast organism commonly found as part of the normal **flora** (microorganism inhabitants) of the ear canal and skin of dogs and cats. There are several species of *Malassezia*. The most common one found on dogs and cats is *Malassezia pachydermatis* (formerly known as *Pityrosporum pachydermatis*). Seven strains of *M. pachydermatis* have been identified; these are named type Ia through type Ig. More than one species or strain may be found on an individual pet. Some strains require higher levels of lipids (oily substances) to support their growth; however, all are capable of causing disease. As with **staphylococci** and *Demodex*, small numbers of *Malassezia* organisms may be present on the skin without causing signs of disease. However, under favorable conditions for their growth, *Malassezia* organisms in the skin or ear canal may multiply and then produce enzymes that damage tissue, often causing severe **inflammation** (pain, swelling, redness, and heat). Additionally, **allergic reactions** to *Malassezia* are common. These allergic reactions may produce severe inflammation in the skin and ear canals.

Many factors can predispose a pet to overgrowth of these organisms and subsequent *Malassezia* dermatitis. (Ear diseases are discussed in Chapter 12.) It is important to identify and then eliminate these underlying factors, to prevent reoccurrence of *Malassezia* dermatitis. Predisposing factors may include:

- **Skin folds (these trap sebum and moisture)**
- **High humidity (infections are most common during the summer)**
- **Food allergies (skin inflammation favors growth of yeast)**
- **Atopy (skin inflammation; also, allergy to *Malassezia*)**
- **Immunodeficiency (especially IgA deficiency in dogs, feline immunodeficiency virus and feline leukemia virus infections in cats)**
- **Genetics (Basset Hounds, Beagles, Cocker Spaniels, English Setters, Dachshunds, Shih Tzus, and West Highland White Terriers have increased risk of infection)**
- **Hypothyroidism (abnormally low production of thyroid hormone) and other endocrine-related skin diseases (changes in skin lipids and impaired immune function)**
- **Keratinization defects and seborrhea (oily skin; yeasts proliferate when skin is oily)**
- **Staphylococcal pyoderma (skin infection) (staphylococci and yeast have a symbiotic relationship—infection with one favors the growth of the other organism)**

Clinical Signs and Symptoms

Malassezia dermatitis is a common problem in dogs. A majority of affected dogs suffer from severe pruritus (itching). Skin in areas of infection becomes thickened (**lichenification**) and erythematous (red), with areas of

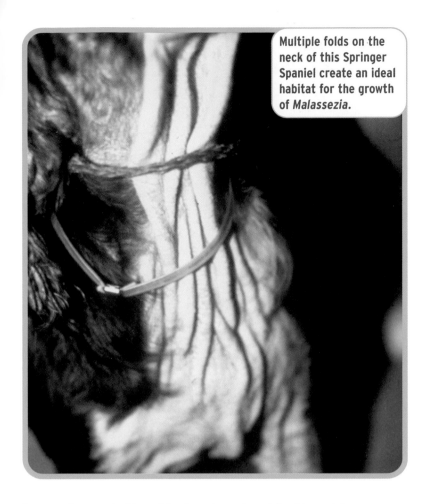

Multiple folds on the neck of this Springer Spaniel create an ideal habitat for the growth of *Malassezia*.

hyperpigmentation (dark-colored or black) and is greasy or waxy, scaly, and crusty. Affected dogs often have an offensive, rancid-fat odor. The bases of the nails may become reddish-brown, with a dark waxy **exudate** (fluid that has seeped from the skin) in the nailfold. The areas affected often include the axillae ("armpits"), **inguinal** region (groin), front of the neck, skin folds, ears, lips, muzzle, between the toes, and the skin around the anus. Some dogs have episodes of frantic clawing at their nose and lips. Those with ear disease often shake their head and scratch their ears.

Malassezia is an infrequent cause of skin and ear disease in cats. Yeast cells are present in some cats with feline acne (see "Chin Pyoderma" in Chapter 5), **otitis externa** (see Chapter 12), nailbed infections (**paronychia**), and seborrhea. Reoccurring, generalized *Malassezia* der-

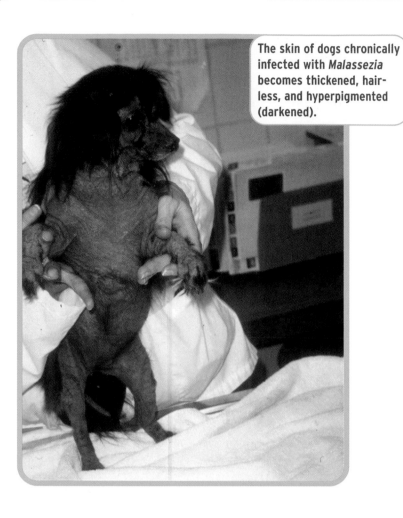

The skin of dogs chronically infected with *Malassezia* becomes thickened, hairless, and hyperpigmented (darkened).

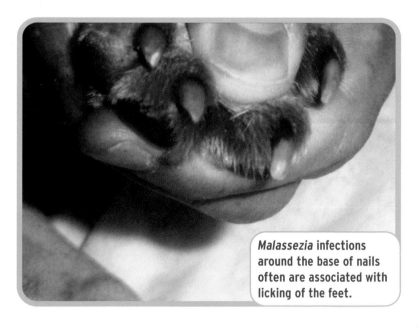

Malassezia infections around the base of nails often are associated with licking of the feet.

matitis may appear as an erythematous (red), crusty, and scaly skin disease. It has been reported occasionally in cats with feline immunodeficiency virus infections and those with certain internal malignancies (cancers involving the thymus and pancreas).

Malassezia dermatitis has been reported in low-birth-weight infants in an intensive care hospital unit. Infections in these infants were traced to the hands of workers who owned dogs and cats with *Malassezia* infections. So although *Malassezia* infection is not highly contagious, wash your hands thoroughly after handling an affected pet, to avoid transmitting the infection to anyone else.

Diagnosis

Malassezia infections should be suspected in pets that have red, scaly, bad-smelling skin or ears and those with chronic itching or thickened, hyperpigmented (darkened) skin. The most useful diagnostic tool is **cytology** (microscopic examination of cells). Swabs may be taken from affected areas and rolled on a glass slide, or a clear piece of tape may be pressed on the skin and transferred to a glass slide. The slide is then stained and examined under a microscope. *Malassezia* organisms appear as small budding yeast cells—resembling miniature snowmen or footprints. Yeast cells also may be found on skin biopsy samples and cultures. These tests are more expensive than direct cytology. Many allergy tests include *Malassezia* in the **allergens** (substances that cause allergic reactions) used to evaluate dogs and cats for the presence of allergen-specific **immunoglobulin E** (IgE) **antibodies** (see Chapter 4 for information on allergy testing). A good response to treatment will confirm the role of *Malassezia* in a pet's skin disease.

Because *Malassezia* dermatitis is almost always a secondary problem (occurring after or resulting from another illness), additional diagnostic testing is needed to identify the primary disease predisposing the pet to overgrowth of yeast. Depending on the pet's age and history and other clinical findings, tests for endocrine diseases, **allergies**, **immunodeficiency** (inability to fight infections), primary keratinization defects, nutritional imbalances, and other infections may be required to identify the primary cause of the skin disease.

Treatment

Focal lesions (limited to a particular area) of *Malassezia* infection may be present in feline acne and in skin fold pyoderma of dogs. These focal lesions can often be treated with topical antifungal therapy (administered directly to the affected area). **Astringent** wipes or pads containing acetic acid and boric acid (Malacetic Wipes) or miconazole and chlorhexidine (Malaseb Pledgets) may be used daily for cleaning these areas and often are effective in treating mild infections. More severe infections may require the use of creams or lotions containing miconazole or clotrimazole.

Mild cases of multifocal *Malassezia* dermatitis occasionally respond to topical antifungal therapy as the sole treatment. More severely affected pets commonly require systemic (taken internally) antifungal drugs but also benefit from topical therapy. The pet should be bathed in a degreasing shampoo to remove surface lipids, which serve as food sources for yeast. Benzoyl peroxide shampoos are excellent degreasers and also may suppress sebum production from **sebaceous** glands. The degreasing shampoo should be followed with an antifungal shampoo—for example, ones containing ketoconazole (dogs only), miconazole, chlorhexidine, and/or selenium sulfide (dogs only). Selenium sulfide has both degreasing and antifungal properties; however, it causes irritation in some dogs and is toxic to cats.

After the pet is bathed, a lotion or rinse containing miconazole and/or chlorhexidine may be applied for residual antifungal activity. Two topical products with excellent activity against *Malassezia* are lime-sulfur (2%) and enilconazole (0.2%) dips. Lime-sulfur has antipruritic, antifungal, antibacterial, and antiparasitic activity. It also emits a strong offensive odor, stains jewelry, stains bathtubs (stain may be removed with bleaching), and stains hair coats of white dogs yellow. Enilconazole is not licensed for use in the United States. Shampoos and applications of lotions or dips should be continued every 3 to 7 days until lesions have healed and follow-up skin cytology shows negative test results for yeast. Systemic treatment should be added if the yeast infection is severe or has not healed after a month of topical treatment.

Systemic treatment is recommended for all dogs with moderate to severe skin lesions as well as for those with milder lesions that do not heal with topical treatment alone. Itraconazole is my drug of choice for treating smaller dogs; it usually is given once daily until results on follow-up skin cytology are negative for yeast. By comparison, ketoconazole is less expensive and just as effective in treating *Malassezia* infections, but it has more frequent side effects—for example, poor appetite, vomiting, and liver damage. Blood tests should be taken before treatment with systemic antifungal medications is started, and blood tests should be repeated 2 to 4 weeks later to evaluate the pet for liver disease. Griseofulvin is ineffective against *Malassezia*. Terbinafine has been shown to be effective against yeast; however, it is expensive and is rarely used unless the pet can't tolerate either ketoconazole or itraconazole. Systemic antifungal therapy should be continued for at least 1 week after all lesions have resolved and no organisms are found during skin cytological examination.

Most dogs with *Malassezia* dermatitis also have staphylococcal pyoderma at the same time. So appropriate antibiotic therapy (see "Staphylococcal Pyoderma" in Chapter 5) also should be given until both infections are eliminated. Your veterinarian will search for underlying diseases that predispose the pet to infection, and appropriate corrective measures will be recommended to resolve those problems. The likelihood of recovery is good if underlying causes can be identified and corrected. When the underlying cause cannot be identified or corrected, regular use of antifungal shampoos and intermittent systemic antifungal therapy often are required to minimize lesions and keep the pet comfortable.

Subcutaneous and Systemic Fungal Infections

Subcutaneous mycoses are fungal infections with invasion into nonkeratinized tissues. These usually are acquired through penetrating injuries (plant awns or thorns, bite wounds, or other puncture wounds). Subcutaneous **mycoses** are rare infections that are started by traumatic implantation of a fungus from soil or plants into the pet's subcutaneous tissues. The most common subcutaneous mycosis in dogs and cats is sporotrichosis. *Sporothrix schenckii* infections result in the formation of nodules within the skin that ulcerate and drain a brownish red fluid. This **exudate** (discharge) may contain large numbers of infectious organisms and poses a health hazard to people. Gloves should always be worn by anyone handling a pet with sporotrichosis. Your veterinarian will make the diagnosis by finding the organisms on cytological examination of the fluid or with fungal cultures or skin biopsy of the lesions. Oral iodides are the traditional treatment of choice; in many pets, however, clinical signs of iodinism (excess iodine) develop, which may limit its use. Itraconazole also is effective in treating most pets with sporotrichosis. Treatment should be continued for a minimum of 1 month after all lesions have resolved.

Systemic mycoses are fungal infections that usually involve multiple body tissues. Organisms causing systemic mycoses are fungal organisms found in soil rich in organic material; some are associated with exposure to bat feces, and others with exposure to bird droppings. Most of these organisms are **endemic** in certain geographical areas (naturally occurring in those regions). Skin is one body tissue that can be affected by systemic mycoses; when affected, the skin provides a readily available source of material for cytology, culture, or biopsy to identify the organism causing disease in a patient. It is much easier to obtain samples from skin than from lungs, liver, or the gastrointestinal tract!

The four organisms involved in systemic mycoses are *Blastomyces dermatitidis*, *Histoplasma capsulatum*, *Cryptococcus neoformans*, and *Coccidioides immitis*. *Blastomyces dermatitidis* inhabits the moisture-rich acidic or sandy soils along the Missouri, Mississippi, Illinois, Tennessee, Ohio, and St. Lawrence rivers and also the southern Great Lakes region. Disease caused by *Blastomyces* is called blastomycosis and most commonly involves young, large-breed dogs. Hounds and dogs of sporting breeds allowed to run free outdoors have the highest risk of acquiring this infection. Blastomycosis is rare in cats and smaller breeds of dogs. The most common and severe form of blastomycosis is fungal pneumonia from infection of the lungs. Clinical signs include coughing, difficulty breathing, and tendency to tire quickly with exercise. Other organs frequently infected include the eyes (may result in inflammation, glaucoma, and blindness), bones (may result in lameness), lymph nodes, brain, and skin. Skin lesions usually are **nodules** (masses) that may develop **ulcers** and draining tracts with a **purulent** (pus-like) discharge. Your veterinarian can confirm the diagnosis by finding *Blastomyces* organisms in the discharge (they appear as thick-walled, budding yeast forms, 5 to 20 micrometers in diameter, on cytology) or tissue biopsies. Radiographs (x-ray films) of the dog's chest will show changes typical of a fungal pneumonia (changes in the lungs and enlargement of lymph nodes in the chest). Special blood tests can be performed to detect the presence of antibodies against *Blastomyces*. The drug of choice for treatment is itraconazole. Treatment should be continued for a minimum of 60 days and for at least 1 month after all signs of disease have disappeared. Keto-conazole may be used when itraconazole is deemed too expensive; however, it has a higher incidence of side effects, is less effective, and relapses are more common. In selected cases (usually those with severe pneumonia or when there is no improvement after treatment with itra-conazole), an intravenous form of the drug amphotericin B may be recommended. Amphotericin B is expensive and can cause irreversible kidney damage. The long-term out-look for dogs with systemic forms of blastomycoses is uncertain, because pneumonia or involvement of the brain may be fatal. In both dogs and cats, occasionally a local-ized, subcutaneous form of blastomycosis may develop after a penetrating injury to the skin (usually on a foot or leg). Localized cases have a good likelihood of recovery and can be treated with itraconazole or amputation. Amputation may be recommended if a localized infection

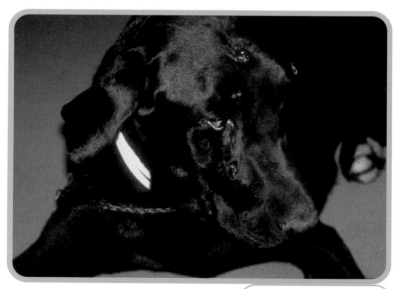

Nodular lesions on the head and face of this young Labrador Retriever were caused by *Blastomyces dermatitidis* infection.

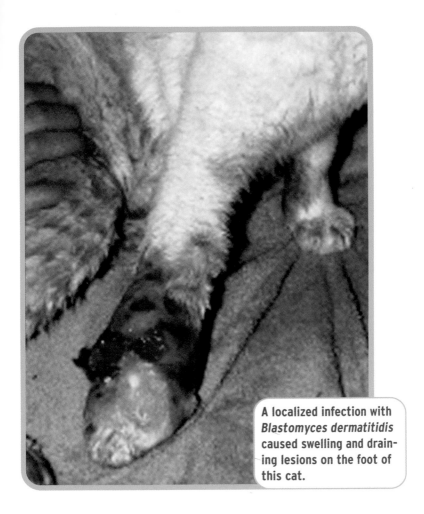

A localized infection with *Blastomyces dermatitidis* caused swelling and draining lesions on the foot of this cat.

involves the bone, because bone infections are much more difficult to treat than infections of other tissues.

Histoplasma capsulatum is a fungal organism that thrives in soil contaminated with bat feces or bird droppings. It is commonly found in chicken houses and under favorite bird roosting sites. *Histoplasma* is endemic in Midwestern and Southern states and is especially common along the Mississippi, Missouri, and Ohio rivers. Young to middle-aged dogs and young cats are at highest risk of infection. Pointers, Weimaraners, and Brittany Spaniels may be more likely to develop clinical signs of histoplasmosis. Infection may be acquired by ingestion (swallowing of contaminated material), resulting in signs involving mainly the gastrointestinal system (for example, poor appetite, vomiting, diarrhea, and weight loss) and liver (for example, jaundice–yellowed skin). Infection also may be acquired by inhalation, resulting in signs related to the respiratory system such as coughing, dyspnea (difficulty breathing), and exercise intolerance. Infection may spread from the respiratory or gastrointestinal systems to involve the lymph nodes, eyes, bone marrow, bones, and skin. Skin lesions usually appear as multiple small nodules that may open (ulcerate) and drain pus. Diagnosis is made by finding the organisms inside **white blood cells** (where they are seen as yeast forms 2 to 4 micrometers in diameter) on cytology or biopsies. Radiographs (x-ray films) show a fungal pneumonia in pets with the respiratory form of the disease. Special blood tests can be used to detect the presence of antibodies against *Histoplasma*. Itraconazole is the drug of choice for most cases, although intravenous amphotericin B may be recommended for dogs with severe gastrointestinal disease, which are unable to absorb oral medications. Treatment with itraconazole should be continued for at least 1 month after the pet seems fully recovered.

Cryptococcus neoformans is found in pigeon droppings and contaminated soil. It rarely causes disease in dogs but is the most common systemic mycosis (fungus-caused disease) in cats. Siamese cats may be predisposed to infection with *Cryptococcus*. **Immunosuppression**, including that due to feline immunodeficiency virus and leukemia virus infections, causes cats to be at increased risk and to develop more severe forms of the disease. The skin form of cryptococcosis is common. Skin lesions usually are in the form of **papules** and nodules on the face, ears (**pinnae**), and legs. Nodules often open (ulcerate) and drain pus. The nose also is frequently involved. Clinical signs of nasal infection include sneezing, nasal discharge, and in some cases, a **polyp**-like mass visible inside or protruding from the nostrils. Nodules also may be found inside the cat's mouth and on its lips, gums, tongue, and palate. Lymph nodes often are enlarged and may rupture and drain pus. Infection may spread to involve the eyes, causing blindness, and to the brain, causing seizures, weakness, incoordination, and eventually death. Cryptococcosis only rarely develops in dogs. Disease in dogs may involve the nasal cavity, eyes, or skin and also may spread to the brain. To diagnose *Cryptococcus* in both dogs and cats, your veterinarian will look for numerous thin-walled yeast cells, 2 to 20 micrometers in diameter, surrounded by a thick capsule in **impression smears**, **fine-needle aspirates**, or biopsies of the lesions. Buds of *Cryptococcus* yeast have a narrow base, which helps distinguish them from the broad-based buds of *Blastomyces*. Specialized blood tests can be used to detect cryptococcal capsular **antigens**. Infected cats also should be tested for feline immunodeficiency and leukemia virus infections. The drug of choice for treatment is itraconazole. Relapses are common, so treatment should continue for 2 months after clinical signs have cleared up and results of cryptococcal capsular antigen tests are negative. These tests should be monitored for another 6 months for early detection of relapses.

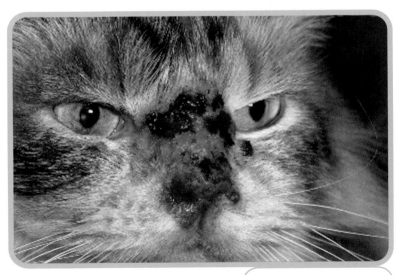

Skin lesions caused by *Cryptococcus neoformans* infection involving the nose and face of a cat.

Coccidioides immitis is a fungus found in the sandy, alkaline, semi-arid soil of deserts of the Southwestern United States, Mexico, and South America. Coccidioidomycosis also is known as Valley fever. Young male dogs are most likely to be infected. Boxers and Doberman Pinschers have an increased incidence of multiorgan disease. Dust storms, earthquakes, and digging in the soil spread the fungal spores. Clinical signs of coccidiomycosis may include:

- **Fever**
- **Coughing**
- **Dyspnea (difficulty breathing)**
- **Bone swelling**
- **Joint enlargement**
- **Lameness**
- **Weakness**
- **Back and neck pain**
- **Seizures**
- **Eye inflammation**
- **Enlarged lymph nodes**
- **Skin nodules (masses) that open and drain pus**

Diagnosis is made by finding large spherules characteristic of *C. immitis* on impression smears, in fine needle aspirates, or in biopsy material from of lesions. Specialized blood tests can be used to measure antibody titers to *C. immitis*. Radiographs (x-ray films) may show a fungal pneumonia and bone lesions. Coccidioidomycosis is the slowest of all the mycoses to respond to treatment, and the chance for recovery is fair to poor. Long-term therapy (minimum of 1 year) with oral itraconazole is the treatment of choice. Treatment should be continued until follow-up antibody titers for *C. immitis* are negative. Alternative antifungal drugs that may be used include ketoconazole, fluconazole, and amphotericin B.

Fungal-Like Infections: *Pythium* and *Lagenidium* Infections

Pythium insidiosum and *Lagenidium* species are fungus-like organisms classified as oomycetes. These organisms are found in water in the southeastern United States. Organisms are most common in swamps but also may be found in wetlands and ponds. Disease caused by these organisms has been referred to as "swamp cancer," "Florida leeches," and "canker." Oomycete infections are endemic (occur naturally) in states that border the Gulf of Mexico. These infections have been reported also in Indiana, Illinois, Kentucky, Tennessee, Missouri, Arizona, and Texas. Young male German Shepherd dogs and retriever-type dogs have the highest incidence of pythiosis. Lagenidiosis has been reported in young to middle-aged dogs, and no particular breed seems more likely to become infected.

Pythiosis may involve the gastrointestinal tract or skin. Skin lesions in pythiosis often begin as papules that develop into hemorrhagic **bullae** (blood blisters) and nodules that ulcerate and drain a purulent fluid (pus). These lesions usually begin on a leg or the tail and spread rapidly. The area often is pruritic (itchy), and the dog may mutilate the area with intense licking and chewing. Cats are sometimes affected with pythiosis; subcutaneous masses may develop on the base of the tail, in the groin, or around the eyes.

Lagenidiosis results in skin lesions similar to those associated with pythiosis. Lagenidiosis may spread to involve the lungs and other internal organs. Diagnosis may be based on history, clinical signs, and finding broad, irregularly branching hyphae (thread-like filaments) in skin biopsy samples.

Confirmation of the specific organism involved may be based on culture (a special culture medium is required) or specialized testing to detect the antigens of *Pythium* and *Lagenidium* in biopsy samples. Specialized blood tests also can be used to detect antibodies to *Pythium insidiosum*.

The treatment of choice for cutaneous forms of pythiosis and lagenidiosis is surgical removal of the affected tissue and a wide surrounding area (this usually requires limb or tail amputation) followed by the combination of

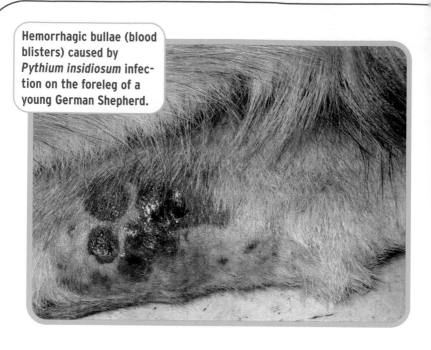

Hemorrhagic bullae (blood blisters) caused by *Pythium insidiosum* infection on the foreleg of a young German Shepherd.

itraconazole and terbinafine for a minimum of 2 months. Horses and cows also can be infected with these organisms. A vaccine for *Pythium* has shown promise in horses but to date has been ineffective in dogs. Chance of recovery is good with early surgery for pythiosis, but recovery is less certain in lagenidiosis or in pythiosis that has become widespread or involves lesions that cannot be surgically removed. Pets should be kept away from water sources known to harbor these organisms.

Summary

Fungal organisms are ubiquitous in the environment. Fortunately, only a few species produce disease in cats and dogs. Perhaps because of its constant exposure to the environment, the skin is the organ with the greatest risk of infection by fungal organisms. Treatment often is expensive and must be continued for long periods of time to prevent relapses. It is important to know and understand the factors that increase the risk of becoming infected by fungi and to minimize the exposure of pets to areas where the different infectious fungi are found.

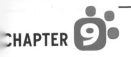

IMMUNE-MEDIATED SKIN DISEASES

Certain diseases develop when the body makes **antibodies** or cell-destroying **lymphocytes** against itself. These diseases are disorders of the body's immune system and are known as immune-mediated diseases. The normal role of the immune system is to tell "self" from "nonself" and then to destroy any "nonself" particles (known as **antigens**) that enter the body. "Self" includes everything in the body that is supposed to be there; "nonself" is everything else. When the immune system thinks certain components of the body do not belong to "self" and instead considers them foreign, it attacks and destroys them. The immune system's destruction of body components causes various problems, depending on which body system is affected. Antibodies against body components belonging to "self" are called **autoantibodies.**

The skin and **adnexa**—the hair, the nails, and the oil glands of the skin (also known as **sebaceous** glands)—often are affected in immune-mediated diseases. Parts of the skin that are targeted for the type of immune-mediated destruction just described include proteins found on cell membranes and skin pigment (**melanin**). Antigens associated with blood vessels and fat under the skin are sometimes the targets of immune-mediated disease as well.

The clinical signs of immune-mediated skin disease vary according to which part of the skin is being attacked. Most of these diseases are identified by certain characteristics found in skin biopsy specimens. Blood tests also are available to help diagnose some immune-mediated diseases.

257

Pemphigus Complex

The **pemphigus** complex is a group of diseases characterized by blisters, pustules, and crusts on the skin and includes six distinct diseases: pemphigus foliaceus, pemphigus erythematosus, pemphigus vulgaris, pemphigus vegetans, paraneoplastic pemphigus, and canine benign familial chronic pemphigus. These diseases occur in your pet when antibodies are produced against specific antigens on the cells in the skin's outer layer; these cells are called **keratinocytes**. Structures that attach keratinocytes to each other are damaged, and this results in blisters (**vesicles**) and raised, pus-filled bumps (**pustules**) in the epidermis (the skin's outer layer). The destruction of the attachments between cells is called **acantholysis** and results in the separation of the epidermal cells. When this happens, blisters form containing fluid and free-floating, detached epidermal cells. These free-floating cells are called **acantholytic keratinocytes**. **Neutrophils** (white blood cells) are attracted to the blisters; when these cells arrive, the blisters turn into pustules containing the acantholytic keratinocytes. The types of pemphigus differ in the location of these blisters and pustules on the body and also in which layer of the skin they are found (superficial, middle, or deep). For example, blisters form in the superficial epidermal layers in pemphigus foliaceus and deep in the epidermis in pemphigus vulgaris.

Pemphigus Foliaceus

Pemphigus foliaceus is the most common form of pemphigus in dogs and cats. The owner of a dog with this disease usually first sees pustules, crusts, and hair loss over the bridge of the dog's nose and around the eyes. The dog's ears often become involved; when this happens, inflammation of the ear and outer ear canal (**otitis externa**) develops—accompanied by pus (**purulent** discharge) or sores (**ulcers**). The footpads may become thickened and cracked. The disease spreads to other areas of the body.

In cats, the nailbed often is affected; this results in **paronychia** (pus at the base of the claws). The skin around the nipples also may be affected.

Pemphigus foliaceus is most common in middle-aged dogs and cats, but it may develop at any age. Akitas, Chow Chows , Dachshunds, Newfoundlands, Doberman Pinschers, and Labrador Retrievers are affected more often than dogs of other breeds. The disease may develop on its own, but it also may be triggered by drugs (especially certain antibiotics), infections (viral or fungal), or long-term skin diseases.

Pemphigus foliaceus looks a lot like some other diseases. Recurrent bacterial **pyoderma**, **dermatophytosis**

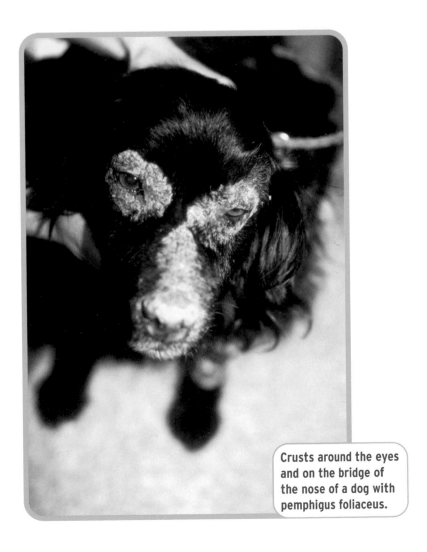

Crusts around the eyes and on the bridge of the nose of a dog with pemphigus foliaceus.

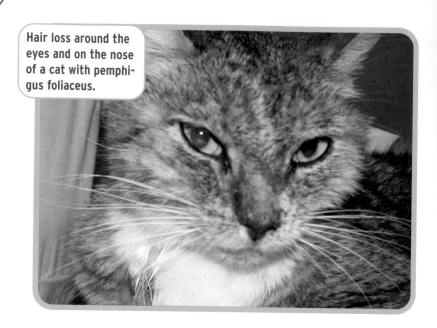

Hair loss around the eyes and on the nose of a cat with pemphigus foliaceus.

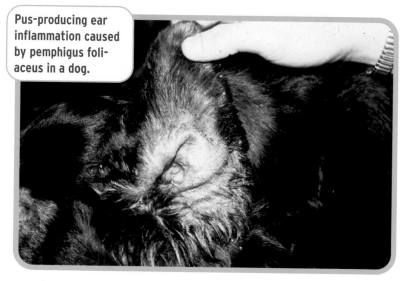

Pus-producing ear inflammation caused by pemphigus foliaceus in a dog.

(ringworm), **demodicosis** (a type of mange), **seborrhea** (scaly skin disease), **zinc-responsive dermatosis** (discussed in Chapter 10 under "Zinc-Responsive Dermatoses"), adverse drug reactions, and other immune-mediated skin diseases all must be ruled out before your veterinarian will be able to diagnose pemphigus foliaceus. The vet will usually base the diagnosis on the findings on skin biopsy and other tests examining the cells of the skin.

How your veterinarian chooses to treat your pet's pemphigus foliaceus will depend on how severe the disease is.

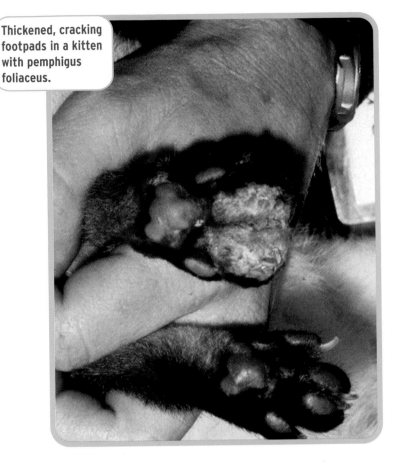

Thickened, cracking footpads in a kitten with pemphigus foliaceus.

The disease often is accompanied by bacterial skin or ear infections, which should be treated with antibiotics (your veterinarian will be careful in selecting an antibiotic, because some antibiotics are suspected of causing pemphigus) and **topical** therapy (bathing to remove crusts and scales and help control the infection). Mild or isolated **lesions** may be treated with topical **corticosteroids** or tacrolimus applied directly to the skin. Mild pemphigus foliaceus may also respond to a combination of tetracycline and niacinamide. Most cases of pemphigus foliaceus require oral immunosuppressive therapy (see under "Medications for Immune-Mediated Diseases," page 279). Once the disease is in remission, the medications are slowly tapered until the lowest dose required to prevent a relapse is found. Most animals with pemphigus will require lifelong immunosuppressive therapy, but a few are able to stop treatment after months or years.

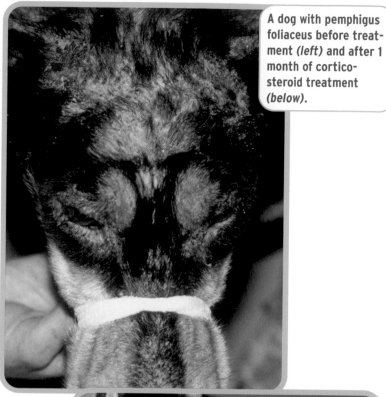

A dog with pemphigus foliaceus before treatment *(left)* and after 1 month of corticosteroid treatment *(below)*.

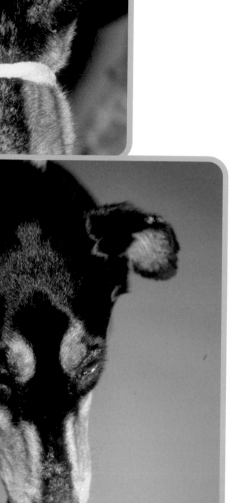

Pemphigus Erythematosus

Pemphigus erythematosus shares many features with pemphigus foliaceus and a few with discoid lupus erythematosus (discussed later in the chapter). Lesions, which usually are found only on the head, include pustules, scales, and crusts on the nose, the skin around the eyes, and the external part of the ear (**pinna**). The nose often loses its color (depigmentation), and the normal "cobblestone" appearance may be lost as well. German Shepherd dogs and Collies seem to be more likely to get pemphigus erythematosus, and sun exposure makes the lesions worse.

Your veterinarian will diagnose pemphigus erythematosus by first ruling out other possible causes of the lesions—bacterial pyoderma, **ringworm**, demodicosis, **dermatomyositis**, **discoid lupus erythematosus**, drug reactions, and zinc-responsive dermatosis.

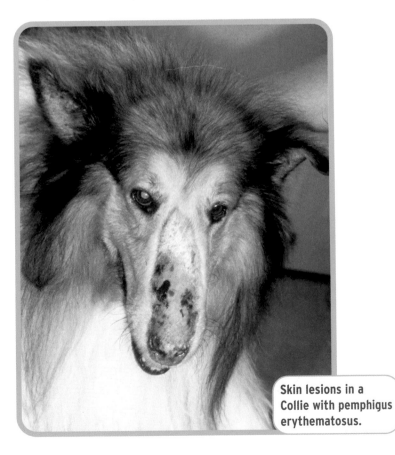

Skin lesions in a Collie with pemphigus erythematosus.

Pemphigus erythematosus usually covers less of the body and is less severe than other immune-mediated diseases, so only local therapy may be required. **Ultraviolet radiation** makes the lesions worse, so it's important to protect your pet from sunlight (keep the pet indoors and use goggles and sunscreens). Topical corticosteroids or tacrolimus may be used for spot treatment of lesions. Severe cases may be treated with tetracycline and niacinamide or with oral corticosteroids. Vitamin E also may help ease the skin inflammation associated with pemphigus erythematosus. Affected dogs generally require treatment for the remainder of their lives.

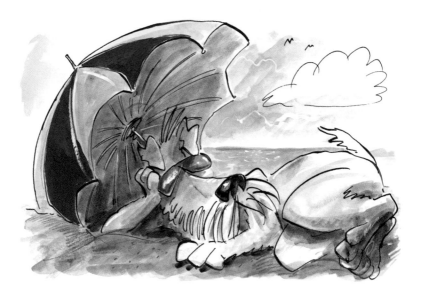

Pemphigus Vulgaris

Self-destructive antibodies (autoantibodies) in pemphigus vulgaris target the **intercellular adhesion molecules** located above the **stratum basale** (the deepest layer of the epidermis) (see "Structure of the Skin" in Chapter 1). Lesions often are found in areas where mucous membranes meet the skin—inside the mouth and on the eyelids, anus, prepuce (penile sheath), and vulva. Lesions also are found in the ears and around the base of the nails. Skin lesions may spread to the axillae ("armpits") and groin. They often appear as pustules or vesicles that

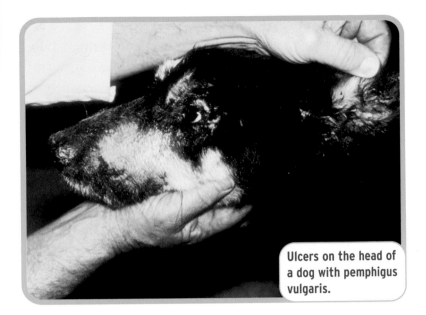

Ulcers on the head of a dog with pemphigus vulgaris.

rupture, leaving sores. Lesions on haired skin become crusted, and bacterial infection is common.

Your veterinarian will diagnose pemphigus vulgaris first by ruling out other diseases and then by finding characteristic changes in skin biopsy specimens.

Pemphigus vulgaris is the worst of the pemphigus diseases. Sores in the mouth may be so painful that the pet will not eat. Skin infections are common and may be severe. Untreated, pemphigus vulgaris usually is fatal. Because it is such a serious disease, pemphigus vulgaris typically is treated aggressively with oral immunosuppressive therapy (see under "Medications for Immune-Mediated Diseases," page 279). Skin infections should be treated with oral antibiotics and **antiseptic** shampoos or rinses. The prognosis for pets affected with pemphigus vulgaris is fair. Most will respond favorably to treatment, but few are cured. So life-long therapy usually will be needed to prevent new lesions from developing.

Paraneoplastic Pemphigus

Paraneoplastic pemphigus develops when antigens produced by cancer cells are similar to antigens found in the skin. Anticancer antibodies then attack both skin and cancer cells. Pemphigus in dogs has been reported to occur when antibodies cross-react between keratinocytes and a variety of cancers. **Immunosuppression** to decrease antibody formation may cause the cancer to spread, so the outlook for a pet with paraneoplastic pemphigus is poor unless the cancer can be cured (through surgical removal, for example).

Lupus Complex

Lupus was first recognized in people in the 13th century. The term *lupus* means "wolf" and was used to describe the wolflike facial appearance due to the coarsening of features and inflammation of the skin seen in affected people. A typical finding is a facial rash called a "butterfly rash" because of its general shape in the center of the face–around both eyes, down the nose, and around the lips. A variety of antigens and tissues may be targeted by antibodies in the lupus diseases (the lupus complex), including red blood cells, **platelets**, **leukocytes**, and skin cells, as well as the pancreas, **adrenal gland**, muscles, joints, nerves, and thyroid gland. Lupus has been called the "great imitator" because it can involve many different tissues and show a variety of clinical signs.

Skin lesions in lupus are made worse by sun exposure. Features of lupus in skin biopsy specimens include premature death (**apoptosis**) of keratinocytes and the presence of lymphocytes and **plasma cells** along the dermal-epidermal border within the skin (referred to as a **lupus band** of cells).

Discoid Lupus Erythematosus

Discoid lupus erythematosus is a common cause of loss of nasal pigmentation in dogs. It is rare in cats. Signs include depigmentation, scaling, crusting, erosion, and ulceration of the nose, which loses its normal "cobblestone" appearance. Sometimes ulcers develop inside the nose, damaging blood vessels and resulting in nosebleeds. The lesions may spread to the bridge of the nose and the lips.

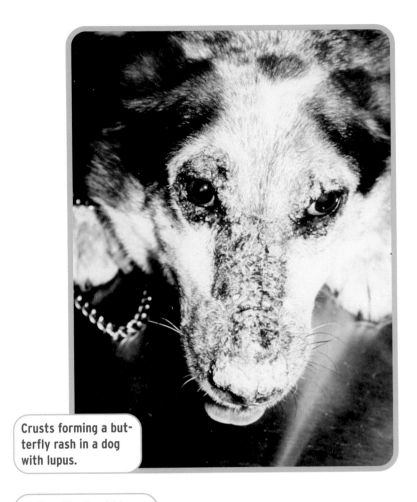

Crusts forming a butterfly rash in a dog with lupus.

Collie with discoid lupus erythematosus. Note the depigmentation and ulceration of the nose.

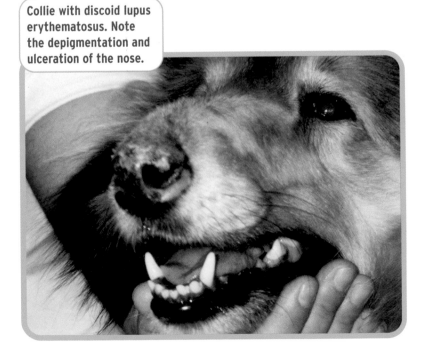

Several breeds are at greater risk of developing discoid lupus erythematosus, including Collies, Shetland Sheepdogs, German Shepherd Dogs, Siberian Huskies, Brittany Spaniels, and German Shorthaired Pointers. Sunlight makes the lesions worse, so the disease is at its worst during the summer months.

In mild cases, avoiding sun exposure and applying topical corticosteroids or tacrolimus may be enough to control the disease. Some dogs have shown improvement when given omega-3 fatty acids; others have gotten relief with oral vitamin E (400 to 800 IU/day). Another alternative is to give a combination of oral tetracycline and niacinamide, which has been reported to be effective in as many as 70% of cases. Dogs with severe lesions and those with frequent nosebleeds may require treatment with **systemic** corticosteroids or other immunosuppressive drugs (see under "Medications for Immune-Mediated Diseases," page 279). Lesion severity may wax and wane, but most affected pets will require lifelong therapy to prevent new lesions from developing.

Systemic Lupus Erythematosus

Systemic lupus erythematosus (SLE) is a multisystem disease in which the body makes antibodies against a variety of its own components. The signs vary according to which body system or systems are affected in a particular dog or cat, but they include redness and inflammation of the skin and scaling, crusting, ulceration, and scarring of the face, ears, feet, and legs. Mouth ulcers may cause the dog or cat to stop eating, or they may become infected, resulting in bad breath. Other signs include chronic fever, stiff gait or limping, arthritis with joint swelling, anemia and weakness, bleeding disorders, kidney failure, behavior problems, neurological problems, and even heart failure.

Diseases that appear similar to SLE include infections, cancer, drug reactions, and other immune-mediated diseases. Your veterinarian will make a diagnosis by finding at least two of the signs listed in the accompanying box, ruling out other causes, and seeing test results that support the diagnosis. Blood tests may reveal anemia or low numbers of platelets. Analysis of your pet's urine (urinalysis) may show that protein is being lost in the urine because of kidney damage. Two tests that are used to further support a diagnosis of SLE are the antinuclear antibody test and the lupus erythematosus cell test. These tests reveal the presence of certain autoantibodies that are often found in SLE. Skin biopsies often show the presence of a lupus band (plasma cells and lymphocytes below the junction of the dermis and epidermis) and signs of breakdown in the cells of the lowest level of the epidermis (see "Structure of the Skin" in Chapter 1).

Clinical Signs of Systemic Lupus Erythematosus

- **Anemia (from immune-mediated destruction of red blood cells)**
- **Bleeding disorders (often from immune-mediated destruction of blood platelets)**
- **Fever**
- **Heart failure**
- **Kidney disease**
- **Enlarged lymph nodes**
- **Muscle pain (caused by inflammation)**
- **Nervous system disorders (incoordination, weakness or paralysis, seizures)**
- **Polyarthritis (lameness, swollen joints)**
- **Secondary infections (caused by immune dysfunction and destruction of white blood cells)**
- **Skin lesions (rashes, hair loss, scaling/ crusting, loss of skin pigment, ulcers)**

Antibiotic therapy helps control infections of the skin and bladder in a pet with SLE. Whole-body (systemic) corticosteroids usually are required to control the signs of SLE. Additional immunosuppressive drugs may be required in severe cases (see under "Medications for Immune-Mediated Diseases," page 279). Your veterinarian may also suggest using a shampoo to reduce scaling, as well as an antiseptic rinse to help prevent infection. The prognosis for pets affected with SLE varies depending on the body organs affected by the disease. Skin forms of SLE are not as severe as the forms affecting the blood cells and kidneys and generally respond favorably to treatment. Lifelong treatment usually is required to prevent reoccurrence of lesions.

Symmetric Lupoid Onychodystrophy

Symmetric lupoid onychodystrophy is a form of lupus that involves the cells from which the nails grow. Inflammation is concentrated at the base of the nails, resulting in swelling of the nailfold, pain, lameness, and separation of the nail from the underlying skin. Eventually the nails may fall out. Bacterial infections may develop under the nails, resulting in pus and a bad odor. Once a nail has fallen out, the new nail that grows in its place may be deformed, brittle, and dry.

Some breeds are at greater risk for development of symmetric lupoid onychodystrophy, including German Shepherds, Rottweilers, and Standard Schnauzers. Both male and female dogs are affected. Most dogs with this condition are 3 to 8 years old, although the age at onset ranges from just a few months to more than 10 years. To diagnose symmetric lupoid onychodystrophy, your veterinarian will have to rule out other immune-mediated diseases, **vasculitis** (inflammation of the blood vessels), drug reactions, cancers of the nail or bone, fungal infections, nutritional deficiencies, **metabolic epidermal necrosis** (skin death caused by a metabolic problem such

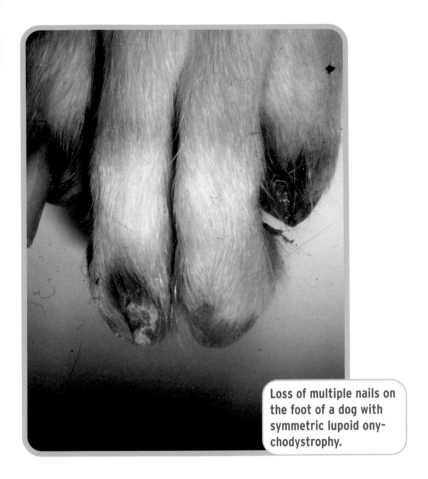

Loss of multiple nails on the foot of a dog with symmetric lupoid onychodystrophy.

as with liver disease or cancer), and trauma. The only way for the veterinarian to diagnose this condition beyond a doubt is to amputate an affected toe so that the nail cells can be examined under a microscope. Usually a dewclaw is taken for study because its removal won't affect how the dog walks or runs.

The first step in treatment is to remove all loose nails. Doing this will ease your pet's pain (a loose nail causes pain with each step the pet takes) and help lessen the risk of bacterial infection (organisms thrive under a loose nail). Your veterinarian will want to use a general anesthetic to prevent pain during nail removal and may prescribe pain relievers for several days after the surgery. Antiseptic foot soaks and antibiotics are helpful in treating bacterial infections of the nailbed. Omega-3 fatty acids help ease inflammation in many cases of symmetric lupoid onychodystrophy. Food allergies may be involved, so your vet may recommend a restrictive food trial, in which several foods are removed from your pet's diet to see whether the condition becomes less severe. If your pet does not improve with these treatments, the veterinarian may prescribe a combination of tetracycline and niacinamide to ease inflammation in the feet. Pentoxifylline also has been recommended to decrease inflammation and get more oxygen into the nailbed. Severe cases may require oral immunosuppressive treatment (see under "Medications for Immune-Mediated Diseases," page 279). Declawing (onychectomy) has been recommended for dogs with chronic foot pain that is difficult to control with medications.

Miscellaneous Immune-Mediated Skin Diseases

Several other immune-mediated skin diseases are occasionally found in dogs and cats. Once other diseases have been ruled out, diagnosis is based on skin biopsy.

Bullous Pemphigoid

In bullous pemphigoid, autoantibodies are produced against specific parts of the **basement membrane zone** ("BP antigens"). Antibody-mediated destruction of the basement membrane causes blisters that rupture, leaving sores. Commonly affected areas include junctions between mucous membranes and skin (around the lips, eyes, anus, vulva, and prepuce), footpads, and inside the mouth. The armpits, head, neck, and abdomen also may be affected. Disorders that resemble bullous pemphigoid and must be ruled out before it can be diagnosed include other immune-mediated skin diseases (especially SLE and pemphigus vulgaris), drug reactions, bacterial and fungal infections, metabolic epidermal necrosis, and certain can-

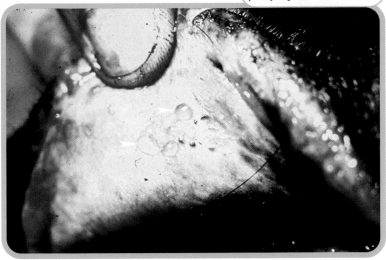

Vesicles on the upper lip of a dog with bullous pemphigoid.

cers. Once other diseases are ruled out, the veterinarian will look for subepidermal blisters on skin biopsy specimens to make the diagnosis. Acantholytic keratinocytes are not seen in bullous pemphigoid.

Your veterinarian will prescribe antiseptic shampoos and rinses, plus oral antibiotics to treat skin and mouth infections. Systemic corticosteroids are needed to control blister formation. Additional oral immunosuppressive drugs may be prescribed for cases that are difficult to control with corticosteroids alone (see under "Medications for Immune-Mediated Diseases," page 279). Tetracycline plus niacinamide may be useful in mild cases. A majority of pets diagnosed with bullous pemphigoid require lifelong treatment to prevent reoccurrence of lesions.

Immune-Mediated Vasculitis

Immune-mediated **vasculitis** usually results when antibodies and antigens combine to form **antibody-antigen complexes** (also known as **immune complexes**) that are deposited in small blood vessels. This can occur in SLE

273

and in some infections and cancers. One form of immune-mediated vasculitis that's becoming more and more common involves a reaction to killed rabies vaccine. Such reactions, which can take 3 to 6 months after vaccination to develop, are most common in Poodles, Maltese, and Yorkshire and Silky Terriers. The reaction starts with hair loss over the place where the vaccine was given. The skin becomes much darker once the hair has fallen out. Lesions may last months or even years. The veterinarian will make the diagnosis after learning that the affected dog has a history of receiving rabies vaccines and after observing deposits of vaccine, invasion of blood vessels by lymphocytes, and breakdown of hair follicles in skin biopsy specimens.

Immune-mediated vasculitis is a cosmetic disease. Topical tacrolimus or oral pentoxifylline may ease inflammation and encourage new hair to grow. The veterinarian will check the dog's antibodies to rabies and wait to give another vaccine until the antibody level (titer) has dropped below the protective level. (The vet may have to obtain approval from the city or county regulatory board to perform a rabies titer evaluation instead of the regular vaccination.)

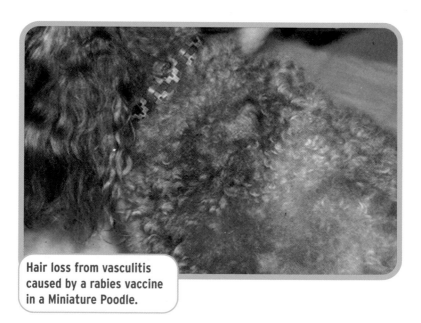

Hair loss from vasculitis caused by a rabies vaccine in a Miniature Poodle.

Plasma Cell Pododermatitis

Plasma cell pododermatitis is a disease of the footpads of cats. The exact cause is not known. Several footpads at a time usually are involved; they become soft, swollen, and "mushy." Sores may develop, causing bleeding from the footpads. These lesions often are painful, and a cat with this condition may be lame and try to avoid walking. Some cats also have plasma cell stomatitis (inflammation and ulceration inside the mouth), and a few have renal **amyloidosis** (presence of deposits of a starchlike protein in the kidneys). Diseases and lesions that resemble plasma cell pododermatitis include contact dermatitis (inflammation caused by contact with an irritant), trauma, bacterial or fungal infection of the feet, **eosinophilic granulomas** (knotty accumulations of immune cells and connective tissue) of the footpads, viral infections, metabolic epidermal necrosis, cancers, and other immune-mediated diseases such as pemphigus foliaceus or SLE. Biopsy of the footpads is required for diagnosis. Microscopic examination of the biopsy sample shows large numbers of **plasma cells** invading the feet. If the cat is not lame, a wait-and-see attitude may be appropri-

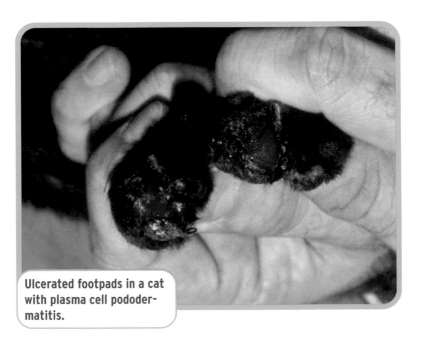

Ulcerated footpads in a cat with plasma cell pododermatitis.

ate because some lesions disappear on their own. Treatment with doxycycline is effective in some cases; others respond better to systemic glucocorticoids. Still other treatment alternatives are cyclosporine and topical tacrolimus. Any bacterial infection should be treated with topical or oral antibiotics.

Sterile Nodular Panniculitis

Panniculitis is an inflammation of the fat under the skin. Lesions appear as nodules beneath the skin. They usually start as firm swellings that become more fluid when enzymes released from inflammatory cells (**neutrophils** and **macrophages**) turn the fat to liquid. The nodules may rupture and discharge a yellowish, oily fluid. Lesions may occur anywhere on the body. Some affected dogs have a fever and poor appetite and are reluctant to move around when new lesions are developing. The lesions may wax and wane in severity.

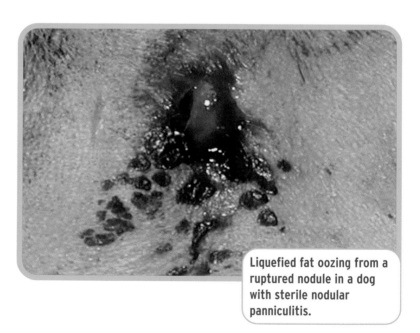

Liquefied fat oozing from a ruptured nodule in a dog with sterile nodular panniculitis.

Diseases that appear similar include infectious causes of panniculitis (bacteria and fungi), foreign bodies, vaccine reactions, SLE, other forms of sterile nodules, **hematomas** (pockets of blood under the skin), and various cancers. Diagnosis requires tissue biopsies (these must be deep enough to obtain subcutaneous fat). Samples should be submitted for evaluation of cells under a microscope and for cultures for microorganisms. Many treatments are effective, including high doses of vitamin E, a combination of tetracycline and niacinamide, pentoxifylline, oral corticosteroids, and other immunosuppressive drugs (azathioprine for dogs, chlorambucil for cats).

Uveodermatological Syndrome

Uveodermatological syndrome involves autoantibodies produced against **melanin** (the black pigment in the skin

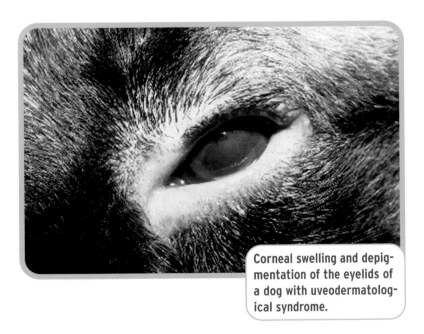

Corneal swelling and depigmentation of the eyelids of a dog with uveodermatological syndrome.

and hair). Melanin also is found in the uvea, the inner lining of the eyeball. Genetic factors may be involved; Akitas, Samoyeds, Siberian Huskies, Irish Setters, and Chow Chows are the breeds most commonly affected. Eye problems usually are noticed first; the animal may suddenly be sensitive to light and may have inflammation of the eyeball, cornea, and lining of the eyelids. Eye involvement can lead to blindness. Other clinical signs include loss of pigment in the eyelids, nose, and lips. Sores are sometimes seen. If the condition is not treated, depigmentation may eventually involve the scrotum or vulva, anus, footpads, and hard palate. In a few cases, generalized skin and haircoat depigmentation has been reported. Diseases that resemble uveodermatological syndrome include other immune-mediated diseases and other causes of uveitis. Skin biopsy specimens from depigmented areas contain a mixture of inflammatory cells below the border of the dermis and epidermis.

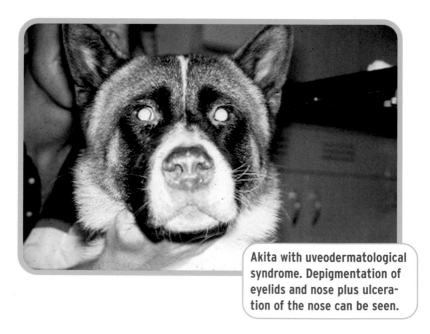

Akita with uveodermatological syndrome. Depigmentation of eyelids and nose plus ulceration of the nose can be seen.

Your vet will no doubt recommend early, aggressive treatment to prevent glaucoma and blindness. Corticosteroid eye drops are usually recommended, along with a **cycloplegic** solution to dilate the pupil and relieve pain. Immunosuppressive doses of oral corticosteroids are given until the inflammation has subsided; then the dose is slowly tapered. In some cases, treatment with azathioprine is required to get the disease into remission. The long-term prognosis is excellent when the disease is diagnosed and treated early.

Medications for Immune-Mediated Diseases

Drugs used to treat autoimmune skin diseases vary from **topical** drugs (medications applied directly to the skin) to powerful **systemic** immunosuppressants (usually given orally), depending on the severity of the disease. Topical treatments are used for milder diseases and include creams or ointments containing **corticosteroids** or tacrolimus. Corticosteroids have anti-inflammatory effects; high levels of corticosteroids are immunosuppressive. Tacrolimus is used for its immunosuppressive qualities. You should wash your hands after applying topical medications to your pet's skin, and you need to wear latex or vinyl gloves when applying tacrolimus, because it is a possible carcinogen.

Tetracycline is an antibiotic that also works to decrease inflammation in the skin. It is most effective when used in combination with niacinamide, a form of vitamin B$_3$. It is important to use niacinamide and not niacin, because high doses of niacin may cause cutaneous flushing. Tetracycline should not be used in dogs and cats younger than 6 months of age, as it may interfere with tooth enamel formation and cause discoloration of developing teeth. Niacinamide should not be used in dogs with a history of seizures or epilepsy. Doxycycline is an antibiotic that is closely related to tetracycline and often is used as a substitute for tetracycline in young dogs and cats.

Vitamin E is an antioxidant that stabilizes cell membranes and decreases inflammation in the skin. It often is prescribed as part of the treatment of discoid lupus erythematosus and panniculitis. Vitamin E also may be used in treating other immune-mediated diseases. Vitamin E is very safe, with no known side effects.

Pentoxifylline is an oral medication used to treat some autoimmune diseases that affect the blood vessels or that produce inflammation in the skin. Pentoxifylline improves blood flow to tissues and decreases the production of inflammatory chemicals in the skin. It is particularly useful in treating discoid lupus erythematosus and panniculitis.

More severe diseases require oral immunosuppressive therapy. **Corticosteroids** are used alone or in combination with one of three immunosuppressant agents: azathioprine (marketed as Imuran), chlorambucil (Leukeran), or cyclosporine (Cytoxan). High doses of corticosteroids can cause signs of **iatrogenic** (caused by a medical procedure or treatment) **Cushing's disease** (see "Hyperadrenocorticism [Cushing's Disease]" in Chapter 7), including panting, muscle weakness, abdominal bloating, thinning of the skin, hair loss, **steroid hepatopathy** (liver disease caused by the steroids), increased appetite, increased drinking and urination, and urinary tract infections. If side effects are severe or if the disease doesn't respond to corticosteroids, your veterinarian will add one of the other drugs, which will allow the dose of corticosteroids to be reduced. In dogs, the most commonly added drug is azathioprine. In cats, chlorambucil is used most often. If these drugs are not effective or if your pet can't tolerate them, cyclosporine may be used. Once the disease is in remission, the medications are slowly tapered until the lowest dose required to prevent a relapse is found. Treatment usually is necessary for a minimum of 6 months, and for some diseases, it may be lifelong.

During oral immunosuppressive treatment, your pet will need to be seen by your veterinarian regularly to monitor for side effects. Blood tests will be run to look for dangerous bone marrow suppression and other adverse effects. During treatment, your pet is more susceptible to infections; your veterinarian will run tests to monitor for infections, such as checking urine samples for signs of bladder infection. Rechecks may be needed every 2 to 4 weeks during the early months of treatment. After the disease is in remission, recheck appointments will be needed every 3 to 4 months.

Summary

Many skin diseases are caused by a dysfunction of the immune system in which autoantibodies attack parts of the skin and related structures such as the hair and nails, causing destructive inflammation. Diagnosis almost always requires skin biopsy and sometimes special tests. Treatment often requires large doses of steroids or other immunosuppressive drugs. Without treatment, many of these diseases can leave a pet susceptible to skin infections severe enough to cause death. You and your veterinarian must work together to find the lowest dosages that will keep the disease in remission, because side effects from these medications are common. Your veterinarian probably will continue therapy for many months after the disease appears to have disappeared, to help avoid relapses—in fact, treatment for many immune-mediated diseases must be continued for life.

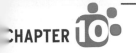

PEDIATRIC, CONGENITAL, AND HEREDITARY SKIN DISEASES

The skin is the second-largest organ of the body (after the skeleton) and makes up 25% of the weight of a newborn kitten or puppy; therefore it is not surprising that problems sometimes occur when the skin is developing. Pediatric skin diseases are those affecting young puppies and kittens. Pediatric diseases may be caused by genetic factors, an immature immune system, or external factors (e.g., nutrition, housing, parasites, toxins, infections). Congenital diseases are those affecting the pet at birth. Congenital diseases may be due to genetic factors or caused by nongenetic factors affecting the development of a fetus (e.g., drugs or toxins to which the mother was exposed during pregnancy). Hereditary disorders are those caused by genetic factors; the genes responsible for these disorders are passed on from one generation to the next. Knowing whether the cause of a disease is genetic or nongenetic is important because animals with genetic diseases should not be bred. Dogs have 39 pairs of chromosomes made up of genes for different traits, cats have 19 pairs, and humans have 23 pairs. One pair of chromosomes is involved in the determination of sex: the X and Y chromosomes (two X chromosomes in female subjects, one X and one Y chromosome in male subjects). The chromosomes that do not determine sex are referred to as *autosomes*. A trait is autosomal dominant if it appears in an individual having only one gene for that trait. A trait is autosomal recessive if it appears only in individuals having two genes for that trait. An animal exhibits an autosomal recessive trait only if it has inherited a gene for that trait from both of its parents.

Acanthosis Nigricans

Acanthosis nigricans appears as hyperpigmented (black), thickened skin in the **axillae** (armpits). The pet may appear to have chunks of tar stuck in its armpits. The lesions may spread to involve the forelegs, front of the neck, chest, abdomen, groin, **perineum** (the area between the anus and genitals), hocks, and also the skin around the eyes and on the ears. These skin abnormalities increase the likelihood that the animal will contract infections from bacteria and yeast (**Malassezia**). Acanthosis nigricans may be a hereditary disorder in Dachshunds. The hereditary form of acanthosis nigricans is called *primary acanthosis nigricans* to distinguish it from nonhereditary **secondary** forms (forms arising as a result of another condition) of acanthosis nigricans. Primary (hereditary) acanthosis nigricans develops in Dachshunds younger than 1 year of age. Early cases may not require treatment but should be watched for the development of secondary skin infections. If skin **cytology** shows the presence of bacteria or **yeast** organisms, your veterinarian will treat the infections with **topical** or **systemic** antibiotics and antifungal agents. As the lesions become worse, topical **antiseborrheic** shampoos and lotions may help. Vitamin E (200 IU twice daily) may help to decrease **inflammation** and thickening of the skin. Topical and systemic **corticosteroids** are useful in controlling signs in dogs with severe cases.

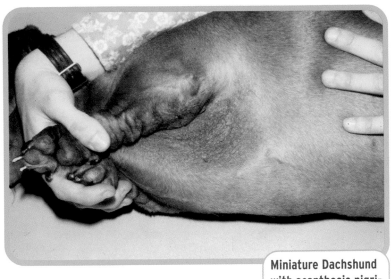

Most dogs with acanthosis nigricans have a nonhereditary disease that develops as a result of another condition. Hyperpigmentation of the armpits and skin thickening develop as a result of friction (e.g., skin folds, rubbing of leg against chest), scratching (e.g., from **atopy**, food allergies, contact **allergies**), **endocrine** diseases (e.g., from **hypothyroidism**, **Cushing's disease**), or **dermatitis** caused by yeast infection. For these dogs the underlying cause of the disease should be found and corrected if possible.

Acral Mutilation Syndrome

Acral mutilation syndrome is a hereditary disorder affecting German Shorthaired Pointers and English Pointers. Puppies suffering from this affliction are normal at birth, but at 3 to 5 months of age, they begin to chew their toes. This compulsion worsens to the point at which the puppies sometimes chew off their own feet. Acral mutilation syndrome is caused by a breakdown of sensory cells along the spinal cord. The puppies do not feel pain as a result of their self-mutilation and continue to walk on the stubs of their feet. Attempts to prevent further mutilation usually are unsuccessful because the puppies will chew through bandages and casts; euthanasia generally is considered to be the most humane option. Because acral mutilation syndrome is inherited as an autosomal recessive disorder, parents and siblings of affected dogs should not be used for breeding.

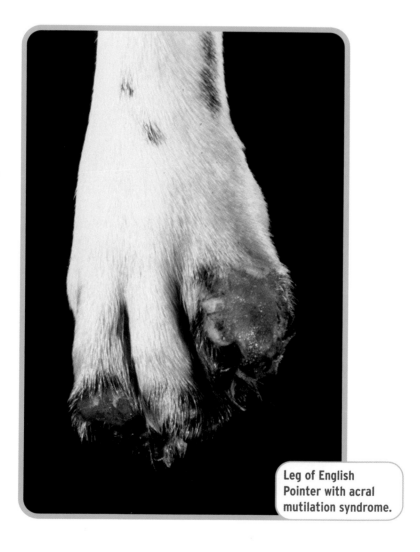

Leg of English Pointer with acral mutilation syndrome.

Color Mutant Alopecia and Black Hair Follicular Dysplasia

Also called color dilution **alopecia** or "blue Doberman syndrome," color mutant alopecia is a hereditary disorder affecting blue and fawn-colored dogs. Blue (grey) coat color is due to the clumping of black pigments within hair shafts. Fawn coat color is due to the clumping of brown pigments within hair shafts. This clumping of pigment granules weakens the hair shafts, causing early breakage and loss of hair. Affected dogs are at increased risk for bacterial skin infections, which increase hair loss. Antibiotics are useful in treating secondary bacterial infections. Moisturizing or **antiseptic** shampoos may be helpful in treating **seborrhea** caused by this condition. Affected dogs are otherwise healthy and will live healthy lives despite their sparse hair coat.

Black hair **follicular dysplasia** is a syndrome with some similarities to color dilution alopecia in that abnormal clumping of **melanin** pigment is seen within hair shafts of

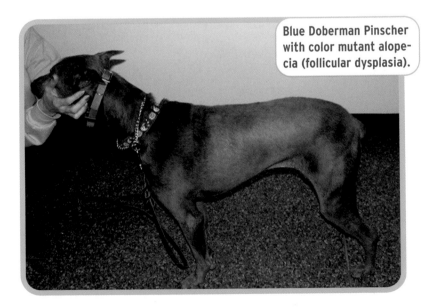

Blue Doberman Pinscher with color mutant alopecia (follicular dysplasia).

black areas. Hairs in black areas break off, whereas hairs in nonpigmented white areas are completely normal. Black hair follicular dysplasia has been reported in the following breeds:

- **Chihuahuas**
- **Terriers**
- **Bearded Collies**
- **Border Collies**
- **Basset Hounds**
- **Papillons**
- **Salukis**
- **Beagles**
- **Parson Russell Terriers**
- **American Cocker Spaniels**
- **Schipperkes**
- **Cavalier King Charles Spaniels**
- **Dachshunds**
- **Gordon Setters**
- **Pointers**
- **Mixed-breed dogs**

Black hair follicular dysplasia; note that white areas are normal, whereas black areas have broken hair shafts and scaling.

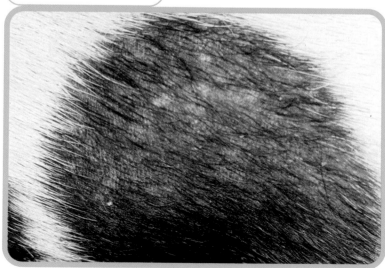

Congenital Hypotrichosis

Congenital **hypotrichosis** is due to disorders in the development of **hair follicles**. Congenital hypotrichosis may affect the entire skin or only certain areas of the body.

Several breeds of dogs and cats were deliberately bred to be hairless, including Mexican Hairless dogs, Chinese Crested dogs, Inca Hairless dogs, American Hairless terriers, Turkish Naked dog, and Sphinx cats. Some of these pets are prone to developing bacterial infections and seborrhea; these animals will benefit from regular use of antiseptic or antiseborrheic shampoos. Protecting hairless pets from excessive sunlight exposure is wise because they can live normal lives with proper skin care.

Focal (localized) areas of congenital hypotrichosis occur in a number of breeds. Male animals are affected more often than female animals. Breeds that occasionally are affected by focal areas of congenital hypotrichosis include the following:

- **German Shepherd Dogs**
- **American Cocker Spaniels**

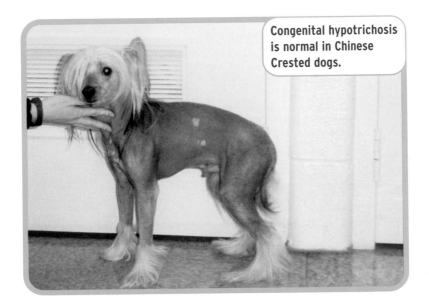

Congenital hypotrichosis is normal in Chinese Crested dogs.

- Belgian Shepherds
- Toy Poodles
- Miniature Poodles
- Whippets
- Beagles
- French Bulldogs
- Rottweilers
- Yorkshire Terriers
- Labrador Retrievers
- Bichon Frises
- Lhasa Apsos
- Basset Hounds

Most affected dogs are born with noticeable areas of hair loss that may enlarge during the first month of life. Hairless areas are often well-delineated from surrounding normal areas. Affected areas commonly include the top of the head, the earflaps, the back, and the chest. Some affected dogs also experience abnormalities in tooth development. Focal hypotrichosis is a cosmetic disorder, and the only precaution needed is to protect the affected areas from excessive sunlight exposure. Affected animals and their parents and siblings should not be bred.

A more generalized form of congenital hypotrichosis has been reported in Birman, Burmese, Devon Rex, and Siamese cats. Affected kittens have a thin, downy coat at birth that is lost in the first few weeks of life. In Birman and Siamese breeds, the mode of inheritance is an autosomal recessive gene. Affected Birman kittens also lack claws, whiskers, and tongue papillae and are unlikely to thrive.

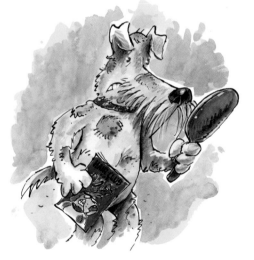

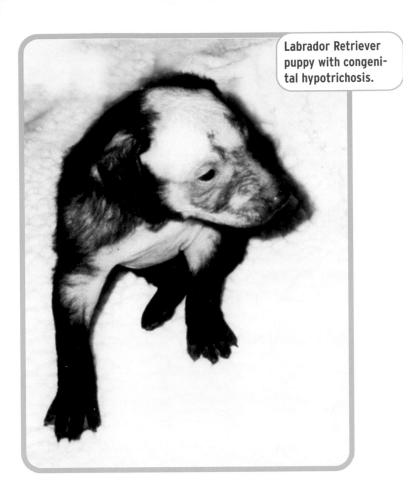

Dermatomyositis

Dermatomyositis (DM) is a hereditary inflammatory disease affecting the skin and muscles of collies, Shetland Sheepdogs, and their crosses. It also has been reported in Chow Chows, German Shepherd Dogs, Beauceron Shepherds, Welsh Corgis, Lakeland Terriers, and Kuvaszs. Skin lesions include hair loss; erythema; scaling; and crusting of the face, ears, legs, and tail tip. Muscle-related symptoms include sloppy eating and drinking, a high-stepping gait, and noticeable wasting and weakness. Studies using Collies showed that this disease is inherited as an autosomal dominant disorder, with incomplete **penetrance**. The incomplete penetrance results in a wide range of degrees of severity, ranging from unnoticeable to very obvious. Skin and muscle **biopsies** are helpful in confirming a diagnosis of DM. DM can be treated in several ways. Vitamin E may be used topically and systemically (given orally) to lessen inflammation. Pentoxifylline decreases inflammation and also improves tissue oxygenation. The brand-name version of pentoxifylline, Trental (Aventis, Kansas City, Mo.), should be used because generic forms are less effective in dogs and also cause more side effects (e.g., vomiting and diarrhea). Trental always should be given with food to decrease gastrointestinal side effects. Topical and systemic corticosteroids may be helpful in dogs that do not respond well to

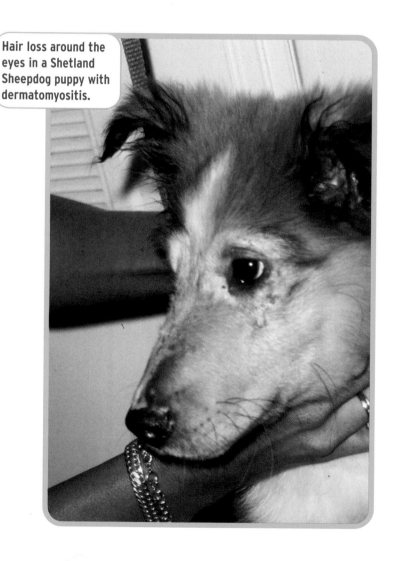

Hair loss around the eyes in a Shetland Sheepdog puppy with dermatomyositis.

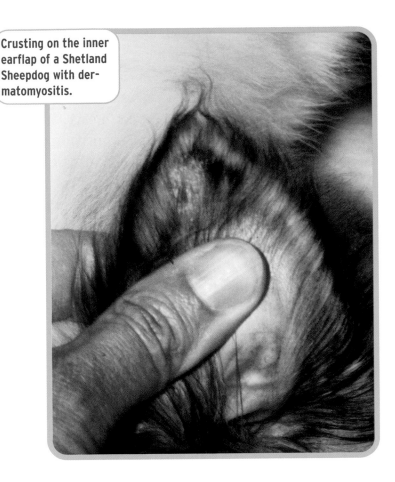

vitamin E and Trental. Caution should be exercised when administering corticosteroids; use the lowest dose possible to minimize the risk of causing **iatrogenic** Cushing's disease. Azathioprine also has been used to treat DM; use it with caution because it can cause liver damage, pancreatitis, and bone marrow suppression. The long-term outlook for this disease is unpredictable; DM may wax and wane in severity. Regardless of severity, affected animals and their relatives should not be used for breeding.

Ehlers-Danlos Syndrome

Also known as "rubber puppy disease," Ehlers-Danlos syndrome (EDS) includes a group of rare genetic **connective tissue** disorders. In humans, nine forms of EDS have been identified; they are classified according to the way they are inherited and the underlying defect in the body. Other names for the condition are *dermatosparaxis* and *cutaneous asthenia*. These disorders are caused by defects in the production of structural proteins within the skin. Defective formation of structural proteins weakens the affected tissues. The skin is often hyperelastic ("stretchy") and fragile (tears easily). Affected pets may tear their skin during normal grooming. Minor trauma may result in large, gaping wounds that are slow to heal. EDS has been reported in the following breeds:

- **Beagles**
- **Boxers**
- **Dachshunds**
- **English Setters**
- **English Springer Spaniels**
- **Fila Brasilieros**
- **Garafino Shepherds**
- **German Shepherd Dogs**
- **Greyhounds**
- **Irish Setters**
- **Keeshonds**
- **Manchester Terriers**
- **Red Kelpis**
- **Saint Bernards**
- **Soft-Coated Wheaten Terriers**
- **Toy Poodles**
- **Welsh Corgis**
- **Mixed-breed dogs**
- **Domestic Longhair cats**
- **Domestic Shorthair cats**
- **Himalayan cats**

Diagnosis is based on the presence of excessive skin elasticity and skin biopsies showing structural defects of **collagen** fibers (**electron microscopy** is helpful in evaluating EDS). Care of affected pets includes protection from trauma, declawing of affected cats and other cats living in the household, and prompt treatment of any wounds. Affected animals and their relatives should not be bred.

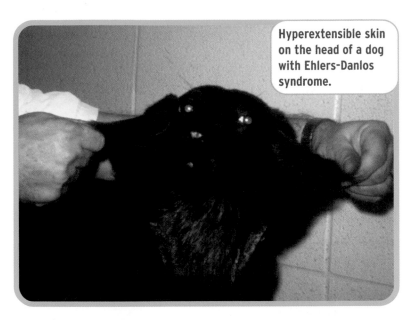

Hyperextensible skin on the head of a dog with Ehlers-Danlos syndrome.

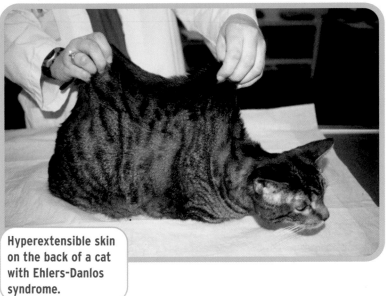

Hyperextensible skin on the back of a cat with Ehlers-Danlos syndrome.

Epidermolysis Bullosa

Epidermolysis bullosa (EB) includes a group of disorders involving structural defects where the **epidermis** (outer skin layer) and the **dermis** (deeper skin layer) meet. These diseases are divided into four main subtypes—EB simplex, EB acquisita (see Chapter 9), junctional EB, and dystrophic EB—on the basis of differences that are seen using electron microscopy. EB simplex has been reported in Collies and Shetland Sheepdogs. EB acquisita affects Great Danes. Junctional EB has been reported in Toy Poodles, Beaucerons, German Shorthaired Pointers, mixed-breed dogs, and Siamese cats. Dystrophic EB occurs in Akitas, Beaucerons, Golden Retrievers, Domestic Shorthair cats, and Persian cats.

All forms of EB result in similar skin lesions. **Vesicles** (small fluid-filled blisters) are rarely seen because they are fragile and rupture easily; visible lesions include erosions and **ulcers** located on bony, prominent parts of the face and pressure points on the legs, the earflaps (pinnae), and the footpads. Some pets have lesions inside their mouths or around their nails (which may be shed). Treatment involves minimizing trauma to the skin and treating the symptoms of any skin infections that develop. Affected animals and their relatives should not be bred.

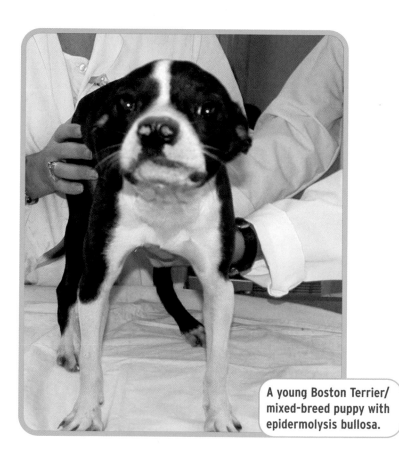

A young Boston Terrier/ mixed-breed puppy with epidermolysis bullosa.

Follicular Dysplasia

Follicular dysplasia simply means "abnormal development of hair follicles." Follicular dysplasias may be color-linked, as described in the previous section on color mutant alopecia and black hair follicular dysplasia, or noncolor-linked, as in alopecia X and canine recurrent flank alopecia (see Chapter 7). These disorders are diagnosed on the basis of skin **biopsy** findings, after other diseases that affect hair follicle development have been ruled out.

Ichthyosis

Ichthyosis is a rare inherited disorder of **keratinization**. Several forms of ichthyosis have been described in humans. Each type of ichthyosis differs in the way in which it is inherited and the specific biochemical defect. Abnormalities in **keratin** formation result in severe scaling, and in some cases, keratin forms thick crusts and skin projections. Any area of the body may be affected. The footpads and **planum nasale** (hairless tip of the nose) often develop thick accumulations of keratin. Affected dogs often have lesions at birth, and several puppies or kittens in a litter may be affected. Ichthyosis seems to be most common in West Highland White Terriers, but it has been reported in many other breeds and in mixed-breed dogs. Treatment of the symptoms with **antiseborrheic** shampoos and moisturizers may be helpful. Some pets have shown improvement after treatment with high doses of Vitamin A; others improved when they were treated with synthetic **retinoids** (compounds related to Vitamin A). As with other hereditary diseases, no cure for ichthyosis exists. Affected animals and their relatives should not be bred.

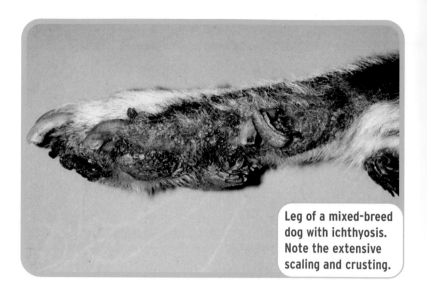

Leg of a mixed-breed dog with ichthyosis. Note the extensive scaling and crusting.

Idiopathic Facial Dermatitis of Cats

Also referred to as "dirty face syndrome," **idiopathic** facial **dermatitis** affects young Persian cats. It begins to appear in cats between 4 months and 4 years of age, the average age of onset being 12 months. The problem affects the head and neck region and consists of a black discharge that mats the hairs around the eyes, mouth, chin, and nasal folds of the face. Bacterial and yeast infections are common secondary conditions. Treatment is aimed at relieving itchiness and minimizing secondary infections. Gentle cleansing with medicated wipes (Malacetic Wipes, Dermapet or Malaseb Pledgets, DVM Pharmaceuticals, Inc.) may be helpful in some cases. No cure has been identified; affected cats and their relatives should not be bred.

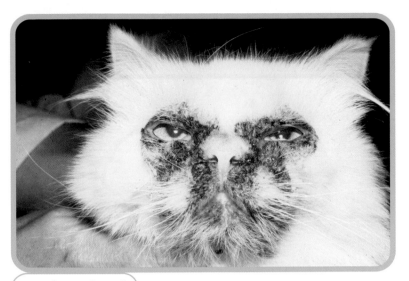

Face of a Persian cat with "dirty face syndrome" (idiopathic facial dermatitis).

Juvenile Pyoderma (Juvenile Cellulitis, Puppy Strangles)

Juvenile pyoderma, also called *juvenile cellulitis* or *puppy strangles,* is a pediatric skin disease discussed in Chapter 5. It is a severe skin disease that mainly involves the head, with purulent (puslike) discharge and swelling of the skin. Lymph nodes under the jaw become enlarged and may rupture and drain pus. Treatment includes warm compresses and the use of antibiotics and corticosteroids. After recovery, most dogs live normal lives. Although the precise cause of this disorder is unknown, it is thought to be caused by multiple factors, genetics being only one.

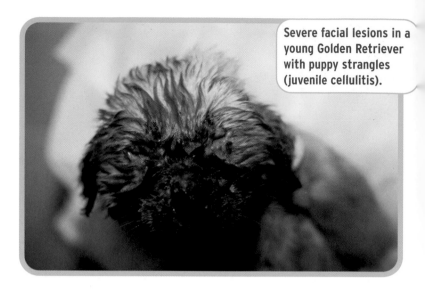

Severe facial lesions in a young Golden Retriever with puppy strangles (juvenile cellulitis).

Lethal Acrodermatitis

Lethal acrodermatitis is an autosomal recessive syndrome that affects Bull Terriers. Affected dogs metabolize zinc and copper in abnormal ways. Affected puppies often have a white or lightly colored skin and hair coat. Signs linked to lethal acrodermatitis include the following:

- **Weakness**
- **High-arched palate**
- **Slow growth**
- **Flat feet with splayed toes**
- **Thick, cracked footpads**
- **Deformed nails with pus in the nailfold**
- **Crusts and ulcers on the feet, legs, and paws**
- **Bacterial or fungal skin infections**
- **Respiratory infections**
- **Diarrhea**

Clinical signs often appear by the time the animal is 7 weeks of age. Skin biopsies show marked **parakeratosis** (an abnormality of the cells of the **stratum corneum**)—a feature linked to zinc deficiencies. **Serum** levels of zinc and copper are below normal. There is no effective treatment, and most affected puppies die as a result of infections before they are 7 months old. The littermates and parents of affected dogs should not be used for breeding.

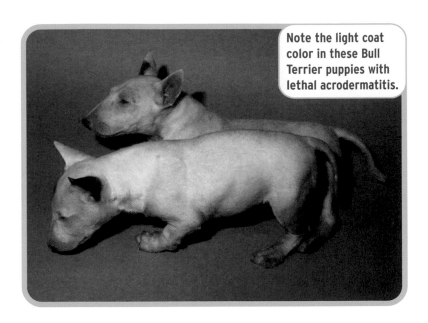

Note the light coat color in these Bull Terrier puppies with lethal acrodermatitis.

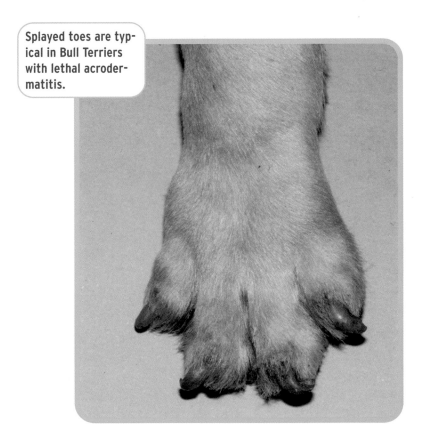

Splayed toes are typical in Bull Terriers with lethal acrodermatitis.

Mucinosis

Mucinosis is the result of excessive amounts of **mucin** in the skin. Mucin, also known as "ground substance," is the polysaccharide-rich, gummy fluid found between fibers in the dermis of the skin. Extra amounts of mucin result in thickening of the skin with exaggeration of skin folds, particularly on the head, underside, and legs. Mucin-filled blisters sometimes form within the skin. **Idiopathic** cutaneous mucinosis occurs as a hereditary disorder of Chinese Shar-Peis. Mucinosis also may be seen in some pets with **hypothyroidism** or **acromegaly** (a disorder caused by high levels of growth hormone in adult animals). Diagnosis is made by ruling out other causes of mucinosis (e.g., by testing the dog for hypothyroidism). Idiopathic cutaneous mucinosis is most common in young Chinese Shar-Peis. It often improves as the pet gets older. Mucinosis is primarily a cosmetic disorder and does not require treatment unless the skin folds are causing breathing difficulties or **pyoderma** develops in the skin folds. Systemic corticosteroids can be given to decrease mucin production in severely affected pets.

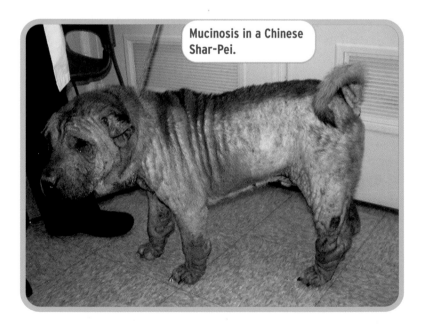

Mucinosis in a Chinese Shar-Pei.

Pattern Baldness

Pattern baldness is a form of delayed (tardive) **alopecia** in which puppies are born with normal hair coats and lose hair in various areas as young adults. Dachshunds, Boston Terriers, Chihuahuas, Whippets, Greyhounds, Italian Greyhounds, and Manchester Terriers develop hair loss on their earflaps and over the top of their heads. Pattern baldness is more common in female animals than male ones. American Water Spaniels and Portuguese Water Dogs develop alopecia on the front of their necks, thighs, and tail. Greyhounds may develop a slowly worsening alopecia over their rear legs that extends to the abdomen; this has been referred to as "idiopathic bald thigh syndrome of Greyhounds." No specific treatment is needed to address these cosmetic disorders. **Melatonin** may help to stimulate new hair growth in some pets.

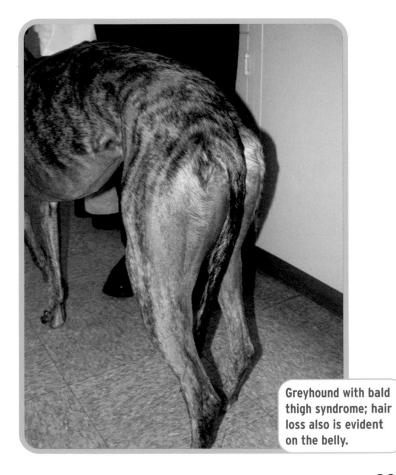

Greyhound with bald thigh syndrome; hair loss also is evident on the belly.

Primary Keratinization Defects (Primary Seborrhea)

Keratinization is the process of transforming the living cells arising from the bottom layer of the epidermis into the horny dead cells on the surface of the skin. **Keratinization defects** arise when problems occur during this transformation process. Keratinization disorders often interfere with the normal functions of the skin, resulting in increased vulnerability to infections, excessive water loss through the skin, and increased scaliness of the skin.

Primary seborrhea is an inherited keratinization disorder that causes increased scaliness or excessive **sebum** production. Oily forms are called **seborrhea oleosa,** and dry, scaly forms are called **seborrhea sicca**. Breeds commonly affected with seborrhea oleosa include the American Cocker Spaniel, English Springer Spaniel, West Highland White Terrier, and Basset Hound. Seborrhea sicca is common in Doberman Pinschers and Irish Setters. Generally, signs begin at a young age and worsen over time. Affected dogs may have a dull, flaky hair coat (seborrhea sicca) or patches of greasy scales and crusts (seborrhea oleosa). Many dogs with primary seborrhea have excessive **cerumen** (earwax) production. The skin abnormalities make bacterial and yeast infections more likely (secondary infections). The dog may have a strong, offensive odor. Footpads are often thick, and the nails may be unusually brittle. Diagnosis of primary seborrhea is made by ruling out the causes of secondary seborrhea (e.g., **allergies**, **endocrine** diseases, **ectoparasites**, nutritional deficiencies, environmental effects) and by observing changes found on skin biopsies. Management of dogs with primary seborrhea includes treatment of secondary skin and ear infections and regular bathing with antiseborrheic shampoos (see Chapter 2). Fatty acid supple-

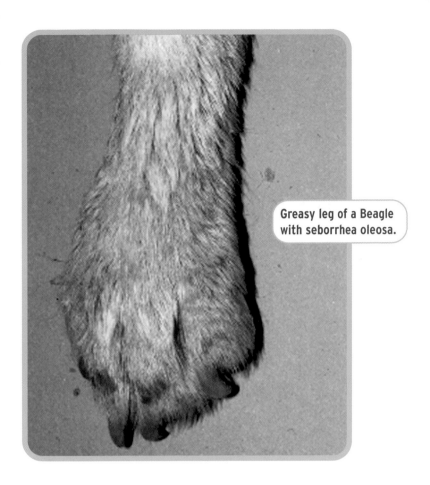

Greasy leg of a Beagle with seborrhea oleosa.

ments sometimes are helpful in treating dogs with seborrhea sicca. Synthetic retinoids sometimes are helpful in treating dogs with seborrhea oleosa.

Vitamin A-responsive seborrhea occurs in Cocker Spaniels and also occasionally in Labrador Retrievers. Clinical signs include the buildup of keratin around the base of hairs and in empty hair follicles. The skin develops fronds of keratin and resembles the skin of toads. Diagnosis is based on ruling out other causes of seborrhea and the pet's positive response to high doses of vitamin A. Veterinarians monitor dogs treated with vitamin A for possible side effects, including increases in serum cholesterol or triglycerides, decreases in tear production, and increases in liver enzymes.

Persian cats sometimes are affected by a primary hereditary seborrhea oleosa (PHSO). Affected kittens may have a dirty appearance that is first noticeable when they are 2 to 3 days old. Initially, the hair coat is curly and pasted together with **sebaceous** (oily) discharges. The whole body becomes scaly and oily, emitting a rancid odor. Regular bathing with antiseborrheic shampoos may decrease the odor and counter the pet's tendency to develop skin infections. Keeping the hair coat clipped short is also helpful. Synthetic retinoids sometimes are beneficial, but there is no cure for PHSO.

Sebaceous Adenitis

The exact causes of sebaceous **adenitis** are not yet known, although genes play a role. The disease is inherited as an autosomal recessive disorder in Standard Poodles. Other breeds frequently affected with sebaceous adenitis include Akitas, Samoyeds, and Vizslas. Sebaceous adenitis starts with an inflammation of the sebaceous glands and may lead to complete destruction of the glands. Visible symptoms include excessive dandruff or scaling, hair loss, a musty odor, and secondary skin infections. Hairs in affected areas may epilate (pull out) easily and often have a coating of dead cells and sebum around their base (these have been called *follicular casts* or **keratosebaceous casts**). Lesions often develop in a **serpiginous** (wavy-bordered) pattern that may look as if someone has poured hot wax over the dog's head or back.

Diagnosis includes ruling out other causes of folliculitis and hair loss and taking multiple skin biopsies. The distinctive signs of sebaceous adenitis are inflammation and destruction of sebaceous glands. A variety of treatments may be used depending on the severity of the condition. Secondary bacterial and yeast infections should be treated with appropriate antibiotics and antifungal drugs. Antiseborrheic shampoos may help to decrease scaling. A mixture of propylene glycol and water may be sprayed on the coat daily until improvement is seen and then two to three times per week for maintenance. Intensive oil treat-

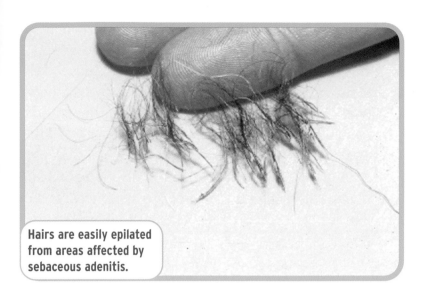

Hairs are easily epilated from areas affected by sebaceous adenitis.

The serpiginous pattern of hair loss on the head of this dog is typical of short-coated breeds affected by sebaceous adenitis.

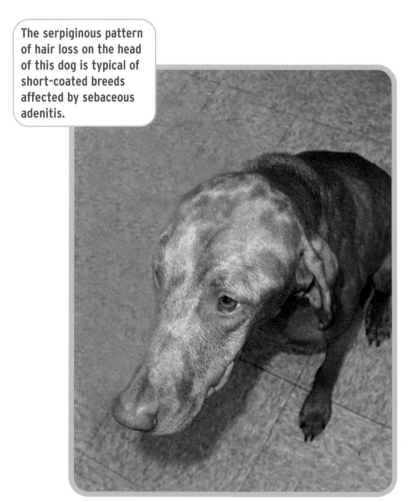

ments are helpful in restoring moisture to the skin and hair coat. The entire body is soaked in mineral oil or an emulsified bath oil for several hours. The oil is then removed by bathing the animal in a degreasing shampoo followed by a **humectant** spray. Oral fatty acid supplements and high doses of vitamin A sometimes are helpful. If the skin biopsies show an inflammatory reaction around sebaceous glands, treatment with a combination of tetracycline and niacinamide may decrease symptoms associated with the disease. Other medications that have been helpful in affected dogs include oral corticosteroids, synthetic retinoids, and cyclosporine. The Orthopedic Foundation for Animals maintains a sebaceous adenitis registry to help breeders track the genetic patterns of this disease (www.offa.org/sageninfo.html).

Zinc-Responsive Dermatoses

Normal keratinization requires adequate levels of zinc. Keratinization problems occur when diets do not include enough zinc or zinc is not absorbed well because of either genetic abnormalities or diets containing high levels of calcium or **phytates,** which interfere with zinc absorption. Clinical signs linked to inadequate levels of zinc in the skin include thickening of the skin over pressure points; thickening and cracking of the footpads; and crusting, scaling, and hair loss involving the skin around the mouth, eyes, chin, ears, feet, and genitals. Bacterial and yeast skin infections are common secondary complications of the disease. Skin biopsies show abnormalities in keratinization, most notably the retention of nuclei in the cells of the upper layers of the skin (this is called **parakeratosis**). Breeds commonly affected by a zinc-responsive dermatosis include Siberian Huskies and Alaskan Malamutes; these breeds may have impaired zinc absorption or requirements for zinc that exceed levels found in most commercial dog foods. Young, rapidly growing large-breed dogs also may develop a zinc-responsive dermatosis. High levels of calcium or phytates from plant proteins in the diet may keep these animals from absorbing enough zinc to meet the needs of rapid growth.

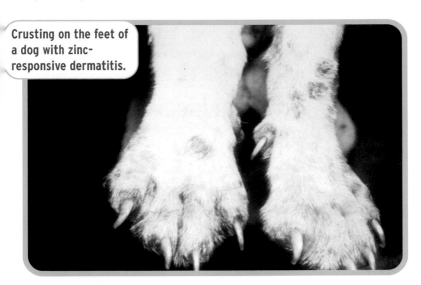

Crusting on the feet of a dog with zinc-responsive dermatitis.

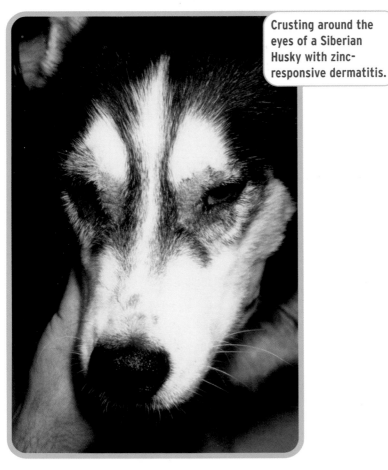

Crusting around the eyes of a Siberian Husky with zinc-responsive dermatitis.

Treatment of zinc-responsive dermatosis includes oral zinc supplements (zinc methionine, zinc gluconate, or zinc sulfate); correction of any dietary imbalances; cessation of any calcium supplements; and treatment with antiseborrheic shampoos, antibiotics, and antifungal medications to address secondary skin problems. Skin lesions in Alaskan Malamutes and Siberian Huskies may wax and wane. In some cases, a variety of zinc supplements must be tried before the most effective formulation can be identified.

Summary

This chapter covers a variety of diseases associated with specific breeds of dogs and cats, most of which are genetic problems. For most of these conditions, multiple factors, including a combination of genetics, environment, nutrition, and secondary infections, are involved in the type and severity of the clinical symptoms seen. Care should be taken to refrain from selecting animals for breeding that have a history of hereditary skin disease or relatives with such diseases. Selective breeding will help to decrease the number of pets with hereditary skin diseases in the future. The treatment of hereditary skin diseases usually involves lifelong management of symptoms because few of these diseases can be cured.

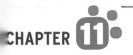
BEHAVIOR- RELATED SKIN DISEASES

Psychogenic skin diseases are self-induced lesions caused by underlying behavioral problems. In some cases, the skin lesions result from simple boredom or attention-seeking behavior; in others, the underlying problem is caused by anxiety or an **obsessive-compulsive disorder** (OCD). It is helpful to understand several terms used to describe behavior-related disorders:

- *Stereotypic behaviors:* **These are excessive, consistent, repetitious motions that have no obvious purpose and that interfere with normal activities and behavior. The motions may originate in normal behaviors. Examples include repetitive, excessive licking, sucking, chewing, biting, scratching, and hair pulling.**
- *Anxiety:* **This is the apprehensive anticipation of impending doom. In animals, the most common type of anxiety is separation anxiety, in which the pet becomes frantic when left alone. Behaviors typical of separation anxiety include howling, urination and defecation, and destructive behavior toward objects in the environment or the pet's own body (e.g., scratching, licking, chewing, biting, and self-mutilation).**
- *Obsessions:* **Repeated thoughts or impulses that are considered inappropriate and that may result in great anxiety.**
- *Obsessive-compulsive disorders:* **These disorders are characterized by repetitive, stereotypic, ritualistic behaviors that interfere with normal daily activities and functioning.**

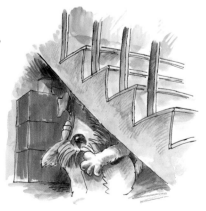

You may wonder why some pets have stereotypic, ritualistic behaviors and why these behaviors tend to reinforce themselves and become repetitive. A number of factors seem to contribute to the development of these behaviors: (1) genetics—breeds that are emotional and fearful have a higher risk of developing psychogenic skin diseases, (2) lifestyle—pets that spend long periods of time confined or in a boring environment, and (3) stressors—events that produce anxiety. Indulging in a stereotypic behavior is thought to release chemicals called **endorphins** in the brain. The release of endorphins

Factors Contributing to Behavior-Related Disorders in Cats and Dogs

Factor	Examples
Genetic predispositions: individuals or breeds that are emotional and nervous or fearful	Abyssinian cats, Siamese cats, Burmese cats, other Oriental cat breeds; Doberman Pinschers, Great Danes, Irish Setters, Labrador Retrievers, German Shepherd Dogs; individual pets of any breed with a nervous temperament
Lifestyle: boring	Long periods spent confined in a crate or cage, continually tied, small-pen housing, lack of human or animal companionship
Stressors: events or conditions that may provoke stereotypic behaviors	Inadequate socialization, inadequate exercise, change of environment, overcrowding, territorial disputes, status disputes, addition or loss of family members or pets, change in daily routine, hospitalization or boarding kennel confinement

Important Information for Management of Psychogenic Skin Diseases

- Source of the pet (those adopted from shelters or rescue groups are at higher risk)
- Chronologic progression of the problem
- Frequency and length of the problem
- Seasonal associations (if any)
- Medical history
- Dietary history
- Previous and current medications
- Response to any previously prescribed medications
- Previous skin or ear infections (or both)
- Were any skin lesions present before the start of the behavior?
- Parasite control measures (is this pet receiving flea control products? Are other pets in the household receiving flea control products?)
- Have other pets in the household experienced dermatologic or behavioral problems?
- Have any people in the household experienced skin problems?
- Does the problem behavior occur when people are around?
- How hard is it to interrupt the problem behavior?
- Describe the pet's sleeping habits.
- Describe a typical day for this pet (e.g., activities, periods alone, contact with other pets).
- Have any changes occurred in the pet's daily routine?
- Have any changes occurred in the pet's contact with people or other pets?
- What training has this pet received?

confers a sense of peace and happiness, helping the pet cope with stress; by providing positive reinforcement, endorphins also encourage the pet to continue the stereotypic behavior. Over time, the pet may become chemically addicted to the endorphins released during stereotypic behavior.

Syndromes caused by stereotypic behavior in dogs and cats include the following:

- **Acral lick dermatitis**
- **Feline psychogenic alopecia and dermatitis**
- **Tail sucking**
- **Tail biting**
- **Flank sucking**
- **Foot licking**
- **Self-nursing**
- **Anal licking**
- **Preputial licking**

True neurologic disease may be present in a few pets with these signs; however, most cases appear to represent a type of OCD.

Lick Granuloma (Acral Lick Dermatitis)

The term *acral* refers to the legs and feet. Acral lick dermatitis (ALD), also known as a lick granuloma, is a self-induced lesion on the front surface of a leg. Continual licking at one area of the leg produces hair loss, erosions or **ulcers**, and thickening of the skin. A typical lesion of ALD is a thick, red, hairless, oval plaque found over the front surface of one leg. Occasionally, more than one leg may be affected. The most common sites are over the carpus ("wrist"), metacarpus (the foot), the lower foreleg, and just below or above the hock on the rear leg.

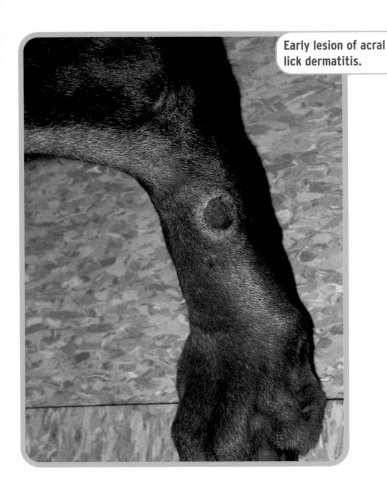

Early lesion of acral lick dermatitis.

Breeds most likely to develop ALD include the Doberman Pinscher, Great Dane, Labrador Retriever, Irish Setter, Golden Retriever, and German Shepherd Dog. Male dogs are affected twice as often as female dogs. Although dogs may develop ALD at any age, most are older than 5 years of age when they are taken for veterinary treatment.

Other conditions that may appear similar to ALD include tumors (mast cell tumors, **histiocytomas**, fibrosarcomas, melanomas, and squamous cell carcinomas; see Chapter 13), granulomas (pressure point, **calcinosis circumscripta**, fungal, mycobacterial, foreign body), deep infections (bacterial, fungal), **demodicosis**, and trauma-induced wounds. Veterinarians use diagnostic tests such as **skin scrapings**, bacterial and fungal cultures, skin **cytology**, and skin **biopsies** to confirm the

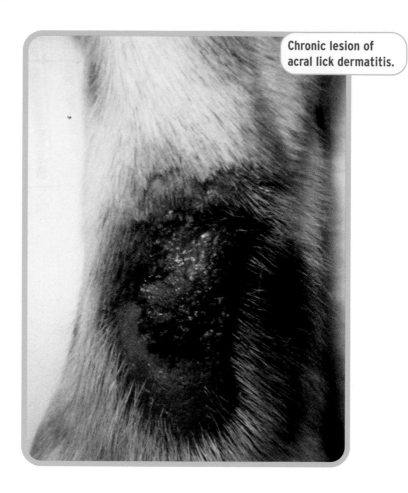

diagnosis. In addition to ruling out these conditions, veterinarians will also examine the dog for underlying arthritis or joint disease, bone infections, and nerve damage because dogs sometimes feel compelled to lick areas of their bodies where they feel discomfort. Radiographs (x-rays) and arthrocentesis (removal of joint fluid for analysis) can be helpful in ruling out orthopedic disorders. A veterinary neurologist should be consulted if nerve damage caused by prior trauma or surgery is suspected. Before condemning the dog with ALD to a diagnosis of OCD, a veterinarian should always check the dog for causes of itching, such as **atopy**, food allergies, allergic contact dermatitis, **ectoparasites**, and infections.

Treatment of ALD involves many possible approaches. The lesions frequently are infected and should be treated as a deep **pyoderma**; **systemic** antibiotics should be continued for a minimum of 2 weeks after all signs of infection have disappeared, which may require 10 to 12 weeks of antibiotic treatment. The dog should also be treated for any underlying skin disease (for example, control underlying allergies and ectoparasites).

Treatment Strategies for Acral Lick Dermatitis

Category	Examples
Correct underlying cause	Boredom: Increased playtime, new playmate, less confinement, environmental enrichment, obedience training (providing the pet with a job to do) Stress: Counterconditioning, removal of dominant or competing animal
Provide behavior-modification training	Counterconditioning, desensitization training, electroshock training (remotely operated shock collar)
Treat the lesion	Antibiotics, topical corticosteroids, topical nonsteroidal anti-inflammatory agents (DMSO, flunixin meglumine), bitter-tasting topicals, topical capsaicin, laser surgery, cryosurgery, surgical removal
Alter skin sensation	Topical capsaicin, laser surgery, acupuncture, antihistamines, corticosteroids
Treat the mind	Anxiolytics, antidepressants, serotonin reuptake inhibitors, opioids, sedatives, tranquilizers, dopamine antagonists, progestagens

If your veterinarian is unable to diagnose an underlying disease, the next step is to identify and eliminate the stressors in the pet's life. This may involve providing more human companionship, decreasing confinement, increasing activity (more walks and games with the pet), separating the pet from more dominant animals, providing a suitable playmate, and providing environmental enrichment (toys, music, television). Behavior-modification strategies may be helpful for dogs suffering from separation anxiety; consult with a canine behavioral specialist for recommendations. Behavior-modification strategies include the use of counterconditioning and desensitization techniques, rewarding the dog for new behaviors while gradually exposing it to situations that have triggered excessive licking in the past. Electroshock therapy has been used as another means of stopping licking behavior—a remotely controlled electric-shock collar is placed on the dog, and a brief shock is delivered each time the dog starts to lick its leg. Acupuncture has been reported to help some pets.

Your veterinarian may use a variety of strategies to treat the lesion. As previously noted, any bacterial infections that have developed in the wound must be treated with appropriate antibiotic therapy. Likewise, any fungal or yeast infections should be treated with antifungal medications to eliminate infections as contributors to the lesion. Anti-inflammatory medications, including **corticosteroids** applied topically or injected directly into the wound, may be helpful in relieving any itching that stimulates licking. Bitter-tasting **topical** medications may discourage licking. One of the best topical agents to stop licking is capsaicin, a concentrated extract of jalapeño peppers. In addition to its bitter taste, capsaicin cream blocks nerve transmission; after an initial burning sensation, nerves are deadened for several hours and therefore cannot transmit impulses to the brain that stimulate endorphin release. This blockage of endorphin short-circuits the positive feedback loop caused by licking. **Laser surgery** may encourage healing by removing the excessive fibrous tissue and thickened skin. In addition to stimulating healing, carbon dioxide (CO_2) lasers sterilize the lesions and deaden nerve endings. The deadening effect produced by CO_2 lasers lasts much longer than that produced by capsaicin (weeks versus hours). In contrast to CO_2 laser surgery, traditional surgical removal of lesions generally is not a good option for the treatment of ALD. There simply is not enough excess skin on the legs to cover the site of a removed ALD lesion. Moreover, if the underlying cause of the licking behavior is not addressed, the dog may quickly mutilate the surgical site. **Cryosurgery** functions similarly to CO_2 lasers in deadening nerve endings and removing the thickened tissue associated with ALD. Cryosurgery must be performed with caution to prevent damage to underlying tendons and blood vessels. Cryosurgery should be performed only by veterinary surgeons familiar with its use.

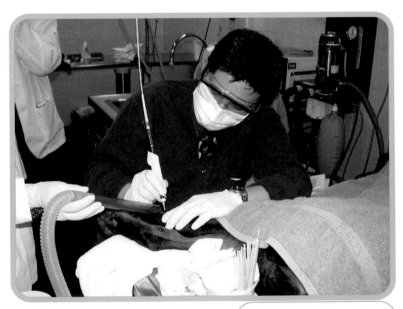

Carbon dioxide laser being used to encourage healing of an acral lick dermatitis lesion. (The laser removes excess scar tissue and deadens nerve sensations from the area.)

Elizabethan collars, harnesses, muzzles, bandages, and casts may be used to keep the dog from licking at lesions. These may help during the initial phase of treatment, when the main goal is to eliminate infections and allow the lesion to heal. Breaking the lick-endorphin release-lick cycle also may be helpful, particularly if the licking behavior began recently.

Psychoactive drugs are sometimes necessary to control the excessive chewing and licking behavior of dogs with ALD. In some cases, these drugs will be needed only for a short time, until the habit is broken through interference with the lick-endorphin release-lick cycle, stress and boredom have been reduced, and behavior-modification therapy has been successful. In other cases, dogs may require long-term treatment. Psychoactive drugs that may be useful in the management of ALD include anxiolytic (antianxiety) drugs, tricyclic antidepressants, selective serotonin reuptake inhibitors, **opioid** antagonists, opioid agonists, and progestagens. Anxiolytic drugs reduce anxiety and therefore may help nervous dogs. Tricyclic antidepressants and selective serotonin reuptake inhibitors (also antidepressants) help pets cope with stress. Opioid antagonists block the effects of endorphins and thus block positive feedback caused by OCD-type behaviors. Opioid ago-

Where We Stand

Because most of these medications have side effects, their use should be carefully monitored by your veterinarian. An awareness of possible drug interactions is critical when psychoactive medications are prescribed; be sure your veterinarian is aware of all treatments being given to your pet and chemicals to which your pet might be exposed (e.g., the use of some insecticides increases the activity of these drugs).

Psychoactive Drugs Used in Treating Psychogenic Dermatitis of Dogs and Cats

Drug Type	Examples	Potential Side Effects
Anti-inflammatory	Antihistamines: chlorpheniramine, diphenhydramine, clemastine, hydroxyzine; Corticosteroids: prednisone, prednisolone, methylprednisolone	Sedation, dry mouth, constipation, paradoxical hyperactivity, seizures; Iatrogenic Cushing's disease
Anxiolytic drugs	Diazepam	Increased appetite, weight gain
Tricyclic antidepressants	Amitriptyline, doxepin, clomipramine	Rapid heart beat, abnormal heart rhythm, dilated pupils, dry mouth, constipation, sedation, weight gain
Selective serotonin reuptake inhibitors	Fluoxetine, paroxetine	Anorexia, vomiting, diarrhea, sedation, agitation, dry mouth
Opioid antagonists	Naltrexone	Nervousness, pruritus, liver damage
Opioid agonists	Hydrocodone	Sedation, constipation, vomiting
Dopamine antagonist	Haloperidol	Hallucinations, muscle twitching, incoordination
Progestagens	Megesterol acetate	Increased appetite, weight gain, diabetes, acromegaly, pyometra, mammary hyperplasia, mammary cancer

nists mimic the action of endorphins, thereby calming the pet and reducing its dependence on self-mutilation to stimulate endorphin release. Progestagens have a calming effect, especially in male dogs.

In summary, ALD is associated with myriad underlying causes and can be difficult to treat. Numerous treatment options are available. Finding an effective treatment for a particular dog may require trial and error and a great deal of patience. Consultations with both veterinary behaviorists and veterinary dermatologists may be helpful.

Psychogenic Alopecia and Dermatitis in Cats

Psychogenic **alopecia** and dermatitis (PAD) in cats is caused by excessive grooming, licking, chewing, and hair pulling as the result of emotional stress. This excessive grooming is a stereotypic behavior. Clinical signs usually are limited to hair loss, but the body areas affected vary. Common areas include the midline of the back, sides, belly, back of the thighs, and forelegs. Hairs remaining in these areas do not epilate (pull out) easily. Broken hairs may be seen. Regrowth may be darker than normal, especially in Siamese and other breeds in which coat color depends on temperature. Occasionally, the cat exhibits an area of skin **inflammation** (rash), ulcerations, or a plaquelike lesion (firm, well-circumscribed, slightly raised lesion with surface erosions). Because many cats are "secret groomers," owners do not always realize when their pets are overgrooming. Checking the cat's stools for hair and watching for symptoms of hairballs (gagging or vomiting balls of hair) may prove that the cat is indeed overgrooming.

In some cats, overgrooming is triggered by a pre-existing disease, such as impacted **anal sacs** or an ear infection. Therefore veterinarians should conduct a thorough physical examination to check the cat for abnormal-

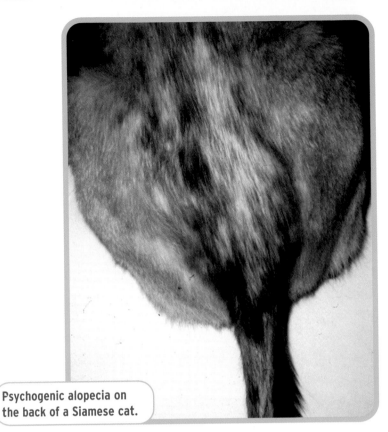

Psychogenic alopecia on the back of a Siamese cat.

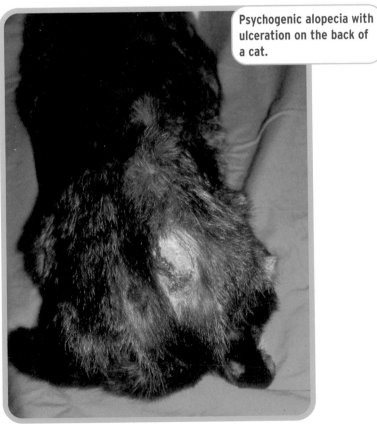

Psychogenic alopecia with ulceration on the back of a cat.

ities that may trigger overgrooming. Any physical problems found during the examination should be corrected.

Before diagnosing a cat with PAD, your veterinarian will rule out other causes of hair loss and overgrooming. Skin scrapings should be collected so that they can be checked for **Demodex** mites and other ectoparasites. The pet's flea control program should be evaluated and improved if necessary. Hairs should be cultured for **dermatophytes** (ringworm). Microscopic evaluation of plucked hairs will reveal fractures if the cat is overgrooming. Restrictive feeding trials should be used to rule out food allergies. **Intradermal skin allergy testing** should be performed to check the cat for atopy. Older cats also should be tested for **hyperthyroidism** and internal malignant tumors (pancreatic or liver cancer). Younger cats should be checked for thymic cancer. Skin biopsies are useful in confirming that hairs are growing, which indicates that the hair loss is not due to **Cushing's disease** or **hypothyroidism**; biop-

Fractured ends of hairs plucked from a cat with psychogenic alopecia.

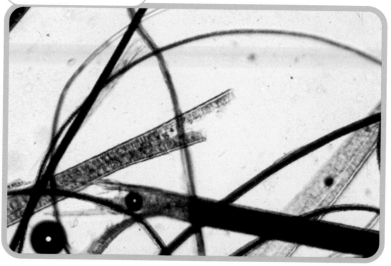

sies also help the veterinarian rule out skin tumors and **eosinophilic granulomas** as the cause of any skin lesions.

Cats of any age and either sex can suffer from PAD. Particularly emotional breeds, such as Siamese, Abyssinian, and other Oriental varieties, may be more prone to the condition than other breeds. The environment should be investigated in the event that a stressful condition is causing PAD. Examples of stressful conditions include the following:

- **Invasion of territory by a new cat**
- **A change in "pecking order" of cats in the household**
- **A barking dog**
- **A new baby**
- **Moving to a new home**
- **Major illness in the family**
- **Changes in family's routine**
- **Loss of a companion animal**
- **Boarding**
- **Hospitalization**

If potential stressors can be identified and eliminated or modified, the cat may improve without medical treatment. In some cases, a 30-day course of antianxiety drugs may be helpful in breaking the habit of overgrooming. If stressors cannot be identified, eliminated, or modified, then the options are long-term treatment or acceptance of the cat's appearance.

Cats that are overgrooming without producing any skin lesions besides hair loss may not require medication. All medications have potential side effects, so it is important to weigh the possible benefits of the drug against its possible side effects. Other factors to consider include the difficulty of medicating the pet (forcing a pill down a cat's throat can be dangerous) and the cost of the medication (many psychoactive drugs are expensive). Elizabethan collars may be used to prove that the hair loss is due to overgrooming rather than another disease (this has been termed an "Elizabethan collar–response test"). However, a

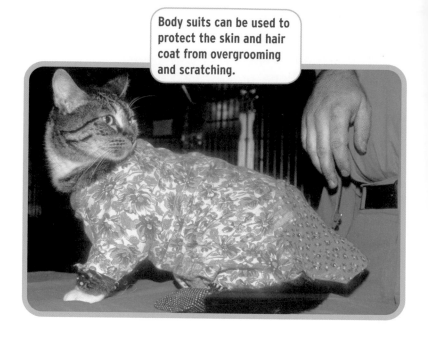

Body suits can be used to protect the skin and hair coat from overgrooming and scratching.

word of caution: Be certain that there are no areas in the cat's environment where the cat could jump or climb and snag its Elizabethan collar on something; if that happens, the cat could die by hanging. Baby "onesies" or home-crafted and sewn bodysuits also may be used to protect most of the body from overgrooming and can help break a lick-endorphin release-lick cycle.

As with canine ALD, some experts believe that PAD may become a self-reinforcing repetitive behavior because of the release of endorphins and other neu-ropeptides (compounds that excite nerve cells). Endorphins may help the cat cope with stress, but they also have a narcotic, addictive effect that can act to rein-force the overgrooming behavior. Opioid and **dopamine** antagonists (blockers) often are effective in decreasing overgrooming, which proves the importance of endor-phins and other neuropeptides in the reinforcement of overgrooming. Drugs that have been reported to be effective in the treatment of PAD include the following:

- **Chlorpheniramine**
- **Diazepam**
- **Phenobarbital**
- **Naloxone**
- **Fluoxetine**
- **Clomipramine**
- **Amitriptyline**
- **Buspirone**
- **Haloperidol**
- **Progestagens**

Because some of these drugs have life-threatening side effects, a veterinarian familiar with their use should closely monitor the pet during treatment.

Tail Sucking and Biting

Tail sucking most commonly is seen in Siamese cats, although it may occur in other breeds. The first 1 or 2 inches of hair at the tip of the tail is usually wet because of persistent sucking; hair loss at the tip of the tail is also common. Tail sucking usually is linked to boredom or long periods of confinement. Cats with chronic diarrhea may develop this habit after spending long periods of time cleaning their tails. Other disorders that may trigger tail sucking include allergies, fleas and other ectoparasites, bite wounds and other injuries to the tail, and **feline urologic syndrome** (FUS). Treatment should focus on the elimination of any contributing factors and reduction of the cat's boredom. Enriching the cat's environment with a variety of toys or a playmate may be effective. Your veterinarian also can prescribe antianxiety drugs or tricyclic antidepressants, although cats receiving one of these should be monitored closely for any side effects.

Tail biting is most common in long-haired dogs with long tails. These dogs chase their tails and then bite the tip. The habit of tail biting often begins when dogs are puppies and may be outgrown with age. Distracting the dog and providing other outlets for play often help interrupt tail chasing. Dogs that continue to chase their tails may have a neurologic disorder and should be checked by a veterinary neurologist. Dogs that have had their tails docked may develop a neuroma at the tail stub. A neuroma is a mass of scar tissue and haphazardly growing nerve fibers. This is a painful condition that results in the dog licking or chewing at the area. Tail-dock neuromas should be removed surgically to eliminate the source of the problem.

Flank Sucking

Flank sucking is most common in Doberman Pinschers, although it may occur in other breeds. The dog will lie on its chest, supported by its elbows, and turn its head to suck on its flank or upper hind leg. It may appear calm and completely absorbed in this activity. Sucking behavior is rarely destructive, but some dogs develop skin infections from the excessive moisture. A combination of genetic factors and boredom is believed to cause flank sucking. Once the behavior becomes established, it becomes a self-reinforcing stereotypic activity. Allergies and ectoparasites should be ruled out as causes of flank itchiness. If present, bacterial or yeast skin infections should be treated with systemic antibiotics or antifungal drugs. Keeping your dog occupied will decrease its boredom and its urge to suck its flank. Frequent walks and obedience training often help. Enriching the pet's environment with toys or a playmate will provide other options for entertainment. Counterconditioning and other behavior-modification programs are helpful; consult with an expert in canine behavior for recommendations. Antianxiety drugs or tricyclic antidepressant medications may be useful in some cases, but their use should be monitored by a veterinarian familiar with possible side effects.

Self-Nursing

Self-nursing is most common in intact female cats and dogs, but it also can occur in neutered and male pets. Usually, the nursing is confined to one nipple. This behavior may start during a pseudopregnancy (false pregnancy). Spaying often is helpful when self-nursing is caused by false pregnancy. Counterconditioning and other behavior-modification programs may be helpful; consult with an expert in animal behavior for recommendations.

Foot Licking

Foot licking usually is caused by atopy, other allergies, pododemodicosis (**Demodex** mites in the feet), or **Malassezia** (yeast) infections of the feet. Cats also may lick their feet excessively as a result of **pemphigus foliaceus**-associated **paronychia** (infections around the base of their claws). Some pets begin licking their feet because they are bored or anxious. In some cases, foot licking becomes an attention-seeking behavior because the owner inadvertently provides positive reinforcement by trying to distract the foot licking pet. The first step in treating

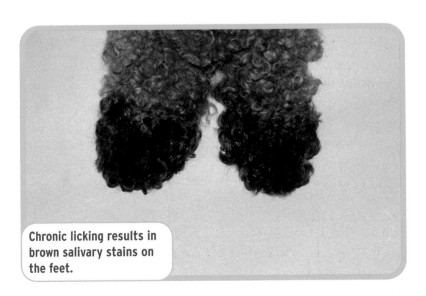

Chronic licking results in brown salivary stains on the feet.

a pet that engages in excessive foot licking is to identify and treat any underlying diseases, such as atopy, other allergies, *Demodex*, pemphigus, and infection. If no underlying cause for the foot licking can be identified, the problem may be a form of OCD. The owner should attempt to eliminate any stressors from the pet's life and provide environmental enrichment. Counterconditioning and other behavior-modification programs may be helpful for some pets; others may require psychoactive drugs. As with other forms of OCD, the severity of the behavior must be weighed against the possible side effects of drugs used in treatment.

Anal Licking

Anal licking is seen most commonly in Poodles, although it may occur in any breed. Many dogs begin licking the anal region because of impacted or infected **anal sacs**. Food allergies and atopy are also common triggers for anal licking.

Many dogs have perianal (surrounding the anus) dermatitis with bacterial or yeast overgrowth. Some pets have **colitis** or chronic diarrhea; a few lick the anal area because of **tapeworm** infestation. In German Shepherd Dogs, anal licking may be one of the first symptoms of **perianal fistulas**. Anal licking becomes an attention-seeking behavior in some dogs. Chronic licking causes the skin to become thickened and hyperpigmented (blackened) and often leads to the development of bacterial and yeast infections. Pets that engage in anal licking should be evaluated by a veterinarian to determine all possible contributing causes. Secondary skin infections should be

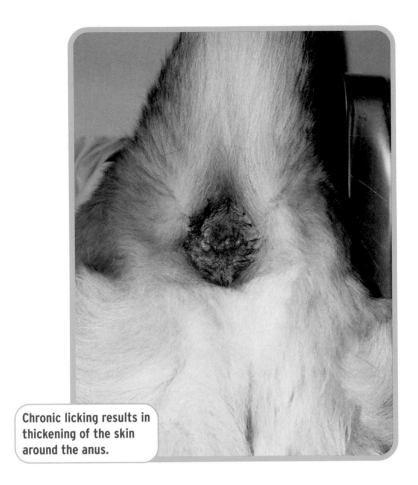

Chronic licking results in thickening of the skin around the anus.

treated. Best results will be achieved when a specific cause can be identified and treated. Counterconditioning and other behavior-modification programs are helpful for some pets; others require treatment with psychoactive drugs. As with other forms of OCD, the severity of the behavior must be weighed against the possible side effects of drugs used in treatment.

Summary

Determining the roles of behavioral disorders and neurologic diseases in the development of skin lesions in dogs and cats is often difficult. In many cases, self-destructive behavior is initiated by an underlying disease and later becomes self-perpetuating because of a positive feedback loop involving the production of endogenous endorphins. In other cases, genetic and environmental factors contribute to the development of stereotypic behaviors. Pets with signs of OCD should be evaluated to identify all possible contributing factors, including underlying diseases, environmental stressors, boredom, and inadvertent positive reinforcements of the behavior. Psychogenic dermatoses can be addressed in various ways. Pet owners should consult animal behaviorists and veterinarians familiar with these diseases for help in choosing the most appropriate treatment options.

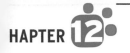
EAR DISEASES

The normal function of the ears is to collect sound waves and transmit them to the eardrum. Sound waves striking the eardrum (**tympanic membrane**) generate nerve impulses that are sent to the brain for hearing. The **pinnae** (earflaps) contain cartilage that rolls into a funnel shape to form the vertical, outer portion of the ear canal; the cartilage turns inward and becomes tube shaped to form the horizontal, inner portion of the L-shaped ear canal. The ear canal is lined by a thin layer of skin that contains **hair follicles, sebaceous glands,** and **ceruminal glands.** Ceruminal glands are modified **apocrine sweat glands.** Earwax is composed of secretions from the ceruminal and sebaceous glands, plus **exfoliating** (shedding) skin cells.

Any disease affecting the skin may involve the ears. The ear pinnae are particularly vulnerable to diseases caused by poor circulation, contact with other animals or the environment, and trauma. In addition, the ear canals are similar to skin folds in that they tend to hold moisture, encouraging the overgrowth of bacterial and **yeast** organisms.

Ear diseases are common problems in dogs and cats. A number of risk factors have been identified. Pets that have one or more factors predisposing them to ear disease should be watched closely for signs of problems. When signs of ear disease are evident, prompt treatment can keep the problem from becoming irreversible, requiring lifelong ongoing treatment and sometimes surgery.

The skin inside a healthy ear is a light pink color; the ear canal normally has a few specks of yellowish-brown wax in it. Diseases affecting the ears result in pain and **inflammation.** The skin inside the ear becomes red and irritated. Excess earwax is produced, and often **white**

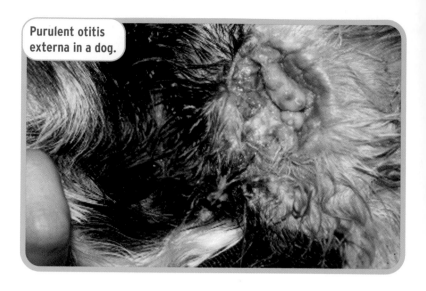

Purulent otitis externa in a dog.

blood cells begin to fill the ear canal, resulting in a foul-smelling yellow, green, or brown discharge within the ear canal. Seek help when you notice any signs of ear problems such as redness, pain, or discharge; head shaking or pawing at the ears; or odor coming from your pet's ears. Your veterinarian will determine the cause of the problem and provide recommendations for proper treatment.

Diseases Affecting the Earflap

Ear pinnae (earflaps) are skin-covered extensions of the **auricular** (ear) cartilage that function to collect sound waves. There is a wide range of sizes and shapes of the ear pinnae among different breeds of dogs. Most diseases affecting the earflaps also affect the skin at other locations of the body; therefore all pets with **lesions** in or on the ears should be thoroughly examined for other signs of disease. The following types of diseases involve the ear pinnae:

- **Hereditary**
- **Environmental**
- **Parasitic**
- **Allergic**
- **Infectious**

- Hormonal (endocrine)
- Immune-mediated
- Neoplastic
- Miscellaneous disorders

Hereditary: Ear "baldness," or **alopecia**, often is caused by a hereditary lack of hair follicles or the presence of tiny, miniature hair follicles. Examples of hereditary disorders causing alopecia on the ear pinnae include pattern baldness, congenital **hypotrichosis**, **follicular dysplasia** (color dilution alopecia, black hair follicle dysplasia), **dermatomyositis**, exfoliative cutaneous **lupus erythematosus**, and primary **keratinization** defects (**seborrhea**). See Chapter 10 for more information about these disorders.

Environmental: Ear pinnae are prone to frostbite because of their thinness and lack of insulation. Frozen ears are pale and blue or purplish black in color. During thawing the skin may become red, swollen, and painful; if the damage is severe, the skin may remain a dark purplish black and slough (shed off). Treatment involves warming the ears and keeping the pet out of extreme cold. Partial amputation of the ears may be needed if the ears have been badly frozen.

Too much exposure to sunlight can result in lesions on the ear pinnae caused by **ultraviolet radiation** (UVB). Lightly pigmented ears and those that are thinly haired

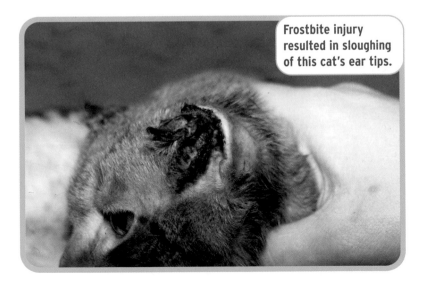

Frostbite injury resulted in sloughing of this cat's ear tips.

are the most prone to UVB damage. White cats are at highest risk of developing lesions, termed **actinic keratoses**, on their ears. Breeds of dogs with increased risk of actinic keratoses include Dalmatians, American Staffordshire Terriers, Beagles, Bassett Hounds, and Bull Terriers. Actinic keratoses first appear as red, scaly lesions on the ear tips or margins or other thinly haired regions such as the thighs or belly. In chronic cases, the lesions become crusted and **plaque**like. These are premalignant lesions that may develop into **tumors** (most commonly into squamous cell carcinomas). **Biopsies** may be necessary to distinguish between premalignant and **malignant** lesions. Treatment involves **laser surgery, cryosurgery**, chemotherapy, or amputation of the affected areas. Sunscreens and **retinoids** (vitamin A or a similar compound) may be helpful in treating mild cases. Protecting at-risk cats and dogs from excessive sunlight exposure is important to prevent UVB damage.

Parasitic: **Sarcoptes** *scabiei* **mites** commonly affect the edges and outer surface of the ear pinnae. These mites produce intense itching and **papules** (small, red bumps). Affected areas often are covered with thick, yellow crusts. Diagnosis and treatment of these mites are reviewed in Chapter 6. *Notoedres cati*, the cause of feline **scabies**, also commonly affects the ear pinnae. These mites are usually easy to find on **skin scrapings**; further information can be reviewed in Chapter 6. Canine **demodicosis**, caused by **Demodex** *canis* mites, may affect the ear pinnae and also sometimes are found in the ear canal. Further information on these mites can be found in Chapter 6. Two species of *Demodex* mites, *Demodex cati* and *Demodex gatoi*, may be found on the ear pinnae or in the ear canals of cats. These are discussed further in Chapter 6.

Chiggers are small, orange-colored mites that usually are picked up from woods and fields during late summer or fall. Chiggers may infest the ears, face, legs, feet, and belly of cats and dogs, causing itching and papules. See

Chapter 6 for more information. Ixodid (hard-bodied) **ticks** may be found on the ear pinnae or within the ear canals of dogs and cats, whereas argasid (soft-bodied) ticks usually affect only the ear canals. More information on ticks is in Chapter 6. **Lice** are subdivided into biting and sucking categories; both types may occasionally affect ear pinnae. See Chapter 6 for additional information on lice affecting cats and dogs. Flies may feed on the ear pinnae of dogs and cats. The ear tips and the outside edge of ear folds are favorite feeding sites. Clinical signs include papules and bloody crusts. See Chapter 6 for information on fly bite dermatitis. Fleas also may produce papules and bloody crusts on ear pinnae. See Chapter 6 for information on fleas and flea control.

Allergic: The skin of the ear pinnae and that lining the ear canals are commonly affected in dogs and cats with allergies. Allergic contact dermatitis may develop as an allergic reaction to physical contact with plants, food bowls, carpets, cleaners, and ear medications; further information can be found in Chapter 4. **Atopic dermatitis** results in redness, skin inflammation, and itching in

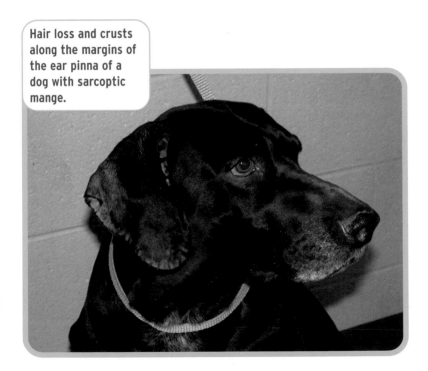

Hair loss and crusts along the margins of the ear pinna of a dog with sarcoptic mange.

response to **allergens** found in the pet's environment. Chapter 4 contains more information on atopy in dogs and cats. Food allergies occur when a pet becomes sensitive to an allergen found in foods. Clinical signs, diagnosis, and management of food allergies can be found in Chapter 4. Mosquito-bite **hypersensitivity** may result in lesions on either the inside or outside surface of the ear pinnae of cats and is reviewed in Chapters 4 and 6.

Infectious: **Mycobacteria** may produce **nodular** (lumpy) lesions on the ear pinnae of cats and dogs. In dogs these lesions sometimes are called "canine leproid granulomas syndrome" or "canine leprosy." Feline leprosy is caused by *Mycobacterium lepraemurium,* but the specific species causing leprosy in dogs has not been determined. Treatment may involve surgical removal or long-term treatment with doxycycline, amoxicillin-clavulanic acid (Clavamox), enrofloxacin (Baytril), and other antibiotics. **Ringworm** may involve the ear pinnae of dogs and cats as either a local area of infection or part of a generalized infection. Information on the diagnosis and treatment of ringworm may be reviewed in Chapter 8. *Malassezia pachydermatis* commonly is involved in **otitis externa** and also may cause dermatitis on the earflaps. See Chapter 8 for additional information on *Malassezia* der-

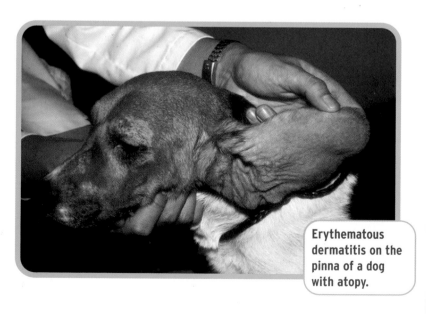

Erythematous dermatitis on the pinna of a dog with atopy.

matitis. Feline cowpox virus can cause lesions on the ear pinnae, neck, and forelegs of cats. This virus is spread by voles and other small rodents. Lesions include papules (small, red bumps), crusts, and hair loss developing 10 to 14 days after the cat is bitten by a **carrier** rodent. Skin biopsies or blood tests are useful in the diagnosis of feline cowpox. Treatment is supportive (e.g., antibiotics to prevent **secondary** bacterial infections). **Leishmaniasis** is a **protozoal** infection that primarily affects dogs and people in the Mediterranean basin. It also has been reported in Mexico, Central America, and in parts of the United States (Oklahoma, Texas, Alabama, Ohio, Michigan, and Maryland). One of the most common signs in dogs is hair loss and dry scales on the earflaps, head, and legs. Skin biopsies or blood tests can be used to diagnose leishmaniasis. A variety of drugs have been used for treatment including meglumine antimonite, allopurinol, aminosidine, amphotericin B, metronidazole, and ketoconazole. The outcome ranges from good to poor, and many affected dogs fail to improve.

Hormonal (endocrine): Hair loss is a common symptom associated with canine **hypothyroidism**, **Cushing's disease**, and other endocrine-related skin diseases of dogs and cats. The ear pinnae may be affected in these disorders. See Chapter 7 for additional information on endocrine-related skin diseases.

Immune-mediated: **Pemphigus foliaceus** (PF) is the most common immune-mediated skin disease of dogs and cats. Ear pinnae and other areas of the head frequently are affected by PF; lesions may include papules, **pustules** (pus-filled lesions), **ulcers**, crusts, and hair loss. Ear canals also are frequently affected and may be ulcerated with **purulent** (pus-like) discharges. Pemphigus erythematosus is another immune-mediated skin disease that commonly involves the face and ear pinnae with lesions that include papules, pustules, crusts, and hair loss. Discoid **lupus erythematosus** generally affects the **nasal planum** and the bridge of the nose; in rare cases, the earflaps may have ulcers and crusts. Systemic lupus erythematosus (SLE) may affect any body organ. Lesions caused by SLE on the ear pinnae include hair loss, ulcers, and crusts. Bullous pemphigoid is another immune-mediated skin disease that may occasionally produce blisters and ulcers on the ear pinnae. Several forms of **vasculitis** in dogs and cats are linked to **antigen-antibody (immune) complexes** lodging in small blood vessels; these cause thrombosis (blood clots blocking the vessels) and result in **necrosis** (tissue death). The margins of the ears are common sites of thrombosis; death of the cells along the edges of the ear may result in a notched appearance to the earflap. **Auricular chondrosis** is a rare immune-mediated disease that affects the cartilage in the ears. Ear pinnae become red, swollen, curled, and painful. Diagnosis is based on biopsies of the ears; these show dying cartilage and **infiltrates** of **lymphocytes** and **plasma cells**. Alopecia areata is an immune-mediated disease affecting hair follicles that results in localized areas of hair loss; ear pinnae are one of the sites that may be affected. Additional information about immune-mediated skin diseases is given in Chapter 9.

Neoplastic (tumors/cancer): Sebaceous gland **adenomas** are one of the most common tumors involving the ear pinnae. These **benign** tumors are particularly common in older poodles and cocker spaniels but may occur in any breed. Surgical removal or laser surgery usually cures the problem. **Histiocytomas** are small, round, raised tumors that may develop on the earflaps of young dogs; these tumors usually resolve on their own within 3 months. Squamous cell carcinomas are most common in lightly pigmented pets, particularly those frequently exposed to UVB radiation (e.g., cats and dogs that like to lie in the sun). These tumors are malignant but usually grow slowly, and surgical removal may cure this disease if performed early. Sunlight damage also may encourage the development of tumors of the blood vessels in the ear pinnae; these are called *hemangiomas* if benign and *hemangiosarcomas* if malignant. Surgical removal usually cures the disease. Mast cell tumors (MCTs) develop in the second layer of skin (dermis) or tissue just underneath the skin (subcutis). In cats, MCTs usually are located on the head and neck, although they may be found on the ear pinnae. In dogs, MCTs usually are located on the rear half of the body, although they can occur anywhere. Cutaneous T-cell lymphoma (CTCL) may cause widespread scaling, crusting, and hair loss. The ear pinnae may be involved and may have **plaques** (raised areas), **nodules**, or ulcers on them. Diagnosis of most tumors is based on skin biopsies. Further information on skin tumors is found in Chapter 13.

Miscellaneous: Multiple apocrine or ceruminal gland **cysts** sometimes are seen in the skin around the opening of the ear canal and within the ear canal itself. These cysts appear as blue blisters or growths on the inner (concave) pinna and within the ear canal. This condition, apocrine **cystadenomatosis**, occurs in cats more often than in dogs. The lesions are benign but may multiply or grow enough to block the ear canals; laser surgery may be used to remove the cysts. Puppy **strangles** (juvenile pyoderma, juvenile cellulitis) often causes swelling of the muzzle, eyelids, earflaps, and **submandibular lymph nodes**. An infection of the outer ear, accompanied by pus-

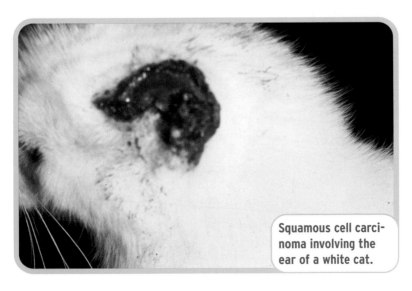

Squamous cell carcinoma involving the ear of a white cat.

filled discharge, also may be present. The diagnosis and treatment of this disease are discussed in Chapter 5. **Zinc-responsive dermatosis** often involves the face and may result in redness, scales, and crusts on the ear pinnae. See Chapter 10 for further information. **Sebaceous adenitis** is a disease associated with the destruction of sebaceous glands and resulting hair loss. Lesions often start on the head and earflaps with scaling, **follicular casts,** and a wavy pattern of hair loss. See Chapter 10 for additional information on this disease. **Aural** (ear) **hematomas** are blood-filled swellings on the inner (concave) side of the ear pinna. Vigorous shaking or scratching at the ear may result in fractures (breaks) within the ear cartilage. Bleeding from a torn blood vessel within the ear cartilage or skin produces a hematoma (blood clot between the cartilage and the skin). Your veterinarian will drain the hematoma and use drains or sutures to prevent the hematoma from returning. The ear usually is bandaged against the head of the dog or cat. To help prevent recurrence, your veterinarian will search for the cause of the head shaking or ear scratching and treat any problems found.

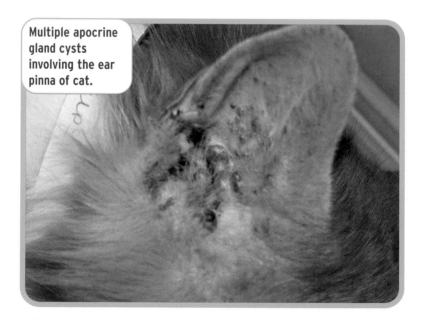

Multiple apocrine gland cysts involving the ear pinna of cat.

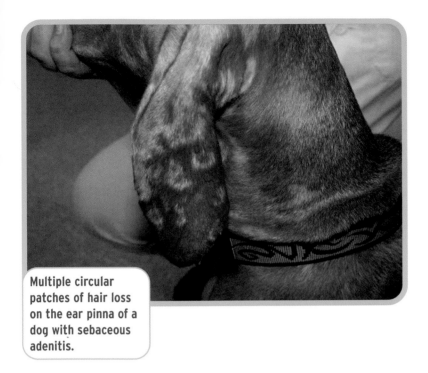

Multiple circular patches of hair loss on the ear pinna of a dog with sebaceous adenitis.

Outer Ear Infections (Otitis Externa)

Otitis externa is the most common disease affecting the ears of dogs and cats. The term *otitis externa* simply means "inflammation of the ear canal"; it describes the location of the disease but does not provide further information regarding the underlying causes of the disease. Identification of the underlying causes is essential for successful treatment and prevention.

Clinical Signs

Early signs of otitis externa are redness of the ear pinna, external meatus (opening of the ear canal), and lining of the ear canal. Other signs may include head shaking, ear scratching, pain when the ears are touched, and a purulent (puslike) or ceruminous (waxy) ear discharge. With recurring or chronic otitis externa, the skin and glands lining the ear canals become **hyperplastic** (thickened, increased in size) and may narrow the ear canal (**stenosis**). In some chronic cases, the cartilage around the ear canal becomes **calcified** and may even turn into bone. Underlying causes of otitis externa commonly are classified as predisposing, primary, and perpetuating causes.

Predisposing Causes

Factors that increase the likelihood that a cat or dog will develop otitis externa are called *predisposing causes*. Recognizing and addressing these factors will help prevent otitis externa.

Anatomic and conformational factors: Breeds with long, drooping ears (spaniels and hounds), narrow ear canals (Chinese Shar-Peis), and excessive hair in the external ear canal (Poodles, Lhasa Apsos, and others) may be prone to otitis externa because these factors decrease air circulation in the ear canal and may help trap moisture. Shaving the hair on the inside (concave surface) of the earflaps and trimming hairs around the opening of the ear canals may be helpful. Whether hairs should be plucked from within the ear canal is a matter that should be discussed with your veterinarian.

Pendulous (hanging) ears predispose dogs to reoccurring otitis externa.

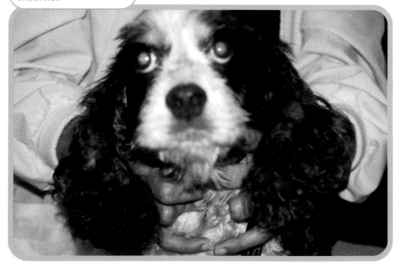

Examples of Conditions Associated With Ear Disease in Cats and Dogs

Predisposing Conditions	Primary Causes	Perpetuating Factors
Conformation Stenotic canals Pendulous ear pinna Excess hair in ears	**Parasites** Ear mites *Demodex* Ticks Others	Bacteria Yeast **Progressive Pathologic Changes** Glandular hyperplasia Epithelial hyperplasia Failure of normal cell movement Stenosis Fibrosis Calcification/ossification **Otitis Media**
Increased Moisture Swimming Bathing Use of water to clean ears High humidity	**Foreign Bodies** Foxtails Other plant awns Dried medications Other objects	
Excessive Earwax	**Allergies** Food/dietary Atopy Contact allergies	
Immune Suppression Disease (endocrine, metabolic, cancer, others) Drugs (corticosteroids, chemotherapy, others)	**Endocrine Diseases** Hypothyroidism Cushing's disease	
	Immune-Mediated Diseases Pemphigus complex Lupus complex	
Iatrogenic Inappropriate ear cleaners (irritants) Hair plucking/depilatory agents Trauma from cotton swabs	**Trauma** Iatrogenic damage Fight injuries	
	Keratinization Disorders Primary seborrhea Sebaceous adenitis	
Obstructive Ear Disease Polyps Ceruminal gland tumors	**Miscellaneous** Puppy strangles Viral infections	

Excessive moisture: Water or high humidity within the ear canals can lead to **maceration** (softening) of the skin surface. Maceration removes the protective barrier of the normal **stratum corneum** (horny layer of the skin) and allows for the proliferation of bacteria and **yeast** in the ears. Pets that swim or receive frequent baths are at highest risk of having excessive moisture in their ear canals. Restricting access to swimming and being careful not to get water in the ears during bathing will help prevent excessive moisture from collecting in the ear canals. Drying agents (**astringents**) also can be used to help keep humidity levels low in the ears.

Excessive cerumen (earwax) production: Overactivity of the ceruminal glands may result from excessive moisture in the ears, hormonal imbalances or deficiencies (hypothyroidism, sex hormone imbalances), or genetic factors (the condition is common in Cocker Spaniels). Buildup of **cerumen** may result in the overgrowth of yeast and bacteria. Correction of underlying causes and regular cleaning of the ears with a **ceruminolytic** agent are necessary to control this problem.

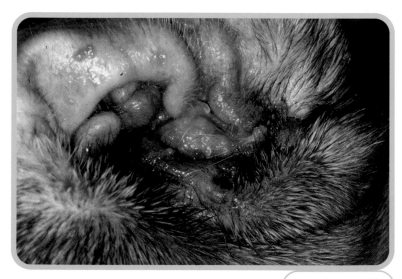

Ceruminous otitis externa.

Iatrogenic factors: Trauma caused by hair plucking or the use of cotton-tipped swabs for ear cleaning may damage the lining of the ear canal and result in inflammation. The use of irritating solutions for ear cleaning also may cause inflammation of the ear canals. If irritation results after ear cleaning or hair plucking, consult your veterinarian for advice on different methods to clean the ears and remove excessive hair.

Obstructive ear disease: **Polyps** or tumors in the ear canals may cause obstruction, preventing air circulation and movement of earwax from the ears. **Nasopharyngeal polyps** are a common cause of obstructive ear disease in young cats. Ceruminal gland tumors are most common in older dogs and cats. Removal of the polyps or tumors is necessary to resolve this problem.

Immunodeficiencies: **Immunodeficiencies** may be hereditary (for example, cyclic hematopoiesis, **IgA** deficiency, lethal acrodermatitis, and others; see Chapter 10 for more information). They also may be a result of endocrine or **metabolic diseases** or cancers. Drugs such as **corticosteroids** and chemotherapy agents may suppress the **immune system** and make pets prone to infections involving the ears and other areas of the body.

Primary Causes

Primary causes of otitis externa are diseases that cause inflammation of the external ear canal. Successful treatment of otitis externa requires identifying and correcting these diseases.

Parasites: The most common parasite causing otitis externa is the ear mite, **Otodectes** *cynotis*. Ear mites are present in up to 50% of cases of otitis externa in cats and 5% to 10% of cases in dogs. Affected ears often have a discharge inside that resembles coffee grounds (dark brown to black, crumbly texture). The veterinarian diagnoses ear mites by using a magnifying **otoscope** or **video-otoscope**, which reveals white mites crawling in the ear canals. Cotton-tipped applicator sticks may be used to remove debris from the ear canals. This material is mixed with mineral oil and examined under a microscope to identify mites. **Demodex** mites also may cause otitis externa. *Demodex canis* is involved in dogs and either *Demodex cati* or *Demodex gatoi* in cats. *Demodex* mites typically are associated with a waxy discharge. The mites can be found by microscopic examination of discharge from the ears mixed with mineral oil. The spinous ear tick, *Otobius megninii*, is another cause of parasitic otitis externa. Spinous ear ticks are most common in south-western regions of the United States, where they infest dogs and occasionally cats. Bugs such as beetles, flies, and mosquitoes occasionally may enter the ear canal and cause otitis externa. **Ectoparasites** that mostly affect the ear pinnae, such as *Sarcoptes scabiei*, *Notoedres cati*, *Cheyletiella* spp., and *Eutrombicula* spp. (chiggers), rarely cause otitis externa.

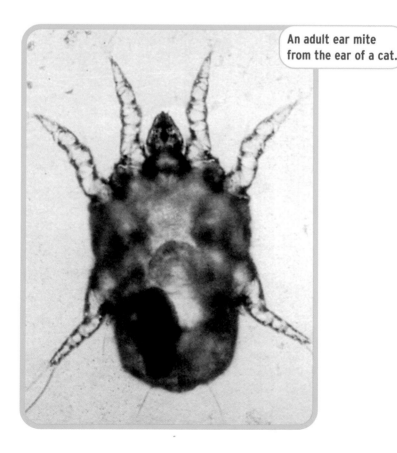

An adult ear mite from the ear of a cat.

Foreign bodies: Foxtail and other plant awns are a common cause of otitis externa. Plant awns may make their way into the deepest part of the ear canal and may penetrate through the **tympanic membrane** (ear drum) to cause **otitis media** (middle ear infection). Other types of material that may cause irritation in the ear canals include the following:

- **Broken hairs**
- **Dirt**
- **Sand**
- **Dried otic (ear) medications**
- **Cerumenoliths (balls of dried cerumen)**
- **Foreign objects placed in the ears by children or others**

These can be seen with a magnifying otoscope or video-otoscope.

Allergies: In my referral practice, more than 80% of cases of chronic otitis externa are due to underlying food allergies or **atopy** (environmental allergies). In most cases, affected dogs or cats show other signs of allergies, such as face rubbing, foot licking, and armpit scratching, and also may have a history of ongoing skin infections. However, otitis externa is the only clinical symptom in approximately 5% of pets with environmental allergies

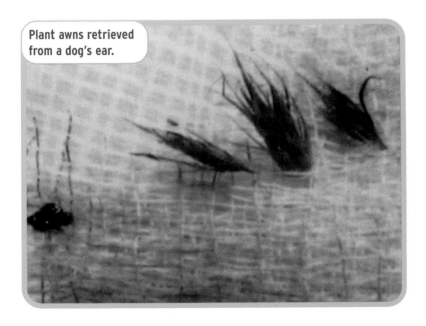

Plant awns retrieved from a dog's ear.

and in up to 25% of pets with food allergies. Allergic contact dermatitis occasionally develops in dogs and cats treated with otic preparations, especially those containing neomycin (a topical antibiotic). The diagnosis and management of allergies is discussed in Chapter 4.

Keratinization disorders (seborrhea): Abnormalities in **keratinization** or **sebum** production may affect both the earflaps and the ear canals. These disorders may be genetic (see Chapter 10) or caused by endocrine diseases (hormonal deficiencies or imbalances; see Chapter 7). Problems with keratinization, the process by which the epidermis forms its outer layer, increase the likelihood that the ear canals will become overgrown with both bacteria and yeast.

Immune-mediated diseases: Pemphigus foliaceus, pemphigus erythematosus, discoid lupus erythematosus, cutaneous vasculitis, and bullous pemphigoid may cause ulceration and inflammation of the ear canals. These diseases almost always affect other locations of the skin or mucous membranes in addition to the ear canals. See Chapter 9 for more information on immune-mediated skin diseases.

Purulent otitis externa in a dog with pemphigus foliaceus.

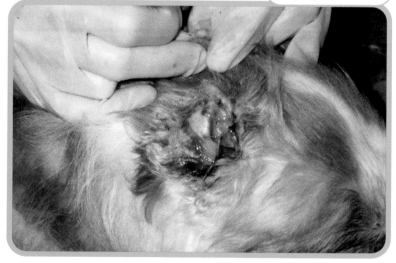

Trauma: Injuries from fights or blunt trauma to the head may cause damage to the earflaps or ear canal.

Miscellaneous: The ear pinnae and canals may be the first site of pus formation in puppies with juvenile pyoderma (strangles). The ears may be affected by cowpox and other viral infections of cats.

Perpetuating Causes

Perpetuating causes do not cause the onset of otitis externa; however, these factors will cause the disease to continue once it has started. Many perpetuating causes become involved in a positive feedback loop in which they act to worsen inflammation, increasing their own growth or severity as a result. For example, growing bacteria produce inflammatory by-products and also trigger the host's defense system to produce inflammation; inflammation helps bacteria to grow, causing more inflammation. This positive feedback results in progressive worsening of the disease. Once present, perpetuating causes of otitis externa must be treated.

Bacteria: The normal ear canal contains several species of bacteria; these are referred to as its normal **flora**. Inflammation of the ear results in **serum** discharge and a warm, moist environment that favors the overgrowth of bacteria. As previously discussed, bacterial overgrowth worsens the inflammation and the infection then increases in its severity. Chronic cases of otitis externa may have overgrowths of strains of bacteria such as *Pseudomonas aeruginosa* or *Proteus mirabilis* that are very difficult to kill with most antibiotics. These infections may cause a "fruity" odor in the ears.

Yeast: Malassezia pachydermatis also is part of the normal flora of the ear canal. Yeast rapidly overgrow in inflamed ears, especially in those with a waxy discharge. The odor caused by yeast infections is often the first sign that excessive yeast is present in the ears.

Otitis media: Otitis media is an inflammation of the middle ear. The most common cause of otitis media in dogs and cats is of the penetration of infection from otitis externa across the tympanic membrane (ear drum). Other possible routes of infection are through the blood or from a nasal or respiratory infection passing up the **Eustachian tube**. Approximately 50% of dogs with chronic otitis externa have otitis media at the same time. **Topical** (locally applied) antibiotics and antifungal agents are rarely effective in treating otitis media. Infection within the middle ear cavity may cause reinfection of the external ear canal.

Progressive proliferative changes: Inflammation and thickening of the skin lining the ear canals keeps cells, earwax, and other debris from being naturally moved out of the ears. Buildup of debris results in an ideal environment for bacterial overgrowth. Ceruminal and sebaceous glands increase in size, which causes further narrowing of the ear canal and trapping of debris and moisture. In addition, epithelial and glandular **hyperplasia** (enlargement) may keep topical medications from entering the ear canals.

Diagnostic Evaluation

The first step in evaluating a pet with ear disease is reviewing the pet's life history for information that provides clues to underlying problems associated with the ear disease. The following table lists important questions that your veterinarian may ask in gathering a complete history for pets with ear disease. Examples of ways in which an animal's history helps to identify underlying problems include the following:

- **A dog that likes to swim or that is bathed frequently may simply be getting too much water in its ears.**
- **A kitten that was recently adopted from a shelter may have a contagious disease such as ear mites or a ringworm infection.**
- **A middle-aged, lethargic Labrador Retriever that also has hair loss may have hypothyroidism.**
- **A dog that has been treated repeatedly with ear drops that used to work but don't any longer may**

have developed a contact allergy to the ingredients in the medication or may have developed an infection that is resistant to that medication.

■ A 3-year-old Dalmatian that is licking its front feet and shaking its head may have atopy.

Important Information to Consider When Evaluating a Pet with Ear Disease

Signalment

Breed (predispositions to underlying factors and primary diseases)

Age (young pets more likely to have ear mites, older pets to have tumors)

Background

Where and when obtained (shelters have increased risk for mites)

Other pets in household (are other pets affected with skin or ear problems?)

Housing and Exercise

Is most of the pet's time spent indoors or outdoors? (sources of allergies, ectoparasites)

Is the pet allowed to roam free? (sources of ectoparasites, plant awns)

Does the pet have regular contact with other pets? (sources of ectoparasites)

Does the pet swim? (moisture predisposes to infections)

Grooming History

Was the pet bathed recently? (source of water in ears)

Has the pet received ear care recently? (plucking or use of ear swabs may have irritated ear canals)

Important Information to Consider When Evaluating a Pet with Ear Disease—cont'd

Dermatologic History

Is the pet itchy? (allergies, ectoparasites)

Does the pet have other skin lesions? (keratinization defects, immune-mediated diseases, fungal diseases, ectoparasites)

Ear History

Has the pet had other episodes of ear disease?
If so, what was the diagnosis?
What treatments have been given?
What was the response?
Are the symptoms this time similar to previous ones?

General History

Does the pet have any other symptoms of disease?
Any changes in appetite or amount of water consumed?
Is the pet on any medications?
What diet is the pet fed? Any treats? Any changes in diet over the past year?

Your veterinarian will conduct a thorough physical examination to find additional clues that might identify primary causes of otitis externa. For example, an enlarged liver may be a sign of underlying Cushing's disease, whereas enlarged lymph nodes are a sign of chronic infections or tumors. A thorough examination of the skin frequently provides clues to help in diagnosing primary causes of otitis externa. The lining of the ear canals is an extension of the skin. Frequently, the same type of changes found in the ears will be found elsewhere on the body. The location and pattern of the lesions often provide clues to help identify the underlying disease. For example, papules and pustules involving the nose, ears, and skin around the eyes, plus thickened, cracked footpads, strongly suggest pemphigus foliaceus. Severe itching accompanied by hair loss and crusts on the ear edges, elbows, and hocks may be a sign of sarcoptic mange. Swelling of the muzzle and ears in conjunction with enlarged submandibular lymph nodes in an 8-week-old Dachshund suggests puppy strangles (juvenile pyoderma).

The next step in the evaluation of a pet with ear disease is to examine the ear pinnae and ear canals. Samples of any discharge present in the ear canals should be collected for microscopic examination and possible culture. Samples for culture should be taken from the deep portion of the ear canal using a sterile cotton-tipped swab. Samples for microscopic examination also are collected using a cotton-tipped swab. The swab is rolled on a glass slide to produce a thin layer of cells and ear debris that can be stained and viewed using a microscope. Important features to be noted in the **cytologic** examination include the numbers and types of bacteria and yeast present, the numbers and type of **white blood cells** present, and whether there are neoplastic cells (cancer cells). Additional ear swabs should be taken to check for parasites within the ear canal. These swabs are rolled in mineral oil placed on a glass slide. The slide is then viewed using a microscope; mites can be seen swimming in the mineral oil.

The entire length of both ear canals should be examined using an otoscope or video-otoscope. Inflamed ears are painful, so sedation or general anesthesia is often required to perform a thorough examination. A variety of primary causes can be diagnosed using an otoscope. These include foreign bodies, some parasites (ticks, ear

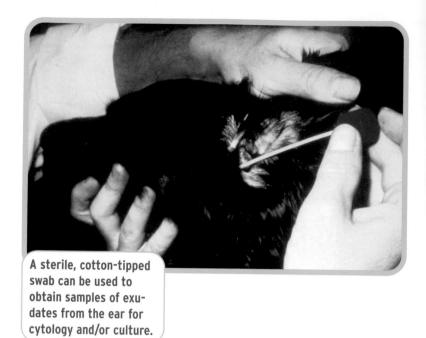

A sterile, cotton-tipped swab can be used to obtain samples of exudates from the ear for cytology and/or culture.

mites, bugs), polyps, and tumors. Predisposing causes of otitis externa that can be identified during otoscopic examination include stenotic (narrowed) canals and hair in the canals. Perpetuating causes of otitis externa that can be diagnosed on otoscopic examination include thickening of the canal epithelium and otitis media (identified by a ruptured or bulging ear drum).

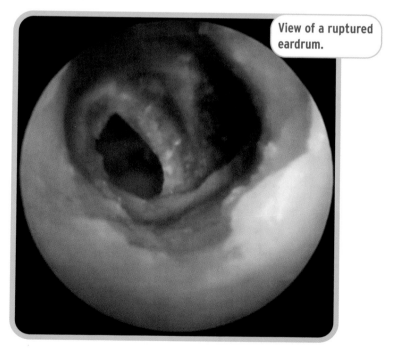

View of a ruptured eardrum.

Biopsies should be taken from any ear masses to check for cancer. Biopsies also should be taken if an immune-mediated disease or a keratinization defect is suspected. **Blood chemistry profiles** and specific hormone assays are needed to diagnose endocrine diseases (see Chapter 7).

Radiographs, **computerized tomography** (CT scan), and **magnetic resonance imaging** (MRI) are useful in evaluating the severity of ear infections. **Electrophysiologic testing** can be used to evaluate hearing. Most veterinary hospitals are equipped to do radiographs. Referral to specialists usually is needed to obtain CT, MRI, and electrophysiologic testing.

Ear Cleaning

Thorough ear cleaning is helpful in resolving ear infections. Cleaning removes nutrient-rich discharges that harbor microorganisms and help them to thrive. Pus-filled discharge is also rich in **proteolytic enzymes** released from white blood cells; these enzymes worsen inflammation of the lining of the ear canals. Therefore removal of discharge from the ears helps in decreasing inflammation. Discharge found in the ears interferes with the ability of antimicrobial medications to physically reach the organisms that the medications are meant to eliminate. Because of this, ears must be clean for medications to work properly. Flushing the ears also may help remove foreign bodies.

Initial ear flushing usually is performed by the veterinarian during the evaluation of the ear canal. Follow-up flushing of the ears often is recommended as part of the pet's at-home care regimen. Owners who are unable

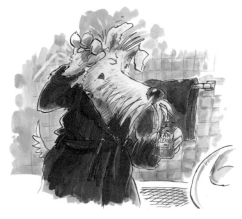

to clean their pets' ears at home may need to take their pets to a veterinarian or grooming facility for ear cleaning every 1 to 2 days until the ear disease is resolved.

It is important to consult your veterinarian to determine the proper type of ear cleanser for your pet. Many types of ear cleansers are available. Most work by breaking up and liquefying earwax so that it can be flushed or wiped out of the ear. *Ceruminolytic activity* refers to the ability of a product to break up earwax. Ceruminolytic products containing dioctyl sodium sulfosuccinate (DSS) or propylene glycol are excellent for cleaning purulent discharges (pus) from ears. Hard, waxy secretions are more difficult to break up and may require the use of ceruminolytic products containing squalene or urea peroxide. Some ceruminolytics, such as ones containing urea peroxide, are very strong and must be thoroughly rinsed from the ear after use to prevent damage to the ear tissues. Many ear cleansers contain **antiseptic** agents to decrease numbers of bacteria and yeast in the ears. Exercise caution when using products containing povidone-iodine because iodine causes irritation in many pets. Chlorhexidine-containing products should not be used in pets with a ruptured eardrum because chlorhexidine can cause deafness. Rinses containing Tris-EDTA (ethylenediaminetetraacetic acid) rupture cell membranes of many bacteria and also are alkalinizing (raise pH), which increases the activity of the aminoglycoside class of topical antibiotics (e.g., neomycin, gentamicin, tobramycin, amikacin). Other rinses contain acetic acid or boric acid to decrease the pH within the ear canal, which discourages the growth of yeast organisms. The best rinse to use for an individual pet depends on the type of discharge present, the types of organisms present in its ear, and any other medications being used in the ear. The final rinse used in cleaning the ear should contain an **astringent** (drying agent). Solutions containing alcohol should not be used in pets with ulcerated or inflamed ears because alcohol can irritate these ears and cause pain.

Ceruminolytic and Drying Agents in Ear-Cleaning Products

Ceruminolytic Agents	Drying Agents
Carbamide peroxide	Acetic acid
Cocamidopropyl phosphatidyl	Aluminum acetate
Dioctyl sodium sulfosuccinate (DSS)	Benzoic acid
Glycerine	Benzyl alcohol
Glycerol	Boric acid
Hydroxypropyl cellulose	Isopropyl alcohol
Isopropyl myristate liquid petroleum	Lactic acid
Lanolin oil	Malic acid
Methylparaben	Salicylic acid
Mineral oil	Silicon dioxide
Oil of eucalyptus	Sulfur, colloidal
Propylparaben	Zinc oxide
Propylene glycol	
Sodium lauryl sulfate	
Squalene	
Surfactants	
Tetrasodium EDTA	
Tween	
Urea peroxide	

The first step in cleaning the ear is to gather the supplies that you will need. These include one or more ear cleansers or rinses, plenty of cotton balls or cotton squares, a large bath towel to put under the pet's head, any prescribed ear medications, scissors, and a trash bag. Start by gently cleaning the inside of the ear pinna. You may wish to use scissors to carefully trim any excess or matted hair from the opening of the ear canal and the inner flap of the pinna. Next, fill the ear canal with the ear cleanser. Gently massage the base of the ear to help spread the cleanser around and break up wax and other debris in the ear canal. For maximal benefit, allow the ear cleanser to remain in the ear canal for approximately 5 minutes. Use cotton balls or squares to gently swab inside the ear to remove liquid and loosened debris. Cotton balls and squares are much safer than cotton-tipped applicator sticks and work just as well. Repeat the applications of the ear cleanser, and wipe with cotton until all debris and discharge have been removed. If a ceruminolytic product is used for cleaning, the final rinse should include a drying (astringent) ear product. Apply any prescribed medication after the ear is clean and dry. Finish by praising your pet and playing with it or giving it a favorite treat.

Treatment

Successful treatment of otitis externa requires identification and management of predisposing, primary, and perpetuating causes of the disease. This section provides information on the management of bacterial and yeast infections (perpetuating causes) and ear inflammation (symptom and perpetuating cause). Other chapters in the book provide information on the management of primary causes that can initiate otitis externa.

Topical therapy is extremely important in the resolution of bacterial and yeast infections. The choice of products to use often is made on the basis of cytologic examination of the discharge from the ears. Antibiotic sensitivity tests are based on blood concentrations of drugs and may not predict the effectiveness of topical ear medications because topical medications can provide much higher drug concentrations than would be possible when the drug is given orally or by injection.

Many ear treatment products contain several active ingredients (antibacterial, antifungal, antiparasitic, anti-inflammatory drugs) in a vehicle (carrier product). Vehicles influence the way the drug dissolves, maintain drug activity, and affect the way the drug is absorbed into the body. Vehicles may be aqueous (water-based), demulcents (solubilizing agents), or **emollients** (**occlusive** agents that carry water-insoluble drugs). Demulcents used in otic (ear) products include polyethylene glycol, propylene glycol, and glycerin. Emollients used in ear products include vegetable oils, animal fats (e.g., lanolin), and hydrocarbons (e.g., petrolatum, mineral oil, paraffin).

Antibacterial agents used in ear medications include aminoglycosides (neomycin, gentamicin, amikacin, tobramycin), fluoroquinolones (enrofloxacin, ciprofloxacin, difloxacin, marbofloxacin), polymyxins (polymyxin B, polymyxin E), silver sulfadiazine, chloramphenicol, and fusidic acid. Antifungal agents used in ear medications include nystatin, thiabendazole, clotrimazole, miconazole, ketoconazole, itraconazole, fluconazole, amphotericin B, and terbinafine. Anti-inflammatory agents used in ear medications include hydrocortisone, dexamethasone, betamethasone, triamcinolone, fluocinolone, and dimethyl sulfoxide (DMSO). Antiparasitic agents in ear medications include carbaryl, pyrethrins, sulfur, and milbemycin. **Systemic** (whole-body) treatment with selamectin, ivermectin, or fipronil also may be used for the elimination of ear mites and other ectoparasites causing otitis.

Treatment of **acute** (first-time) cases of otitis externa often includes an initial ear flush at the veterinarian's office followed by daily or every-other-day ear cleaning at home. A topical ear medication will be prescribed on the basis of cytologic and otoscopic findings. The topical medication usually is prescribed for twice-daily use for a

Active Ingredients in Ear Medications

Antiinflammatory Agents	Antibacterial Agents	Antifungal Agents	Antiseptic Agents	Antiparasitic Agents
Hydrocortisone	Acetic acid	Acetic acid	Chlorhexidine	Pyrethrins
Prednisolone	Boric acid	Boric acid	Povidone-iodine	Carbaryl
Triamcinolone	Chloramphenicol	Clotrimazole		Rotenone
Isoflupredone acetate	Ciprofloxacin	Miconazole		Thiabendazole
Betamethasone	Colistin	Nystatin		Milbemycin
Dexamethasone	Enrofloxacin	Thiabendazole		
Fluocinolone	Gentamicin	Zinc undecylenate		
DMSO	Neomycin			
	Ofloxacin			
	Polymyxin B sulfate			
	Silver sulfadiazine			
	Ticarcillin			
	Tobramycin			
	Tris EDTA			

minimum of 7 to 14 days. The pet should be re-examined by the veterinarian at the end of the treatment plan to check its response and determine whether additional treatment is needed. In some cases, the veterinarian may recommend treatment with oral corticosteroids, oral antibiotics, or oral antifungal agents.

Where We Stand

Topical steroids are useful in relieving ear inflammation and pain caused by environmental and food allergies. However, topical steroids are absorbed into the body through the lining of the ear canals and can have serious side effects, including iatrogenic Cushing's disease. To prevent these serious side effects, (1) avoid using topical steroids every day and (2) use the lowest possible concentration and weakest corticosteroid that will control the pet's signs. Hydrocortisone is the safest corticosteroid for use in eardrops; it is the least likely to cause serious side effects with long-term use. The best solution is to identify the source of your pet's allergies and eliminate your pet's exposure to that allergen.

Long-Term Management

Dogs and cats with chronic or recurring cases of otitis externa should be tested for all possible primary causes of ear inflammation. Long-term management plans are needed when a primary cause cannot be identified or controlled or when the pet has ongoing predisposing or perpetuating causes of otitis externa. Management plans must be tailored for each pet. Many management protocols include regular ear cleaning (frequency may vary from daily to once weekly). The type of product to be used for ear cleaning and any other topical medication to be used on a regular basis depend on the nature of the pet's ear disease:

- Ceruminolytic agents for ceruminous otitis with few organisms
- Hydrocortisone anti-inflammatory agents for chronic inflammation with few organisms
- Antifungal or antiseptic agents for chronic yeast infections
- Antibacterial or antiseptic agents for chronic bacterial infections
- Antiseptics for chronic mixed infections

Middle Ear Infections (Otitis Media)

Otitis media is an inflammatory disease affecting the middle ear cavity. It occurs in as many as 50% of dogs and cats with chronic otitis externa and occasionally develops in pets with no history of external ear disease. Cats may develop otitis media as a side-effect of respiratory disease or because of a **nasopharyngeal polyp** growing in the middle ear cavity. Many pets have otitis media without any outward signs other than, if present, those associated with otitis externa. A few pets with otitis

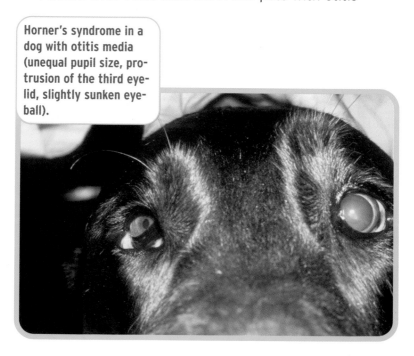

Horner's syndrome in a dog with otitis media (unequal pupil size, protrusion of the third eyelid, slightly sunken eyeball).

media develop **neurologic signs** as a result of nerve damage within the middle ear. These signs may include a head tilt, drooping of one side of the face with an inability to blink the eye on that side (**facial nerve paralysis**), and unequal eye pupil size (**Horner's syndrome**).

A diagnosis of otitis media may be determined by finding a ruptured or bulging eardrum on otoscopic or video-otoscopic examination or through the use of radiographs, CT, or MRI. A **myringotomy** can be performed to obtain samples from the middle ear cavity. The pet is anesthetized for the myringotomy procedure, which involves passing a needle or **catheter** through a small surgical cut in the eardrum and removing fluid and cells from the middle ear cavity for cytologic examination and **culture and sensitivity testing**.

Treatment of otitis media starts with identifying predisposing causes (otitis externa and its various causes, respiratory infections and their causes, polyps or other tumors) and developing a treatment plan to correct the predisposing cause. Management of otitis media usually includes a thorough flushing (cleaning) of the middle ear cavity (**tympanic bulla**), introduction of topical medications into the middle ear cavity, and use of systemic (whole-body) antimicrobials and systemic corticosteroids to reduce inflammation. If nerve paralysis prevents the pet from blinking its eye, topical lubricating agents (eye ointments) should be used to protect the **cornea**. Surgery is required when medical therapy is unsuccessful in resolving otitis media or when a polyp or tumor is present (see Chapter 12).

Inner Ear Infections (Otitis Interna)

Otitis interna is an inflammation affecting the structures of the inner ear—these include the auditory ossicles, cochlea, and the semicircular canals involved in hearing (auditory function) and maintaining balance (vestibular system). Most cases of otitis interna are thought to be a result of otitis media spreading into the inner ear. Other cases are caused by the use of medications that damage the cells of the auditory and vestibular systems. Examples of medications that can cause **ototoxicity** include the following: potent ceruminolytic agents, antiseptics (especially chlorhexidine), antifungal agents (especially amphotericin B), antibiotics (especially aminoglycosides), antineoplastic agents (several chemotherapy drugs), and miscellaneous agents (detergents, potassium bromide, mercury, and others).

Clinical signs of otitis interna include a head tilt toward the affected side, rapid side-to-side eye movements (nystagmus), incoordination, circling or falling to the affected side, vomiting, and deafness (hearing loss may not be noticeable if only one ear is affected). Diagnosis involves thorough physical, otoscopic, and neurologic examinations and the use of radiographic, CT, or MRI evaluations. Treatment involves the identification and correction of the underlying causes.

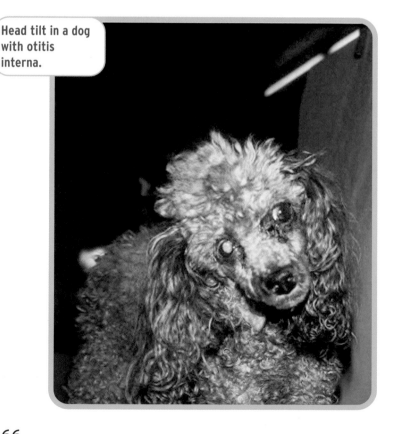

Head tilt in a dog with otitis interna.

Ear Surgery

Surgery may be needed for the treatment of an aural (ear) hematoma, to remove a polyp or tumor, and for management of otitis externa or otitis media when medical therapy fails to resolve the disease. The treatment of aural hematomas was discussed in a previous section of this chapter.

Lateral wall resection: Removal of a V-shaped section of the lateral (outside) wall of the vertical ear canal can be used to improve ventilation in the ear canal. Improved ventilation helps discharge to drain and reduces the humidity and temperature within the ear canal. Lateral ear canal resections may decrease the severity of bacterial and yeast infections, but they will not eliminate inflammation resulting from underlying allergies or keratinization disorders. Improvement is seen in approximately 50% of pets after surgery. The success of this treatment depends on continued medical care of any primary diseases causing otitis externa.

Vertical canal ablation: Removal of the entire vertical portion of the ear canal is performed when disease affects only the vertical portion of the canal. Examples of conditions that may be treated with vertical canal ablation include polyps or tumors affecting only the vertical canal, severe hyperplasia or narrowing restricted to the vertical canal, and trauma-induced damage to the vertical canal.

Total ear canal ablation (TECA): Total ear canal ablation is performed when irreversible changes are present in the ear canal. Calcification, severe narrowing, extreme glandular hyperplasia, and cancer involving the horizontal portion of the ear canal are examples of conditions for which a TECA is recommended. The vertical and horizontal ear canals both are removed during this procedure.

Lateral bulla osteotomy (LBO): An LBO usually is performed at the same time as a TECA. This procedure involves surgical curettage (scraping out) the middle ear cavity (tympanic bulla). LBO removes infected debris from the middle ear cavity and decreases complications caused by recurring infections of the middle ear. Postoperative

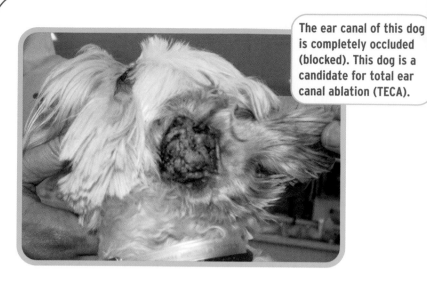

The ear canal of this dog is completely occluded (blocked). This dog is a candidate for total ear canal ablation (TECA).

care usually includes bandaging of the pet's head and several days of **analgesics** (pain-relieving medications). Complications may include nerve damage, deafness, head tilt, and abscesses. It is wise to have ear surgeries performed by a skilled surgeon (a Diplomate of the American College of Veterinary Surgeons). The overall outlook for pets having a TECA/LBO is good. Most pets seem much happier and have an increased willingness to play once they are relieved of the pain caused by chronic ear disease.

Summary

Ear disease is a common problem in dogs and cats. Disease usually is caused by a combination of predisposing, primary, and perpetuating factors. Ear infections are very painful for pets and may even result in changes in behavior. Prompt and aggressive treatment is necessary to prevent an acute infection from becoming a chronic one. If treatment is delayed or not successful, ear infections may spread to involve the middle ear and inner ear. Ear infections can cause a loss of hearing, head tilt, and nerve paralysis. Ongoing cases may require surgery to restore the pet's health and comfort. Because ear diseases usually are caused by more than one factor, consultation with a veterinary dermatologist is often helpful in identifying all the underlying problems and devising a successful treatment plan.

SKIN TUMORS

A **tumor** is defined as any swelling (tumefaction). A **neoplasm** is an abnormal tissue that grows by an increase in the number of cells that is more rapid than normal and that continues after the **stimulus** that initiated the growth ceases. Neoplasms may be **benign** (not likely to spread) or **malignant** (tending to invade tissues locally and spread to other areas of the body). The term *cancer* refers to a malignant neoplasm. Cancer cells often invade normal tissues and **metastasize** (spread) to distant areas of the body. Most cancers occur as tumors (lumps or swellings); however, many lumps are not cancerous. The skin is the most common site affected by neoplasia in dogs and the second most common site in cats.

General Characteristics of Benign and Malignant Tumors

Characteristic	Benign Tumors	Malignant Tumors
Structure	Expansive mass, well-circumscribed or encapsulated, freely movable	Irregular shape, not encapsulated, fixed (attached) to adjacent structures
Rate of growth	Slow	Rapid
Route of growth	Pushes normal tissues aside	Infiltrates adjacent tissues
Dissemination	None (does not spread)	Metastasis common (may spread to lymph nodes, lungs, liver, bones, and/or other sites)

The medical science that concerns the diagnosis and treatment of cancer is called **oncology,** and those who practice it are called **oncologists.** Many veterinary specialty hospitals include veterinary oncologists on staff. Veterinary medical oncologists make the diagnosis, stage the tumor, and prescribe treatment; veterinary surgical oncologists perform surgery to remove the cancer; and veterinary radiation oncologists administer **radiation therapy.** Several of these specialists may be involved in the treatment plan prescribed for a pet.

Non-Neoplastic Skin Masses

Fortunately, many skin tumors are non-neoplastic. Once a veterinarian has determined that the mass is benign, it may be either observed for changes in size and appearance or surgically removed. Follow-up treatments are not necessary for non-neoplastic masses.

Cysts

Cysts are non-neoplastic **nodules** (small lumps) that are lined by **epithelial** (skin) cells and contain a semisolid material composed of a combination of **keratin** (a protein in outer skin cells, hair, and nails), **serum** (the clear, watery portion of blood), and **sebaceous** (oil) or sweat gland secretions. Cysts are benign **lesions.** Problems may arise if a cyst becomes infected or ruptures. When a cyst ruptures, it releases keratin and any other contents into the **dermis** (the deep layer of skin), where these materials incite an intense **inflammatory** response (swelling, redness, heat, and pain). Small cysts may not require treatment; if they become large or seem painful to the pet, these masses should be removed by surgery.

Granulomas

Granulomas are non-neoplastic nodules composed of **macrophages** (white blood cells that devour bacteria and

other foreign material) and fibrous **connective tissue.**
Pyogranulomas are nodules composed of **neutrophils**
(infection-fighting blood cells), macrophages, and fibrous
connective tissue. Granulomas may form around sites of
infection, severe inflammation, foreign bodies, vaccine
sites, ruptured cysts, and hair follicles. Cats develop
eosinophilic granulomas in response to **allergies.**
Treatment is based on the cause of the granuloma.
Infectious granulomas may be treated with long-term
antimicrobial drugs (which fight bacteria and fungi);
other types of granulomas may be treated with antiin-
flammatory drugs, surgically removed, or simply monitored for changes.

Keratoses

Actinic keratoses are benign epithelial growths developing in response to chronic sunlight (ultraviolet B [UVB])
exposure. These lesions sometimes become malignant
epithelial tumors and therefore should be monitored
closely. **Cutaneous** horns may develop as excessive
growths of normal skin cells or may be associated with
viral infections (e.g., **feline leukemia virus** [FeLV], **feline
immunodeficiency virus** [FIV], and **papillomaviruses**).
They are sometimes early forms of skin neoplasms (e.g.,

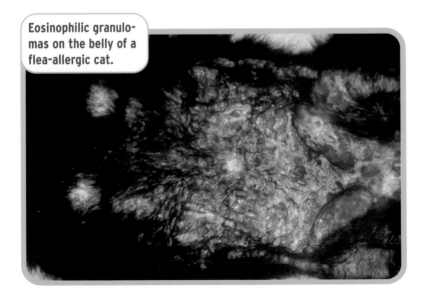

Eosinophilic granulo-
mas on the belly of a
flea-allergic cat.

squamous cell carcinoma, discussed later in this chapter). Skin tags (also called *cutaneous tags*, *acrochordons*, or *fibroepithelial polyps*) are composed of an exophytic* fibrous core surrounded by normal epithelial cells. Fibropruritic nodules develop on the rumps of older dogs; affected dogs usually have a history of chronic flea allergy dermatitis. These lesions, which appear as multiple, hairless, firm nodules, are most common in German Shepherd Dogs and German Shepherd mixed-breed dogs.

Tumors of Epithelial Cells

Cell types normally present in the **epidermis** (outer skin layer) include **keratinocytes** (keratin-producing cells), **melanocytes** (pigment-producing cells), **Langerhans cells** (involved in immune response), and **Merkel cells** (touch receptors). The majority of tumors arising from the epidermis involve keratinocytes.

Papillomas

Papillomas (warts) are growths composed of epithelial cells with variable amounts of connective tissue frame-

*Exophytic refers to a growth that grows outward from an epithelial surface; warts are an example.

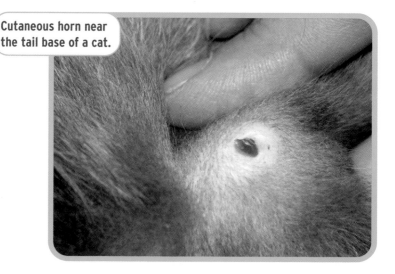

Cutaneous horn near the tail base of a cat.

work. Lesions usually start as white, flat, smooth, shiny **papules** (small, hard bumps) or **plaques** (raised patches) that grow to form whitish grey, pedunculated (having a stalklike base) or cauliflower-like crusted masses that may exceed 1 inch in diameter. Dogs and cats may develop a variety of different papillomas.

Canine oral papillomatosis: Canine oral papillomavirus infections may result in single or multiple masses (warts) located on the face, inner lips, gums, palate, tongue, and occasionally other sites. These lesions are most common in young dogs, and most spontaneously shrink away within 3 months. If the lesions are interfering with eating or do not regress after 3 months, they may be removed by using **laser surgery**, **cryosurgery** (freezing tissue), or traditional surgery. Oral **alpha-interferon** and other antiviral drugs may speed regression of the lesions.

Cutaneous papillomas: Cutaneous papillomas develop on the skin of older dogs, with the highest incidence being in male Cocker Spaniels and Kerry Blue Terriers. These masses, which may be single or multiple, develop on the head, eyelids, and feet. They usually are pedunculated or cauliflower-like and smaller than 1/4 inch in diameter. Cutaneous papillomas in older dogs do not regress; however, these are benign lesions and may be either monitored or surgically removed.

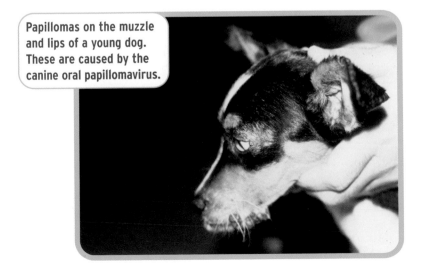

Papillomas on the muzzle and lips of a young dog. These are caused by the canine oral papillomavirus.

Multiple pigmented plaques and multiple pigmented papules: These are other forms of papillomas associated with papillomavirus infections in dogs. The multiple pigmented plaques may be found on the trunk or belly and are most common in Pugs, Miniature Schnauzers, and Chinese Shar-Peis. Some lesions may become malignant squamous cell carcinomas (discussed in the next section); therefore lesions should be monitored for changes in size or appearance. Papillomas also may be found on the footpads of adult dogs, where they appear as firm, hornlike projections. No treatment is necessary unless the lesions are causing lameness.

Feline papillomavirus-2: This usually produces lesions on the undersurface of the tongue of cats. The multiple masses are small, soft, light pink, oval, slightly raised, and flat-topped.

Feline papillomavirus-1: This is associated with masses on the skin of cats. Some masses appear as multiple, pigmented, crusted plaques on the head, neck, back, and belly. In some cats, these plaques develop into premalignant or malignant (squamous cell carcinoma) skin tumors.

Multiple pigmented plaques on the belly of a dog.

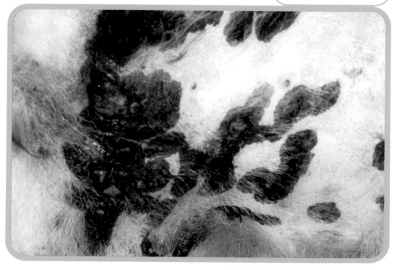

Squamous Cell Carcinoma

Squamous cell carcinomas are malignant tumors originating from keratinocytes in the epidermis. Lesions usually are located on lightly pigmented (white) areas of older dogs and cats. Pets that have spent a lot of time in the sun are at increased risk. Lesions may be raised masses or **ulcers** (sores). Raised tumors often have a cauliflower-like appearance and may be covered in bloody crusts. Ulcerated lesions may have a craterlike appearance. In cats, squamous cell carcinomas are most common on the ear tips of white cats but also may involve the nose, eyelids, and other locations. In dogs, tumors are most common on the feet, legs, nose, lips, scrotum, and trunk. Squamous cell carcinomas of the toes are most common in large-breed, black-coated dogs. Diagnosis usually requires a skin biopsy. The treatment of choice is surgical removal. Further treatment—either radiation therapy or chemotherapy, which may be **topical** (surface), intralesional (injections within the cancer), or **systemic** (whole body, by mouth or injection)—may be recommended in some cases.

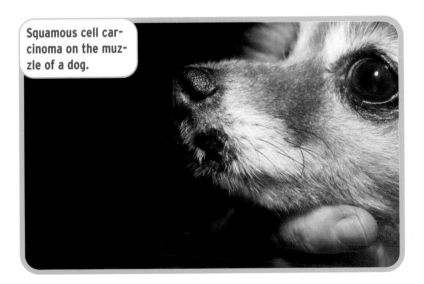

Squamous cell carcinoma on the muzzle of a dog.

Basal Cell Tumors

Basal cell tumors arise from the cells of the **stratum basale** (deepest layer) of the epidermis. When malignant, these tumors are called *basal cell carcinomas*. Basal cell tumors often are pigmented and appear as black, raised, round nodules. In cats, basal cell tumors usually are found on the head, neck, or dorsal back. In dogs, basal cell tumors usually are found on the head, neck, or chest. **Cytology** (analysis of cells) may suggest a basal cell tumor; however, biopsy is required to establish a definitive diagnosis and distinguish benign from malignant tumors. Surgical removal usually is curative.

Merkel Cell Tumors

Merkel cells are classified as **neuroendocrine** cells (having to do with both the nervous system and the production of hormones) that function in touch perception, regulation of blood circulation in the skin, sweat production, keratinocyte proliferation, and hair growth. Merkel cell tumors in dogs usually are malignant, whereas those in cats usually are benign. Diagnosis requires biopsies and special stains to identify the cell type.

Tumors of the Skin Glands and Hair Follicles

A variety of tumors arise from the adnexal (accessory) structures of the skin. These include tumors of the **sebaceous** glands, sweat glands, **hair follicles**, perianal glands, and **ceruminous** (wax) glands. Most of these tumors are benign.

Sebaceous Gland Tumors

Sebaceous (oil) gland tumors usually appear as firm, elevated, wartlike or cauliflower-like growths. They may be yellowish or pigmented, hairless, greasy, or ulcerated (having an open sore). Sebaceous gland tumors usually occur on the head, earflap, eyelids, trunk (main part of body), and legs. They are common in older dogs. The following breeds may be more likely to develop sebaceous gland tumors:

- **Poodles**
- **Cocker Spaniels**
- **Miniature Schnauzers**
- **Dachshunds**
- **Beagles**
- **Irish Setters**
- **Lhasa Apsos**
- **Malamutes**
- **Shih Tzus**
- **Siberian Huskies**
- **Terrier breeds**

Persian cats also may be predisposed to developing these tumors. Nodular sebaceous **hyperplasia**, sebaceous epitheliomas, and sebaceous adenomas are various types of benign sebaceous gland tumors. Malignant ones are called *sebaceous gland carcinomas*. Benign tumors usually grow slowly and do not require treatment unless they become infected or cause discomfort. Laser surgery or surgical removal usually is curative, although new tumors may develop spontaneously at other sites. Synthetic **retinoids** (substances related to vitamin A) may cause tumors to shrink and may be helpful in treating dogs that develop numerous tumors.

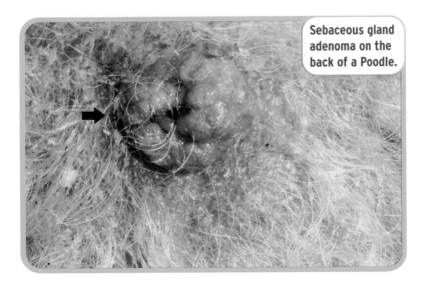

Sebaceous gland adenoma on the back of a Poodle.

Sweat Gland Tumors

Sweat gland tumors arise from the **apocrine** (epitrichial) **sweat glands** of the skin or ears. Solitary tumors appear as raised, hairless, bluish-colored nodules that may be firm or cystic (filled with fluid). Benign tumors are called *apocrine gland adenomas;* malignant ones are called *apocrine gland adenocarcinomas.* The term *apocrine cystadenomatosis* refers to multiple cystlike masses. Apocrine gland tumors are most common on the head, neck, legs, axillary (armpit), and **inguinal** (groin) regions of dogs. Cocker Spaniels, Golden Retrievers, and German Shepherd Dogs may be predisposed to developing sweat gland tumors. In cats, tumors are most common on the head, neck, belly, and legs. The treatment of choice is complete surgical removal.

Hair Follicle Tumors

A variety of tumors can develop from hair follicles. These tumors are given different names depending on their cellular characteristics. These tumors usually are benign, do not invade nearby tissues, and do not spread. They may be monitored without treatment or surgically removed. Removal is recommended for hair follicle

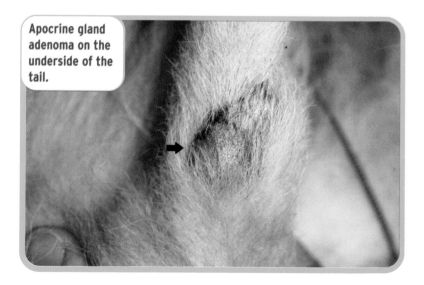

Apocrine gland adenoma on the underside of the tail.

tumors that develop **secondary** infections and those that rupture.

Intracutaneous Cornifying Epitheliomas

Intracutaneous cornifying (corn-forming) epitheliomas are also referred to as *keratoacanthomas* and *infundibular keratinizing acanthomas*. These tumors also originate from hair follicles. A unique feature of intracutaneous cornifying epitheliomas is the presence of a central pore that opens directly to the skin surface. The pore may contain a gray-brown keratinaceous material or a hard, horn-like keratin plug (cutaneous horn). Norwegian Elkhounds have a tendency to develop multiple tumors. Treatment may include observation, surgical removal, and synthetic retinoids. Dogs that have more than one tumor are likely to continue to develop new ones; however, these tumors are benign and do not affect the pet's overall health or longevity.

Perianal Gland Tumors

Perianal (circumanal) gland tumors originate from glands in the skin surrounding the anus and are most common in intact male dogs. The following breeds have an increased incidence of these tumors:

- **Cocker Spaniels**
- **English Bulldogs**
- **Samoyeds**
- **Afghan Hounds**
- **Dachshunds**
- **German Shepherd Dogs**
- **Beagles**
- **Siberian Huskies**
- **Shih Tzus**
- **Lhasa Apsos**

Perianal gland tumors may be single or multiple. Tumors may be located around the anus or on the tail, **perineum** (area between the anus and genitals), prepuce (skin fold covering the penis), thigh, or top of the rump. Castration results in shrinkage of most benign tumors.

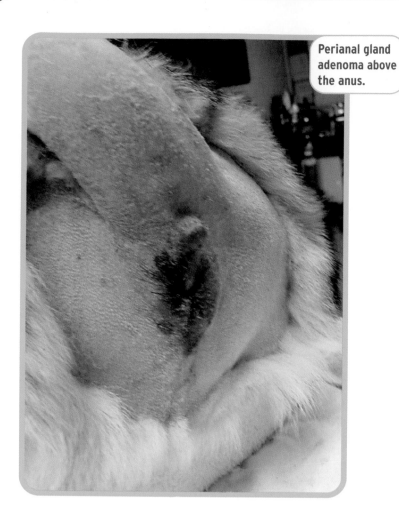

Perianal gland adenoma above the anus.

Malignant tumors should be removed surgically. Additional treatment options include cryosurgery, laser surgery, or radiation therapy.

Ceruminal Gland Tumors

Ceruminal gland tumors are the most common neoplasms found in the ear canals of cats and dogs. They are more common in cats, with approximately half being malignant carcinomas. Most ceruminal gland tumors in dogs are benign. The only effective treatment is surgical removal, usually by lateral ear resection or total ablation of the ear canal (see Chapter 12).

Dermal Tumors

Dermal tumors may arise from any cell type present in the **dermis**, the deep layer of the skin. In this section we will review mast cell tumors and the various types of soft tissue sarcomas.

Mast Cell Tumors

Mast cells originate in the bone marrow and migrate to tissues, where they function as mediators of **inflammation**. Mast cell tumors (MCTs) are common neoplasms affecting both dogs and cats. The following breeds of dogs have an increased incidence of MCT:

- **Boxers**
- **Boston Terriers**
- **Labrador Retrievers**
- **Beagles**
- **Schnauzers**
- **English Bulldogs**
- **Bull Terriers**
- **Staffordshire Terriers**
- **Dachshunds**
- **Pugs**
- **Weimaraners**
- **Chinese Shar-Peis**

Tumors in Chinese Shar-Peis often are malignant and highly aggressive, with both local invasion of other tissues and **metastasis** (spread) to other sites. In cats, MCTs are divided into two types, mastocytic or histiocytic.

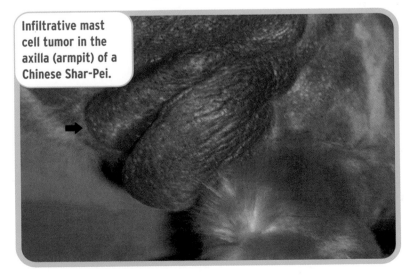

Infiltrative mast cell tumor in the axilla (armpit) of a Chinese Shar-Pei.

Siamese cats have an increased incidence of both types of MCT.

The appearance of MCTs is variable. Many are raised skin lesions that may be haired or alopecic, and some are ulcerated. Handling of the tumor may result in localized swelling and inflammation from the release of inflammatory products from mast cell granules. In dogs, MCTs are most common on the trunk and lower legs. Tumors arising from the nailbed, oral cavity, prepuce, vulva, and perianal region usually grow more quickly and are more likely to metastasize. In cats, MCTs usually are located on the head and neck, although they can be found at other sites. Tumors in cats are rarely malignant.

Treatment options for MCT include surgery, radiation therapy, and systemic chemotherapy. For localized tumors, surgery or surgery plus radiation has a 95% cure rate. The outlook for dogs with aggressive malignant tumors is poor, with an average survival time of 18 weeks after diagnosis. Most MCTs in cats are benign. The histiocytic form of MCT in young Siamese cats may undergo spontaneous remission (disappear without treatment). Older cats of other breeds (non-Siamese) sometimes develop MCTs in their livers or spleens; these should be treated with systemic chemotherapy.

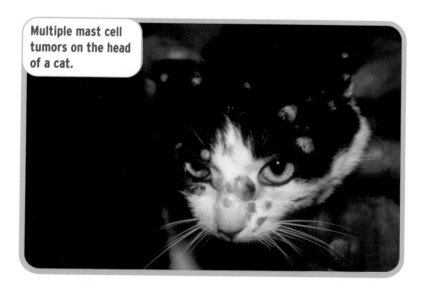

Multiple mast cell tumors on the head of a cat.

Soft Tissue Sarcomas

Soft tissue **sarcomas** may develop from fibrous **connective tissue**, nerves, joint capsules, fat (adipose tissue), lymphatic vessels, blood vessels, myxomatous (containing a jellylike substance) tissues, and muscles in the dermis and **subcutaneous** tissues. These tumors vary in size, physical appearance, location on the body, and biologic behavior. Tumor names that end with -*oma* indicate benign tumors; names that end with -*sarcoma* indicate malignant tumors.

Fibromas/fibrosarcomas: These develop from fibrous connective tissue. Some tumors in cats are associated with **feline sarcoma virus** (FeSV); others are associated with subcutaneous vaccine administration (especially killed rabies vaccines and feline leukemia virus vaccines). No cause has been identified in dogs. Cocker Spaniels, Doberman Pinschers, and Golden Retrievers may be more susceptible to the formation of these tumors. Tumors in dogs usually are located on the legs and trunk. FeSV-associated tumors are most common in cats younger than 5 years of age and may develop on the trunk, lower legs, or earflaps. The treatment of choice for malignant tumors is surgical removal, with wide margins of tissue taken around the tumor. In addition to surgery, radiation therapy or chemotherapy may be recommended.

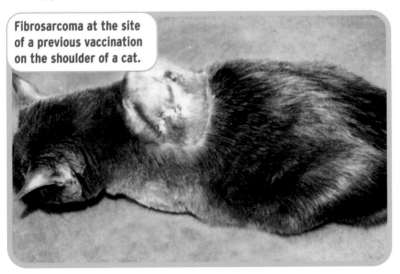

Fibrosarcoma at the site of a previous vaccination on the shoulder of a cat.

Myxomas/myxosarcomas: These develop from **mucin**-producing fibroblasts (cells that produce connective tissue) in the dermis. Doberman Pinschers and German Shepherd Dogs may be predisposed to develop these tumors. They may develop on the back, on the legs, or in the groin. The treatment of choice is surgery, with wide tissue margins taken.

Hemangiopericytomas: These originate from cells surrounding blood vessels. Boxers, German Shepherd Dogs, Cocker Spaniels, Springer Spaniels, Irish Setters, Siberian Huskies, Fox Terriers, Collies, and Beagles are affected more frequently than other breeds. These tumors usually develop on the legs near the stifle (knee) or elbow. Treatment may involve surgical removal or limb amputation.

Hemangiomas/hemangiosarcomas: These develop from cells of the **endothelium**, which line the blood vessels. Lightly pigmented dogs frequently develop hemangiomas and hemangiosarcomas in skin that has been exposed to UVB radiation (sunlight). Boxers, Golden Retrievers, German Shepherd Dogs, English Springer Spaniels, Airedale Terriers, Whippets, Dalmatians, Beagles, American Staffordshire Terriers, Basset Hounds, Salukis, and English Pointers are predisposed to develop these types of tumors. Hemangiomas usually are small, round, firm, or fluctuant (undulating) bluish black nodules located on the lower chest and belly. In cats, hemangiomas are found on the ears, face, neck, and legs. Dermal hemangiosarcomas may appear as red to dark blue plaques or nodules. Subcutaneous (under the skin) hemangiosarcomas are dark red to blue-black, bruiselike, spongy masses. Hemangiomas may be surgically removed or left without treatment unless enlargement or bleeding is noted. Hemangiosarcomas should be surgically removed; however, the long-term outlook is poor because malignant tumors often recur locally and also metastasize.

Lymphohistiocytic Tumors

Histiocyte is a term used to refer to three types of cells: blood **monocytes** (a type of white blood cell), tissue **macrophages** (cells that devour invading microorganisms and cellular debris), and myeloid dendritic cells (cells originating from the bone marrow and involved in immune system responses). **Lymphocytes** originate in lymph nodes, the thymus, the spleen, and other lymphoid tissues. Histiocytes and lymphocytes both are round cells with a single large, round nucleus; this similarity can make differentiation between these cells difficult. Dogs and cats develop many types of lymphohistiocytic tumors.

Cutaneous Histiocytomas

Histiocytomas are benign tumors that originate from epidermal Langerhans cells. These usually appear as a single, rapidly growing, firm, round, raised nodule located on the head, earflap, or leg of a young dog. The tumor usually is hairless and may be ulcerated. Cutaneous histiocytomas usually disappear without treatment within 3 months; for that reason, observation is often recommended. Surgical removal may be recommended if the dog is licking the lesion or causing self-trauma or if the lesion does not regress on its own.

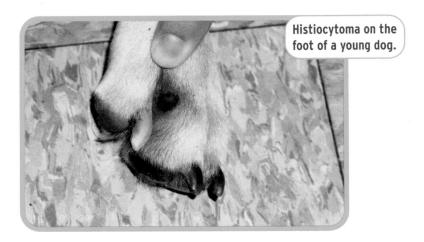

Histiocytoma on the foot of a young dog.

Systemic Histiocytosis

Systemic histiocytosis is a disease of histiocyte cell multiplication involving the skin and internal organs. It is most common in 2- to 8-year-old male dogs. Breeds with an increased incidence of this disease include Bernese Mountain Dogs, Rottweilers, Irish Wolfhounds, Golden Retrievers, and Basset Hounds. Multiple dermal nodules may be present on the head, earflaps, legs, and scrotum, with other nodules found in the nasal mucosa, conjunctiva (lining of eyelids), lymph nodes, spleen, and lungs. Diagnosis requires evaluation of biopsies. The outlook is guarded; treatment may include corticosteroids, cyclosporine A, and leflunomide.

Cutaneous T-Cell Lymphoma (Mycosis Fungoides)

The term *mycosis fungoides* refers to a mushroomlike appearance of nodular lesions caused by cutaneous T-cell lymphomas; many veterinarians use this term to refer to all types of cutaneous T-cell lymphomas, regardless of

Basset Hound with systemic histiocytosis. *Arrows* point to several histiocytic tumor nodules.

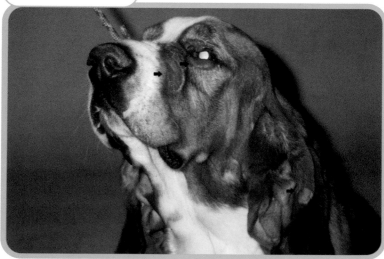

their clinical appearance. Malignant T cells (a type of **lymphocyte**) invade the epidermis of the skin and the hair follicles. Clinical signs are highly variable and include **erythema** (redness), **pruritus** (itching), scaling, crusting, **papules**, plaques, nodules, ulcers, and depigmentation (loss of color) at the junction of skin and mucous membranes (e.g., lips, nose, vulva, prepuce, anus).

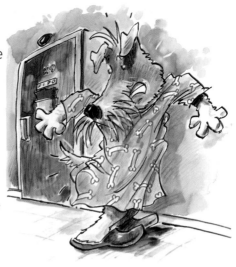

Cats sometimes develop multiple areas of redness, hair loss, and scaling involving their head, neck, and trunk. Diagnosis requires skin biopsies. The outlook is poor; treatment options include topical and systemic corticosteroids, topical retin-A, oral retinoids, interferon-α_{2a}, topical carmustine, oral lomustine, and high doses of **omega-3** and **omega-6 fatty acids.**

Plasmacytoma

Plasmacytomas are composed of **plasma cells** and usually appear as solitary round, raised, reddened nod-

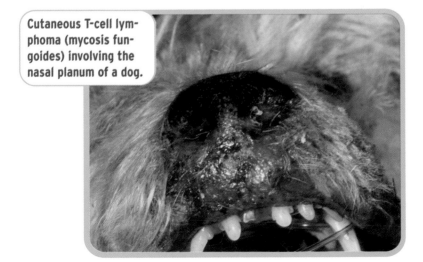

Cutaneous T-cell lymphoma (mycosis fungoides) involving the nasal planum of a dog.

ules on a foot or lip or in the ear canal of an older dog or cat. Cocker Spaniels may be predisposed to developing plasmacytomas. Tumors may ulcerate and bleed easily. Multiple tumors sometimes are present. The treatment of choice is surgical removal, and the outlook is good in most cases. A few feline cases have had systemic disease and metastasis to lymph nodes; these pets have a poor predicted outcome.

Tumors Derived from Melanocytes

Melanocytic tumors are composed of **melanocytes** (cells that produce melanin pigment). The suffix -*cytoma* is used to indicate a benign tumor; however, many people also refer to benign melanocytic tumors as *melanomas.*

Melanocytoma (Melanoma)

Melanocytomas in dogs usually are located on the head (eyelid, muzzle), trunk, or feet (between toes). Predisposed breeds include Cocker Spaniels, Scottish Terriers, Airedale Terriers, Boston Terriers, Springer Spaniels, Boxers, Golden Retrievers, Miniature Schnauzers, Irish Setters, Irish Terriers, Chow Chows, Chihuahuas, and Doberman Pinschers. In cats, tumors usually are located on the head (nose, earflap) or neck. Melanocytomas usually are solitary, round, raised, firm, brown to black in color, and hairless; they may be pedunculated (having a stalklike base) or wartlike. Because benign tumors cannot be distinguished from malignant ones without a biopsy, surgical removal with wide margins is usually recommended.

Malignant Melanoma

Malignant melanomas in dogs often arise from melanocytes in the mouth or at the junction of skin and mucous membranes, such as the lips, eyelids, and base of the nails; others are found on the toes or trunk.

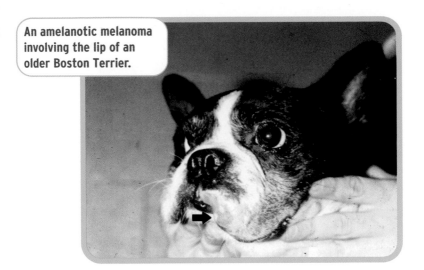

An amelanotic melanoma involving the lip of an older Boston Terrier.

Approximately 50% of melanomas in cats are malignant. Dogs with dark coat colors are more often affected. The following breeds have an increased incidence of malignant melanomas:

- **Cocker Spaniels**
- **Scottish Terriers**
- **Miniature Poodles**
- **Airedale Terriers**
- **Boston Terriers**
- **Standard and Miniature Schnauzers**
- **Gordon Setters**
- **Irish Setters**
- **Golden Retrievers**

Miscellaneous Tumors

A variety of other tumors may involve the skin and subcutaneous tissues.

Lipomas

Lipomas are among the most common tumors affecting dogs; they are less common in cats. These tumors arise from subcutaneous fat (adipose tissue). Single or multiple tumors may be present in a pet. Lipomas are clearly bordered, movable, round or multilobed, soft or firm subcutaneous masses that may range from 1/4 inch to more than 12 inches in diameter. Common locations include the chest, belly, and limbs. Masses suspected of being lipomas should be aspirated (a fine-needle aspiration) to confirm the diagnosis. The contents of FNA resemble drops of oil when placed on a microscope slide. Small lipomas may be monitored without treatment. Cosmetically unacceptable or rapidly enlarging lipomas may be removed surgically.

Transmissible Venereal Tumor

Transmissible venereal tumors (TVT) are sexually transmitted by direct transfer of neoplastic cells from one dog to another, usually during mating. Tumors occasionally are found in the skin of the face or legs. Metastasis is rare but possible. TVTs may spontaneously regress; however, treatment is recommended to prevent metastasis. The drug of choice for treating TVTs is vincristine (a chemotherapeutic drug).

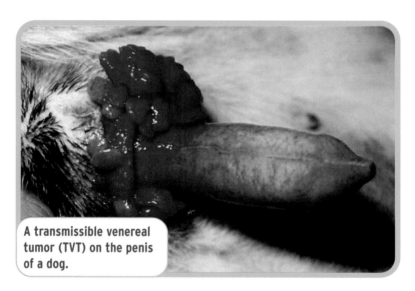

A transmissible venereal tumor (TVT) on the penis of a dog.

Anal Sac Tumors

Apocrine gland tumors of **anal sac** origin are most common in female dogs. Many of these are malignant (apocrine gland adenocarcinomas). Metastasis is common and usually involves nearby lymph nodes. The treatment of choice is surgical removal followed by chemotherapy; however, outlook is poor, with a high likelihood of local reoccurrence and metastatic disease.

Skin Diseases Associated with Remote Tumors (Paraneoplastic)

Some noncutaneous forms of cancer cause **paraneoplastic** skin diseases. Feline paraneoplastic alopecia (hair loss) usually is seen in older cats (9 to 16 years of age). Affected cats are lethargic, have poor appetite, and may undergo a rapid loss of body weight. Hair loss begins around the eyes and on the legs and belly. Hairs epilate (pull out) easily. The skin is thin and scaly. Footpads may be shiny and smooth in appearance.

Thymomas are tumors originating from the thymus (a lymphoid organ in the chest). Cats with thymomas sometimes develop an **exfoliative** (scaly) skin disease that begins on the head and earflaps and can eventually involve the entire body. Thymomas usually are benign, and surgical removal of the tumor is followed by regrowth of a normal hair coat.

Other examples of paraneoplastic skin diseases include **Cushing's disease** (see Chapter 7), Sertoli cell-associated

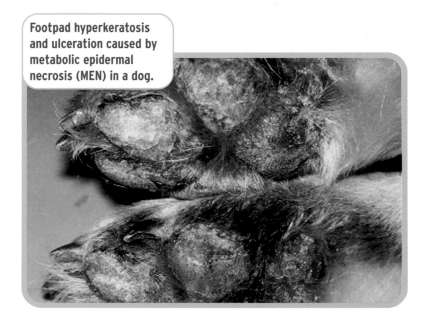

Footpad hyperkeratosis and ulceration caused by metabolic epidermal necrosis (MEN) in a dog.

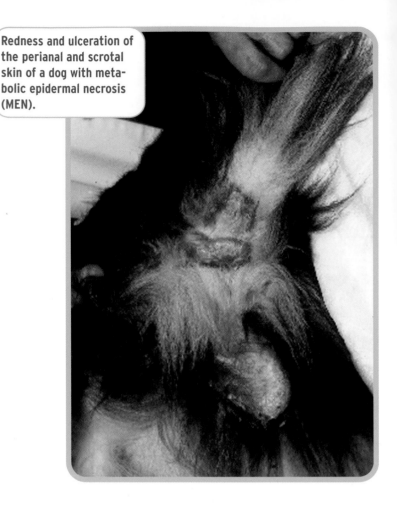

Redness and ulceration of the perianal and scrotal skin of a dog with metabolic epidermal necrosis (MEN).

hyperestrogenism (see Chapter 7), nodular dermatofibrosis (discussed earlier in this chapter), and paraneoplastic pemphigus (see Chapter 9).

Summary

Cancer is the uncontrolled growth of cells within the body. Cancer is common in pets such as dogs and cats; older pets are more likely to be affected. Many types of tumors and tumorlike lesions involve the skin of dogs and cats. Biopsies usually are required to diagnose the cause of a mass. Veterinarians can cure many types of cancer through surgical removal of the mass. Those that cannot be completely removed but have not yet spread to other body sites often can be cured with additional measures (radiation therapy, chemotherapy, immunotherapy).

REFERENCES

Chapter 1

Campbell KL: *Small animal dermatology secrets*, Philadelphia, 2004, Hanley & Belfus.

Scott DW, Miller WH, Griffin CE: *Muller and Kirk's small animal dermatology*, ed 6, Philadelphia, 2001, Saunders.

Solvay Veterinary Inc: *The complete manual of ear care*, Trenton, NJ, 1986, Veterinary Learning Systems Co.

Chapter 2

Bassett BL, Campbell KL: Shampoo therapy in the management of dermatoses. In August JR: *Consultations in feline internal medicine*, Philadelphia, 1994, Saunders.

Campbell KL: *Small animal dermatology secrets*, Philadelphia, 2004, Hanley & Belfus.

Campbell KL, Corbin JE, Campbell JR: *Companion animals: Their biology, care, health and management*, Upper Saddle River, NJ, 2005, Pearson Prentice Hall.

Saunders B: *How to trim, groom, and show your dog*, New York, 1970, Howell Book House.

Scott DW, Miller WH, Griffin CE: *Muller and Kirk's small animal dermatology*, ed 6, Philadelphia, 2001, Saunders.

Chapter 3

Campbell KL: *Small animal dermatology secrets*, Philadelphia, 2004, Hanley & Belfus.

Campbell KL, Corbin JE, Campbell JR: *Companion animals: Their biology, care, health and management*, Upper Saddle River, NJ, 2005, Pearson Prentice Hall.

Melman SA: *Skin diseases of dogs and cats: a guide for pet owners and professionals*, Potomac, Md, 1994, DermaPet Inc.

Scott DW, Miller WH, Griffin CE: *Muller and Kirk's small animal dermatology*, ed 6, Philadelphia, 2001, Saunders.

Chapter 4

Campbell KL: *Small animal dermatology secrets*, Philadelphia, 2004, Hanley & Belfus.

Campbell KL, Corbin JE, Campbell JR: *Companion animals: Their biology, care and management*, Upper Saddle River, NJ, 2005, Pearson Prentice Hall.

Jeffers JG, Meyer EK, Sosis EJ: Responses of dogs with food allergies to single-ingredient dietary provocation, *J Am Vet Med Assoc* 209:608-611, 1996.

Liestra MH, Markwell PJ, Willemse T: Evaluation of selected-protein-source diets for management of dogs with adverse reactions to foods, *J Am Vet Med Assoc* 219:1411-1414, 2001.

Reedy LM, Miller WH, Willemse T: *Allergic skin diseases of dogs and cats*, ed 2, Philadelphia, 1997, Saunders.

Scott DW, Miller WH, Griffin CE: *Muller and Kirk's small animal dermatology*, ed 6, Philadelphia, 2001, Saunders.

Sicherer SH: Clinical implications of cross-reactive food allergens, *J Allergy Clin Immunol* 108:881-890, 2001.

Vieths S, Scheurer SH, Ballmer-Weber B: Current understanding of cross-reactivity of food allergens and pollen, *Ann N Y Acad Sci* 964:47-68, 2002.

Chapter 5

Campbell KL: *Small animal dermatology secrets*, Philadelphia, 2004, Hanley & Belfus.

Medleau L, Hnilica KA: *Small animal dermatology: a color atlas and therapeutic guide*, Philadelphia, 2001, Saunders.

Melman SA: *Skin diseases of dogs and cats: a guide for pet owners and professionals*, Potomac, Md, 1994, DermaPet Inc.

Scott DW, Miller WH, Griffin CE: *Muller and Kirk's small animal dermatology*, ed 6, Philadelphia, 2001, Saunders.

Chapter 6

Barriga OO: *Veterinary parasitology for practitioners*, ed 2, Edina, Minn, 1997, Burgess Publishing.

Campbell KL: *Small animal dermatology secrets*, Philadelphia, 2004, Hanley & Belfus.

Campbell KL, Corbin JE, Campbell JR: *Companion animals: Their biology, care and management*, Upper Saddle River, NJ, 2005, Pearsall Prentice Hall.

Georgi JR, Georgi ME: *Parasitology for veterinarians*, ed 5, Philadelphia, 1990, Saunders.

Ivens VR, Daniel LM, Levine ND: Special Publication 52, *Principal parasites of domestic animals in the United States*, Urbana-Champaign, Ill, 1989, University of Illinois at Urbana-Champaign, Colleges of Agriculture and Veterinary Medicine.

Scott DW, Miller WH, Griffin CE: *Muller and Kirk's small animal dermatology*, ed 6, Philadelphia, 2001, Saunders.

Wall R, Shearer D: *Veterinary ectoparasites*, ed 2, Oxford, UK, 2001, Blackwell Science.

Chapter 7

Campbell KL: *Small animal dermatology secrets*, Philadelphia, 2004, Hanley & Belfus.

Campbell KL, Corbin JE, Campbell JR: *Companion animals: Their biology, care, health and management*, Upper Saddle River, NJ, 2005, Pearson Prentice Hall.

Ettinger SJ, Feldman EC: *Textbook of veterinary internal medicine diseases of the dog and cat*, ed 6, vol 2, Philadelphia, 2005, Saunders.

Feldman EC, Nelson RW: *Canine and feline endocrinology and reproduction*, ed 3, Philadelphia, 2004, Saunders.

Medleau L, Hnilica KA: *Small animal dermatology: a color atlas and therapeutic guide*, Philadelphia, 2001, Saunders.

Melman SA: *Skin diseases of dogs and cats: a guide for pet owners and professionals*, Potomac, Md, 1994, DermaPet Inc.

Scott DW, Miller WH, Griffin CE: *Muller and Kirk's Small Animal Dermatology*, ed 6, Philadelphia, 2001, Saunders,.

Website: http://www.offa.org/thyinfo.html

Chapter 8

Campbell KL: *Small animal dermatology secrets*, Philadelphia, 2004, Hanley & Belfus.

Campbell KL, Corbin JE, Campbell JR: *Companion animals: Their biology, care, health and management*, Upper Saddle River, NJ, 2005, Pearson Prentice Hall.

Medleau L, Hnilica KA: *Small animal dermatology: a color atlas and therapeutic guide*, Philadelphia, 2001, Saunders.

Melman SA: *Skin diseases of dogs and cats: a guide for pet owners and professionals*, Potomac, Md, 1994, DermaPet Inc.

Moriello KA: Treatment of dermatophytosis in dogs and cats: Review of published studies, *Vet Dermatol* 15:99-107, 2004.

Scott DW, Miller WH, Griffin CE: *Muller and Kirk's small animal dermatology*, ed 6, Philadelphia, 2001, Saunders.

Chapter 9

Campbell KL: *Small animal dermatology secrets*, Philadelphia, 2004, Hanley & Belfus.

Medleau L, Hnilica KA: *Small animal dermatology: a color atlas and therapeutic guide*, Philadelphia, 2001, Saunders.

Scott DW, Miller WH, Griffin CE: *Muller and Kirk's small animal dermatology*, ed 6, Philadelphia, 2001, Saunders.

Chapter 10

Campbell KL: *Small animal dermatology secrets*, Philadelphia, 2004, Hanley & Belfus.

Medleau L, Hnilica KA: *Small animal dermatology: a color atlas and therapeutic guide*, Philadelphia, 2001, Saunders.

Melman SA: *Skin diseases of dogs and cats: a guide for pet owners and professionals*, Potomac, Md, 1994, DermaPet Inc.

Orthopedic Foundation for Animals: Sebaceous Adenitis Information. http://www.offa.org/sageinfo.html

Scott DW, Miller WH, Griffin CE: *Muller and Kirk's small animal dermatology*, ed 6, Philadelphia, 2001, Saunders.

Chapter 11

Campbell KL, Corbin JE, Campbell JR: *Companion animals: Their biology, care, health and management*, Upper Saddle River, NJ, 2005, Pearson Prentice Hall.

Melman SA: *Skin diseases of dogs and cats: a guide for pet owners and professionals*, Potomac, Md, 1994, DermaPet Inc.

Patterson AP: Psychocutaneous disorders. In Campbell KL: *Small animal dermatology secrets*, Philadelphia, 2004, Hanley & Belfus.

Patterson S: *Skin diseases of the cat*, London, 2000, Blackwell Science.

Scott DW, Miller WH, Griffin CE: *Muller and Kirk's small animal dermatology*, ed 6, Philadelphia, 2001, Saunders.

Willemse T: Psychogenic alopecia in cats and the role of the opioid and dopaminergic systems. In August JR: *Consultations in feline internal medicine*, ed 3, Philadelphia, 1997, Saunders.

Chapter 12

Gotthelf LN: *Small animal ear diseases: an illustrated guide*, Philadelphia, 2000, Saunders.

Harvey RG, Harari J, Delauche AJ: *Ear diseases of the dog and cat*, Ames, Iowa, 2001, Iowa State Press.

Matousek JL, editor: *Veterinary Clinics of North America Small Animal Practice* 32(2): 379-599. Ear Diseases, Philadelphia, 2004, Saunders.

McKeever PJ, Harvey RG: *Color handbook of skin diseases of the dog and cat*, Ames, Iowa, 1998, Iowa State Press.

Medleau L, Hnilica KA: *Small animal dermatology: a color atlas and therapeutic guide*, Philadelphia, 2001, Saunders.

Scott DW, Miller WH, Griffin CE: *Muller and Kirk's small animal dermatology*, ed 6, Philadelphia, 2001, Saunders.

Chapter 13

Campbell KL: *Small animal dermatology secrets*, Philadelphia, 2004, Hanley & Belfus.

Medleau L, Hnilica KA: *Small animal dermatology: a color atlas and therapeutic guide*, Philadelphia, 2001, Saunders.

Scott DW, Miller WH, Griffin CE: *Muller and Kirk's small animal dermatology*, ed 6, Philadelphia, 2001, Saunders.

Yager JA, Wilcock BP: *Color atlas and text of surgical pathology of the dog and cat dermatopathology and skin tumors*, London, 1994, Wolfe.

Website for the Veterinary Oncology Service at the University of Illinois. http://www.cvm.uiuc.edu/vth/oncology/index.html.

Glossary

abdomen   region of the body between the chest and the hindquarters.

abscess   (plural *abscesses*) a collection of pus in a pocket formed within the tissues.

acantholysis   separation of skin cells from one another resulting from destruction of the intercellular structures that usually hold them together.

acantholytic keratinocytes   skin cells that have been separated from the rest of the epidermis and are floating free in a vesicle, pustule, or crust.

acetate tape   clear tape that is sticky on one side; used by veterinarians to collect cells from the surface of the skin for microscopic examination.

acid-fast stain   used to identify certain types of bacteria (e.g., mycobacteria) that take up the stain.

acne   inflammatory eruption of the hair follicles and the oil and sweat glands of the skin.

acral   relating to the legs and feet.

acromegaly   disease resulting from high levels of growth hormone in a mature animal; the feet, limbs, and head grow abnormally large, and internal organs become enlarged.

actinic   relating to the chemically active rays of ultraviolet radiation, as in sunlight.

actinic keratoses   red, scaly, or crusted skin lesions caused by exposure to ultraviolet radiation.

acute   referring to a health effect that comes on quickly and is of short duration.

Addisonian crisis   a life-threatening drop in blood pressure (cardiovascular collapse) due to inadequate blood volume caused by a lack of corticosteroid hormones and aldosterone normally produced by the adrenal gland.

adenocarcinoma   an epithelial cell cancer; the tumor cells form a glandlike structure.

adenoma a benign tumor of the epithelium; the tumor cells form a glandlike structure.

adenitis inflammation of a gland or lymph node.

adnexa accessory skin structures; in dermatology, refers to hair follicles, the oil and sweat glands, and claws (nails).

adrenal glands paired endocrine glands near the kidneys that produce aldosterone, corticosteroids, sex hormones, and catecholamines (epinephrine, norepinephrine).

allergen a substance that causes allergy.

allergic reaction any response stimulated by an allergen.

allergy an exaggerated reaction by the body to an antigen (such as hypersensitivity).

alopecia lack of hair or hair loss.

alpha-interferon (or *interferon alpha*) a glycoprotein with antiviral activity; produced by white blood cells in response to a viral infection; also produced commercially for the treatment of a variety of infections and tumors.

amyloid any of a group of proteins chemically similar to immunoglobulins.

amyloidosis a disease characterized by accumulations of amyloid in various organs and tissues.

anagen the growth stage of a hair follicle.

anal sacs paired structures near the anus that are lined with sweat and oil glands and produce malodorous secretions.

analgesic pain-relieving compound.

anaphylaxis hypersensitivity to substances such as foreign proteins or drugs; sensitization by an earlier contact with the causative agent is required; may cause respiratory distress (difficulty breathing), cardiovascular collapse ("shock"), and death.

anchoring fibrils microscopic fibers that connect the epidermis to the dermis.

anemia a lower-than-normal number of red blood cells in circulation.

anestrus a period of sexual inactivity; prolonged lack of estrus or heat cycles.

angioedema   leakage of fluid from the blood into the tissues surrounding blood vessels, causing swelling.

anorexia   diminished appetite.

anthelmintic   a compound that will expel or destroy parasitic worms, especially of the intestine.

antibodies   proteins produced by specialized B-lymphocytes after stimulation by an antigen; they bind to that antigen, targeting it for removal by other cells in an immune response; also called *immunoglobulins*.

antigen   protein or carbohydrate capable of stimulating an immune response.

antigen-antibody complexes   molecules that result from binding of an antibody to its specific antigen; may circulate in the blood or may be deposited in tissues such as blood vessels, kidneys, skin, or joints, where they may cause damage.

antihistamine   a compound that counteracts histamine; used to treat allergic reactions.

antimicrobial   a substance that prevents or stops the growth of microbes (bacteria and fungi).

antinuclear antibody (ANA) test   a test used to detect the presence of antibodies against antigens present in normal cell nuclei; used as a screening test in the diagnosis of systemic lupus erythematosus.

antiseborrheic   preventing or relieving excessive secretion of oil and scaling in seborrheic dermatitis.

antiseptic   preventing or stopping the growth of microorganisms.

apocrine sweat glands   (epitrichial sweat glands) sweat glands near the hair follicles of dogs and cats which empty into the hair follicle through a duct.

apoptosis   programmed cell death; often a premature death or loss of cells.

apoptotic keratinocytes   skin cells (keratinocytes) that are prematurely dead or dying.

asthenia   weakness; in dermatology, refers to decreased strength of the dermis, resulting in skin that is easily torn.

astringent   causing shrinkage of tissue; a drying agent.

atopy (atopic dermatitis)   a hereditary allergy produced when the pet is exposed to an offending environmental antigen; signs may include asthma, hay fever, hives, itching, or skin rashes.

atrophy   reduction in size, a wasting away.

aural   pertaining to the ear.

aural hematoma   a collection of blood between the cartilage and skin of the ear flap.

auricular   pertaining to the ear.

auricular chondrosis   abnormality in the cartilage of the ear flap.

autoantibody   antibody developed against a host tissue antigen (against a self-antigen).

autoimmune   refers to an immune reaction directed against the individual's own tissues.

avermectins   a group of drugs that kill both internal and skin parasites.

axilla   "armpit"; junction of a forelimb and the body.

bacteria   (plural of *bacterium*) unicellular microorganisms; may live freely, on decaying matter, or in a mutually beneficial relationship with another organism; also may parasitize another organism, or cause disease in another organism.

basement membrane zone   the junction between the epidermis and the dermis; contains many molecules and fibers that anchor the epidermis to the dermis.

benign   indicating the mild character of an illness or the nonmalignant character of a tumor.

biochemical profile   a series of blood tests to check the function of various body tissues, glands, and organs (see also *blood chemistry panel*).

biopsy   process of removing tissue for diagnostic evaluation.

blastogenesis   transformation of cells into actively dividing ones.

blood chemistry panel   biochemical tests used to evaluate various body organs, including the kidneys, liver, pancreas, adrenal glands, parathyroid gland, and muscles; also called a *biochemical profile*.

bulla a fluid-filled blister in the skin more than 1 cm wide.

calcify to deposit calcium salts or form bone.

calcinosis circumscripta presence of localized deposits of calcium salts in the skin and subcutaneous tissues; may be hereditary in some dogs.

calcinosis cutis presence of deposits of calcium salts in the skin; most commonly seen as one of the signs of Cushing's disease.

calculus an abnormal concretion (hard substance) within the body, usually composed of mineral salts; dental calculus is formed when plaque calcifies.

Canidae a family of the Carnivora; includes dogs, coyotes, wolves, and foxes.

carrier *infectious disease*: bearer and transmitter of a causative agent, especially one who carries the causative agent of a disease (such as typhoid fever) internally but is immune to it; *genetics*: an individual with a specified genetic mutation but who does not show, or only slightly shows, the characteristics encoded by the mutation.

catheter a tube for the passage of fluid from or into a body cavity or blood vessel.

cerumen earwax; composed of secretions from the various glands in the lining of the ear canal.

ceruminal relating to cerumen.

ceruminal glands modified sebaceous glands in the lining of the ear canal that secrete cerumen, or ear wax.

ceruminolytic an agent that breaks up cerumen.

ceruminous relating to cerumen.

Cheyletiella mite that parasitizes cats, dogs, and rabbits and may temporarily infest humans; these white mites live on the surface of the skin.

cheyletiellosis infestation with *Cheyletiella* mites; also called "walking dandruff."

chitin   the horny substance in the outer coat (ectoskeleton) of insects and crabs and present in certain microorganisms, plants, and fungi.

cholinesterase   a family of enzymes that break down acetylcholine; plays an important role in the transmission of nerve signals.

claw   a sharp, slender, usually curved, horny plate growing from the toe of an animal, commonly called a nail.

clinical signs   any abnormalities associated with a disease that can be detected by a physical examination.

colitis   inflammation of the colon (large intestine).

collagen   the main protein in connective tissue fibers.

colonization   the growth of microorganisms in a tissue or on a laboratory growth medium.

color-mutant hair dysplasia   distortion of hair follicles from clumps of melanin in blue- or fawn-colored dogs.

comedo   (plural *comedones*) a dilated hair follicle filled with keratin and sebum; a blackhead.

complete blood cell count (CBC)   measurement of the numbers of red blood cells, platelets, and white blood cells, and of the various types of white blood cells, present in blood.

computed tomography (CT) scan   a process in which x-rays and computer technology are used to produce images showing the internal anatomy in cross-section.

connective tissue   fibers and fibrous tissue that form the structure of the dermis, muscle sheaths, and tendons, and that provide strength to these tissues.

cornea   the transparent outer covering on the front of the globe (eyeball).

corticosteroid   any of various steroid hormones produced by the adrenal cortex; natural and synthetic forms are used medically, especially to fight inflammation.

cortisol   the main corticosteroid produced by the adrenal glands.

cryosurgery   surgery that uses freezing temperature to destroy tissue (often with liquid nitrogen or carbon dioxide).

culture and sensitivity testing laboratory procedure for identifying microorganisms and determining the ability of various antimicrobial agents to inhibit their growth; also referred to as *culture and susceptibility testing.*

Cushing's disease group of disease signs due to excess of corticosteroids, which often include hair loss, excessive thirst, excessive urination, increased appetite, and muscle weakness; caused by oversecretion of corticosteroids by the adrenal gland or by treatment with corticosteroids.

cutaneous relating to the skin.

Cuterebra botfly that resembles a large bumblebee as an adult; larvae are parasites of rodents, lagomorphs (rabbits and hares), and occasionally dogs and cats; larvae develop into spiny grubs, usually in the subcutaneous tissues of the head or neck.

cycloplegic drug that paralyzes the eye muscle that controls the size of the pupil; used in the treatment of some diseases affecting the eye.

cyst an abnormal saclike structure filled with gas, fluid, or semisolid material.

cystadenocarcinoma cancer that grows from glandular epithelium.

cystadenoma/cystadenomatosis benign tumor that grows from glandular epithelium/changes in skin typical of these tumors.

cytological examination the examination of cells under a microscope to identify their cell type and other characteristics.

cytology study of the anatomy, physiology, pathology, and chemistry of the cell; the examination of cells under a microscope to identify their cell type and other characteristics.

definitive diagnosis final diagnosis for a condition.

Demodex microscopic mite that usually lives in hair follicles and sebaceous glands; various species affect different hosts.

demodicosis skin disease resulting from infestation with *Demodex* mites.

dermal pertaining to the dermis.

dermatitis skin disease characterized by inflammation.

dermatomyositis a hereditary disease of Collies and Shetland Sheepdogs that affects the skin and the muscles.

dermatophyte a parasitic fungus that lives on the skin or skin derivatives (such as hair or nails); cause of ringworm.

dermatophytosis skin disease caused by infection with a dermatophyte.

dermis the skin layer under the epidermis; contains connective tissue, blood vessels, and nerves.

desensitize to make a sensitized or hypersensitive individual insensitive or nonreactive to a sensitizing agent, thereby eliminating the signs associated with an allergy.

dewclaw a rudimentary fifth toe on the back of the leg in dogs; does not touch the ground and is functionless.

Diff-Quik a type of stain commonly used for cytological examinations.

differential diagnosis determination of a diagnosis based on a list of diseases that could cause the observed signs; this list helps the veterinarian decide what tests are needed to make a diagnosis.

discoid lupus erythematosus an immune-mediated disease characterized by loss of pigment, crusting, and ulceration of the nose, face, and legs.

dopamine a chemical involved in nerve transmission in the brain; a precursor of several hormones (catecholamines).

ectoparasites parasites that live on the body surfaces.

edema excess accumulation of watery fluid in tissue.

electron microscopy microscopic examination in which the interactions of electrons with the specimen are used to provide information about the structure of the specimen.

electrophoresis the use of electrical fields to move particles; used in some diagnostic tests.

electrophysiologic testing measurement of electrical activity in the evaluation of muscle or nerve function.

elimination diet a restriction in the type of food being fed to an animal to identify the presence of a food allergy.

Elizabethan collar a large plastic cone placed around the neck to prevent an animal from chewing or licking its body.

emollient an agent that softens the skin or soothes irritation.

endemic occurring with predictable regularity within a certain population or region.

endocrine pertaining to glands that produce secretions that pass directly into the blood or lymph and that act on distant tissues; substances secreted by endocrine glands are called hormones.

endocrinopathy disease caused by deficiencies or excesses of hormones in the body; examples of endocrine diseases are diabetes, hypothyroidism, and Cushing's disease.

endorphins substances found in the brain and other parts of the body that are involved in producing a sense of euphoria or well-being.

endothelium cells lining blood or lymphatic vessels.

enzyme-linked immunosorbent assay (ELISA) in allergy testing, a test performed on the patient's serum to measure IgE for a particular antigen.

epidermis the outermost layer of skin.

epilate to pull out a hair.

epinephrine a substance produced by the adrenal glands; involved in the regulation of respiration, circulation, and other important body functions; also called *adrenaline*.

epithelium the cellular layer covering body surfaces; includes the skin and the linings of internal spaces such as the intestinal tract and respiratory tract.

eosinophil   a white blood cell containing granules that stain red with eosin dye; eosinophils are involved in the immune response against parasites and also are involved in type I hypersensitivity reactions (allergies).

eosinophilic granuloma   small nodule (bump) containing eosinophils, macrophages, and connective tissue cells; usually associated with parasites or allergies.

eosinophilic plaque   raised, flat, red skin lesion containing eosinophils; usually associated with allergies.

erythema   reddening of the skin.

eustachian tube   tube that connects the middle ear with the throat; also called the *auditory tube*.

excision   removal (usually surgical).

excisional   referring to complete removal (usually surgical), as in biopsy of a tumor.

excoriation   scratches, usually linear.

exfoliate   to detach and shed the outer layers of the skin.

exfoliative   marked by exfoliation, sloughing, or profuse scaling.

exudate   fluid that has seeped from tissue or capillaries, usually because of inflammation.

facial nerve paralysis   damage to the seventh cranial nerve that results in paralysis and inability to blink the eye on the affected side of the face.

familial   hereditary, found in families.

feline immunodeficiency virus   a viral infection of cats that targets T-lymphocytes and produces immunosuppression; human immunodeficiency virus (HIV) is a related but different virus.

feline leukemia virus   a viral infection of cats that causes immunosuppression and increases the risk of a variety of cancers.

feline sarcoma virus   a virus found in association with feline leukemia virus in cats that causes cancers.

feline urological syndrome   a disorder in cats that causes frequent, painful urination and sometimes bladder obstruction in male cats.

fine needle aspiration use of a small-gauge needle to obtain cells from a tissue or tumor for diagnostic examination.

fistula an abnormal opening from one hollow internal organ to another or to the skin.

fleas small wingless blood-sucking insects with powerful hind legs for jumping; fleas feed on many animals.

flora the microorganisms normally inhabiting a tissue or area.

focal limited to a particular area.

follicular casts accumulations of keratin and sebum around the base of a hair.

follicular dysplasia malformation of hair follicles; some forms are hereditary.

folliculitis inflammation of hair follicles; common causes include *Demodex* mites, *Staphylococcus* bacteria, and dermatophytes (ringworm).

fungal pertaining to fungi.

fungi (plural of *fungus*) any of a group of spore-producing organisms that grow on dead organic matter or are parasitic, usually classified as chlorophyll-lacking plants; include molds, rusts, mildews, smuts, mushrooms, and yeasts.

furunculosis deep infection or inflammation in a hair follicle, often associated with rupture of the hair follicle.

gland an organized group of cells that functions as a secretory or excretory organ.

glucagon a hormone produced by the pancreas that converts glycogen to glucose.

glycogen a carbohydrate that is easily converted to glucose for use as an energy source.

Gram stain a stain for bacteria; useful in identifying bacteria and classifying them as gram-positive or gram-negative.

granuloma a lumpy inflammatory mass, usually made up of scavenger cells and connective tissue.

gynecomastia overdevelopment of the male mammary glands.

hair follicle   the structural unit of a hair; the hair shaft grows from a hair bulb and is encased by a hair follicle with an opening on the surface of the skin.

hamartoma   a malformation that resembles a tumor but grows at the same rate as for normal tissue.

heartworms   *Dirofilaria immitis*; adult parasites live in the heart and arteries of the lungs of dogs and sometimes cats.

hematoma   localized collection of blood outside the vessels, caused by bleeding into a tissue.

hematopoiesis   the production of blood cells.

hemorrhagic   composed of blood; bloody.

hemostat   an instrument used to clamp blood vessels and other tissues.

hemostatic   arrests the flow of blood (stops bleeding).

histamine   a compound that causes dilation of capillaries, contraction of smooth muscle, and secretion of gastric acid; released during allergic reactions.

histiocyte   a cell that engulfs potentially harmful substances and cells; can be one of three cell types: blood monocyte, tissue macrophage, or dendritic myeloid cell.

histiocytoma   a benign growth containing histiocytes.

histology   the science that studies the microscopic structure of tissues and cells in relation to their function.

histopathologic   relating to the study of the cytologic and histologic structure of abnormal or diseased tissue.

histopathology   science that studies the cytologic and histologic structure of abnormal or diseased tissue.

hives   red, raised skin bumps accompanied by itching, often due to a type I hypersensitivity reaction (allergy).

hormone   a substance formed in one organ or part of the body and carried in the blood to another tissue, where it produces an effect.

Horner's syndrome   refers to a group of signs—drooping eyelid, small pupil, and sunken eye—caused by nerve damage.

humectant   moistening compound; an agent that binds water.

hydration   refers to the water content of the body or a tissue.

hyperadrenocorticism   syndrome associated with excessive secretion of corticosteroids; see also *Cushing's disease.*

hypercalcemia   increased blood calcium concentration.

hyperpigmentation   increased concentration of melanin (black pigment) in the skin.

hyperplasia   enlargement of a tissue or organ due to an increase in the number of cells.

hypersensitivity   describes harmful reactions of the immune system, subclassified as types I, II, III, IV. Type I (immediate) hypersensitivity reactions are immediate reactions that develop within 30 minutes in a sensitized host after exposure to an antigen. Examples are anaphylaxis, hives, and atopy. Type II (cytotoxic) hypersensitivity reactions involve the destruction of body cells as a result of antigen-antibody reactions. An example is autoimmune hemolytic anemia. Type III (immune complex) hypersensitivity reactions involve immune complexes. Examples are the arthritis and kidney disease associated with systemic lupus erythematosus. Type IV (delayed) hypersensitivity reactions involve sensitized T-lymphocytes and produce inflammation 24 to 72 hours after exposure to an antigen. An example is the skin's reaction to poison ivy.

hyperthyroidism   syndrome caused by abnormally high levels of thyroid hormones.

hyphae   branching tubular cells formed by fungi; filamentous form of fungi.

hypothyroidism   syndrome caused by abnormally low levels of thyroid hormones.

hypotrichosis   sparse hair coat; fewer hairs than normal.

iatrogenic   caused by the treatment; refers to a response to a medical or surgical treatment, usually unfavorable.

ichthyosis   a congenital disorder of keratin formation that results in dry, scaly skin.

idiopathic   of unknown cause.

IgA   see *immunoglobulin A.*

IgE   see *immunoglobulin E.*

immune complexes   see *antigen-antibody complexes.*

immune-mediated disease   conditions in which the immune response is directed against the animal's own body and is responsible for the clinical signs.

immune system   the system that protects the body from pathogens; consists of the thymus, spleen, lymph nodes, special deposits of lymphoid tissue (as in the gastrointestinal tract and bone marrow), lymphocytes (including B- and T-cells), and antibodies. Its major function is to distinguish self from nonself.

immunodeficiency   a condition resulting from impaired function of the immune system that results in increased susceptibility to disease.

immunoglobulin   see *antibodies.*

immunoglobulin A (IgA)   a type of antibody secreted at body surfaces to protect the body from foreign substances.

immunoglobulin E (IgE)   a type of antibody secreted in response to parasites and in the allergic reactions of patients with atopy.

immunological   relating to the immune response.

immunologist   a scientist who specializes in the study of the immune system.

immunosuppression   inhibition of the immune response by corticosteroids, chemotherapy agents, viruses, poor nutrition, or diseases that destroy or inactivate parts of the immune system.

immunotherapy   method of treatment or prevention of disease that stimulates active or passive immunity; allergen-specific immunotherapy is used to desensitize patients to allergens involved in atopy.

impression smear   the pressing of a glass slide onto a tissue to obtain cells for cytological evaluation.

indolent ulcer   an ulcer on a cat's upper lip; associated with allergies.

infiltrate accumulation of cells or fluids in a tissue.

inflammation a local response to cell injury that is marked by dilated capillaries, white blood cell infiltration, redness, swelling, heat, and pain; helps eliminate damaging substances and injured tissue.

inguinal relating to the groin.

intercellular adhesion molecules molecules that hold cells and structures together.

intermediate host an animal harboring the immature stage(s) of a parasite.

intradermal skin allergy test injection of small amounts of allergens into the skin to test for hypersensitivity reactions.

iodophor topical antiseptic containing iodine.

itch an irritating sensation in the skin that brings on the urge to scratch; also called *pruritus*.

keratin the protein that makes up hair, horn, claws, and feathers.

keratinization the development of keratin or keratinous tissue; cornification.

keratinization defect abnormality in the development of keratin or keratinous tissue; may be primary (hereditary) or secondary (such as that due to nutritional deficiency).

keratinocytes cells of the living epidermis and oral epithelium that produce keratin during transformation to the fully keratinized cells of the stratum corneum, the horny outer skin layer.

keratolytic promoting softening and dissolution of the stratum corneum (the outermost layer of skin cells); a keratolytic shampoo breaks up and removes accumulations of scale during bathing.

keratoplastic promoting normal skin growth and keratinization by slowing the production of new skin cells and decreasing scale production.

keratosebaceous casts see *follicular casts*.

Langerhans cells cells found in the skin that are believed to be involved in the immune response.

larva (plural *larvae*) immature form of insects and worms; do not resemble the adults and must undergo considerable change in form before reaching the adult stage (for example, white grubs in soil or decayed wood are larvae of beetles). Caterpillars, maggots, and screw-worms are larvae.

laser surgery the use of high-energy beams to cut, divide, or dissolve a tissue.

leiomyoma benign tumor of smooth muscle.

leishmaniasis infection with *Leishmania* species of protozoal organisms.

lesion an abnormality resulting from a disease; a wound or injury.

leukocyte any one of several kinds of white blood cells that circulate in the blood; the blood cells responsible for fighting infection.

libido sex drive.

lice (plural of *louse*) host-specific ectoparasites that feed on hair, feathers, epidermal debris, and sometimes the blood of the host.

lichenification thickening of the skin with exaggeration of skin markings; skin takes on the appearance of tree bark.

lupus a term originally used to describe a facial rash with skin erosions; now used to refer to a variety of autoimmune diseases characterized by infiltrates of lymphocytes and plasma cells.

lupus band an infiltrate of lymphocytes and plasma cells located just below the basement membrane zone; associated with diseases in the lupus complex.

lupus erythematosus an autoimmune disease associated with the production of autoantibodies against a variety of tissues.

Lyme disease bacterial infection affecting many parts of the body, caused by *Borrelia burgdorferi*; usually transmitted to animals by immature deer ticks.

lymphocytes (B and T) white blood cells involved in immune reactions. B-lymphocytes have antibody molecules on the surface and become antibody-secreting plasma cells when mature; T-lymphocytes are transformed in the thymus, possess highly specific cell-surface antigen receptors, and include cells that control the initiation (helper T-cells) or suppression (suppressor T-cells) of immunity or that attack and kill antigen-bearing cells (cytotoxic T-cells).

maceration softening or deterioration through the action of a liquid.

macroconidia large spore bodies produced by a fungal colony; dermatophytes are identified by the appearance of their macroconidia.

macrophage a cell found in tissues that devours foreign material and tissue debris by a process called phagocytosis.

maggot a fly larva or grub.

magnetic resonance imaging (MRI) production of an image by use of magnetic fields and the transmission of radio wave energy.

Malassezia yeast that lives in the ears and on the skin of dogs and cats; overgrowth causes inflammation.

malignant referring to invasive and destructive growth and spread (of a tumor).

mange skin disease caused by mites.

mast cells cells found in the connective tissue of the skin, respiratory tract, and gastrointestinal tract; contain intracellular granules filled with histamine and other substances that produce inflammation when released into the tissues; involved in allergic diseases by way of binding of IgE.

melanin a dark-brown to black pigment normally found in cells of the epidermis, eyes, and hair.

melanocytes pigment-producing cells of the skin and hair follicles.

melatonin a hormone produced by the pineal gland.

Merkel cells receptor cells for touch in the skin; also function in regulation of blood circulation in the skin, sweat production, keratinocyte proliferation, and hair growth.

metabolic diseases conditions associated with abnormalities in metabolism (for example, endocrine diseases, diabetes, liver failure, or kidney failure).

metabolic epidermal necrosis death of the cells of the epidermis as a result of a metabolic disease; commonly associated with severe liver disease or glucagon-secreting pancreatic tumors.

metabolism chemical and physical changes in a tissue, including the building of large molecules from small molecules and their breakdown.

metamorphosis in insects, the transition from one developmental stage to another.

metastasis the movement of a disease process or tumor cells from one part of the body to another.

metastatic relating to metastasis.

metastasize to invade by metastasis.

microbiology the science that studies microorganisms.

microorganisms microscopic life forms, including fungi, protozoa, bacteria, and viruses.

microscopic of minute size; visible only under a microscope.

miliary dermatitis a skin disease pattern seen in cats with allergies. The lesions are small, raised, red bumps (papules) that become encrusted and feel like millet seeds on the skin surface.

mite a tiny arthropod of the order Acarina; some species are free-living, but others are parasitic on plants or animals.

miticide an agent that kills mites.

mold a superficial, often woolly fungal growth; can occur on damp or decaying organic matter or on living organisms; spores produced by molds are allergenic to many animals and people.

monoamine oxidase inhibitors drugs that block the activity of enzymes that break down certain neurotransmitters in the brain, resulting in increased levels of the neurotransmitter; these drugs alter brain function and are used as antidepressants.

monoclonal referring to cells originating from a single cell, or to products of monoclonal cells, such as a single type of antibody.

monocyte a white blood cell with a single round nucleus; attacks and destroys harmful substances and cells.

mucin carbohydrate-rich glycoprotein present in connective tissue; also present in secretions of the goblet cells of the intestines and other mucous glandular cells.

mycobacteria organisms belonging to the genus *Mycobacterium* (includes the tuberculosis bacterium and many other acid-fast bacteria).

mycoses diseases produced by fungal infections; they include infections of keratinized elements of the skin (dermatophytosis), infections of subcutaneous (beneath the skin) tissues, and systemic infections, usually involving multiple internal body tissues or organs.

myiasis infestation by maggots (fly larvae).

myringotomy cutting into the tympanic membrane (eardrum).

nasal planum the hairless, leathery skin over the end of the nose of a dog or cat; also called the *planum nasale*.

nasopharyngeal polyps benign masses arising within the nasal cavity or pharynx (throat).

nasopharynx the part of the pharynx (back of the throat) that lies above the soft palate.

necrosis death of cells resulting from irreversible damage due to disease.

nematodes roundworms of the phylum Nematoda; many species are parasites of animals, others are parasites of plants.

neoplasia the process that results in the formation and growth of a neoplasm (tumor).

neoplasm a tumor; an abnormal tissue that grows by a rapid increase in the number of cells and continues to grow after the stimulus that started the growth ceases.

neuroendocrine pertaining to the relationships between the nervous and the endocrine systems; referring to cells that release a hormone into the blood in response to a signal from the nervous system.

neurological signs weakness, paralysis, or changes in behavior caused by abnormalities of the nervous system.

neutrophil a mature white blood cell with a nucleus of variable appearance; functions as a phagocytic cell (devours foreign substances and tissue debris).

nevus (plural *nevi*) a distinctly bordered malformation of the skin, especially one that is colored or hyperpigmented.

nodular having the characteristics of a nodule.

nodule a small, distinct mass of tissue that feels different from the surrounding tissue.

Notoedres a sarcoptic mange mite that affects cats.

nuclear imaging the use of a small dose of a radioactive agent to detect abnormalities in blood flow to a tissue or organ; also called *nuclear scintigraphy*.

nuclear scans the images produced in nuclear imaging.

nymph one of the life stages of many insects; nymphs generally resemble adults but lack full development of wings or genitals.

obsessive-compulsive disorder an anxiety disorder in which repetitive acts are performed to relieve anxiety.

occlusive denotes a bandage or medication that keeps air from reaching a tissue or wound.

omega fatty acids (omega-3 and omega-6) unsaturated fatty acids with varying numbers of double bonds are named based on the location of the first double bond. Omega-3 fatty acids have the first double bond on the third carbon; sources of omega-3 fatty acids include flaxseed oil and fish oils. Omega-6 fatty acids have the first double bond on the sixth carbon; sources of omega-6 fatty acids include vegetable oils and animal fats.

oncologist a specialist in oncology.

oncology the study of the properties of neoplasms (tumors), including their causes, growth, and treatment.

onychodystrophy presence of abnormalities in the claws (nails).

onychomadesis   complete shedding of the nails.

onychomalacia   abnormal softness of the nails.

onychorrhexis   abnormal brittleness and splitting of the free edges of the nails.

onychoschizia   splitting of the nails into layers.

opioid   possessing some of the properties of the opiate narcotics.

organophosphates   a group of phosphorus-containing compounds used as insecticides that interfere with nerve transmission by irreversibly inhibiting cholinesterase.

OTC   over-the-counter; a product that does not require a prescription for purchase.

otic   pertaining to the ear.

otitis externa   inflammation of the ear canal.

otitis interna   inflammation of the inner ear.

otitis media   inflammation of the middle ear cavity.

Otodectes   ear mite of cats and dogs.

otoscope   an instrument for examining the ear canal and eardrum.

ototoxicity   the property of being harmful to the ear.

pancreatitis   inflammation of the pancreas.

panniculitis   inflammation of the subcutaneous fat.

papilloma   a distinct, benign epithelial tumor that usually projects up from the surrounding skin surface; a wartlike mass.

papillomavirus   any of a group of viruses that produce papillomas and warts.

papule   a small, solid, usually conical elevation of the skin; a red, raised skin bump.

parakeratosis   an abnormality in keratinization in which the nuclei are retained in cells of the stratum corneum; also called *parakeratotic hyperkeratosis*.

paraneoplastic   referring to any abnormality associated with a malignant neoplasm but not directly related to invasion by the primary tumor or its metastases.

parasite   an organism that lives, at least for a time, at the expense of a host animal.

parasiticide   a compound that kills parasites.

parathyroid hormone   parathyroid gland secretion involved in the regulation of blood calcium (increases blood calcium concentrations); also called *parathormone*.

paronychia   inflammation of the skin fold around the claw.

pathologist   a doctor who specializes in identifying diseases from laboratory specimens.

pathology   the medical science and practice concerned with the study of all aspects of disease.

pediculosis   infestation with lice.

Pelodera   free-living nematode (roundworm) whose larvae may penetrate the skin of animals that come in contact with infested soil, resulting in inflammation; larvae may be found in the hair follicles of these animals.

pemphigus   immune-mediated blistering diseases with acantholysis (separation of epidermal cells with accumulations of fluid between them).

pemphigus foliaceus   an autoimmune (immune-mediated) disease in which antibodies are directed against the proteins in the skin that hold the cells together, causing blisters or pustules to form.

penetrance   the frequency with which individuals who inherit a gene actually show the inherited trait; how often an inherited trait is clinically evident.

perianal fistula   tract between the subcutaneous tissue and the surface of the skin around the anal region, most common in German Shepherd Dogs.

perineum   the area between the anus and the scrotum or vulva.

periodontal disease   inflammation of the tissues surrounding the teeth; may include inflammation of the gums, pocket formation around the teeth, dental plaque, and calculus and may result in loosening or loss of teeth.

perioral   around the mouth.

phytates   salts or esters of phytic acid found in plants; bind with calcium and magnesium, making them unavailable for absorption from the diet.

pinna (plural *pinnae*) the projecting, mostly cartilage, portion of the external ear; the earflap.

piroplasmosis also called *babesiosis*; disease caused by protozoal parasites transmitted by ticks.

planum nasale see *nasal planum*.

plaque a bacteria-laden film that coats the teeth and the mucous membranes of the mouth.

plasma cells oval cells with an off-center, round nucleus that arise from B-lymphocytes; active in the formation and secretion of antibodies (immunoglobulins).

platelet a constituent of blood that is needed for blood clotting.

pododermatitis inflammation of the skin of the feet.

pollen substance composed of microspores of seed plants; the male germ needed for reproduction; important cause of some allergies.

polyclonal cells derived from two or more cells of different ancestry or genetic makeup, or products of such cells.

polydipsia increased water consumption.

polyp a mass of tissue that bulges outward from the normal surface, sometimes on a slender stalk.

polyphagia increased food intake.

polyuria increased urine output.

porphyrins reddish-brown compounds derived from hemoglobin.

prednisolone a corticosteroid that is used as an anti-inflammatory drug.

prednisone a corticosteroid; requires metabolism in the liver to form prednisolone for anti-inflammatory activity.

proteolytic enzymes enzymes that help break down proteins.

Protozoa a subkingdom of the animal kingdom that includes one-celled and multicellular organisms.

protozoal relating to protozoa.

provocative exposure intentional exposure of an animal to a substance suspected of being responsible for disease, to find out whether the substance causes the condition to worsen.

pruritic threshold   the level of stimulus required to cause itching.

pruritus   see *itch*.

psychoactive drugs   medications with the ability to alter mood, anxiety, behavior, cognitive processes, or mental tension.

psychogenic   of mental origin or causation.

pupa   (plural *pupae*) stage of insect metamorphosis after the larva and before the emergence of the adult form.

purulent   containing, consisting of, or forming pus.

pus   a thick opaque fluid produced as a result of inflammation containing white blood cells and tissue debris.

pustule   a small elevation of the skin containing pus; a pimple.

pyoderma   an inflammatory condition of the skin with pus production.

pyogranuloma   an accumulation of neutrophils and macrophages, often surrounding a foreign body or microorganisms in the skin.

radiation   the transmission of electromagnetic rays for diagnosis or treatment; the rays may be of visible light, short radio waves, ultraviolet rays, or x-rays.

radiation therapy   use of ionizing radiation in the treatment of disease; also called *radiotherapy*.

radioimmunosorbent test (RAST)   in allergy testing, a test performed on the patient's serum to measure IgE for a particular antigen.

radionuclide   an isotope that possesses radioactivity.

renal   pertaining to the kidney.

reservoir   an infected animal (or group of similar animals) that serves as a source from which other animals can be infected.

restrictive diet trial   the feeding of a limited number of ingredients, often one protein source and one carbohydrate source, to reduce the likelihood of an adverse reaction to foods; used in testing for food allergies.

retinoids natural and synthetic forms of retinol (vitamin A₁).

ringworm skin disease caused by infection with dermatophytes (fungal organisms that live in keratinized tissues such as the hair, skin, and claws).

Rocky Mountain spotted fever disease resulting from infection with the rickettsial organism *Rickettsia rickettsii*; transmitted by ticks.

sarcoma a connective tissue neoplasm.

Sarcoptes mite that infests the skin of dogs and other canids and may temporarily infest people.

sarcoptid referring to mites of the family Sarcoptidae, including *Sarcoptes*, *Notoedres*, *Knemidokoptes*, and others.

scabicide a substance that kills *Sarcoptes* mites.

scabies skin disease caused by the burrowing of a sarcoptid mite.

sebaceous relating to sebum; oily, fatty.

sebaceous adenitis inflammation of the sebaceous glands; a hereditary condition in Standard Poodles.

seborrhea overactivity of the sebaceous glands resulting in oily skin and hair; in dogs and cats, also used to refer to scaly skin (excessive dandruff) associated with keratinization defects.

seborrhea oleosa a greasy, oily form of seborrhea.

seborrhea sicca a dry, scaly form of seborrhea.

sebum the substance secreted by the sebaceous (oil-producing) glands.

secondary referring to a condition that arises from another disease rather than being the primary problem; for example, secondary infections are common complications of many skin diseases.

sensitive in immunology, referring to an animal made susceptible to allergic reactions by previous exposure to an antigen.

sensitize to make sensitive, to induce acquired sensitivity, to immunize.

serpiginous creeping, having a wavy, arc-shaped border.

serum the fluid portion of the blood obtained after clots and blood cells are removed.

signalment the age, breed, and gender of an animal.

skin scraping a common diagnostic technique used in dermatology to identify the cause of a skin disease. A surgical blade is used to scrape the surface of the skin and collect cells and any organisms from the skin; the material obtained through this abrasion is transferred to a glass slide and examined under a microscope.

spore a primitive, usually single-celled, dormant or reproductive body produced by plants and some microorganisms such as fungi; capable of developing into a new individual, either directly or after fusion with another spore.

stage a period in the course of a disease; a description of the extent of involvement of a disease process, such as the spread of a cancer.

Staphylococcus (plural *Staphylococci*) gram-positive spherical bacterium (coccus); frequently associated with infections of the skin and hair follicles of dogs and cats.

stenosis narrowing.

steroid hepatopathy changes in the liver produced by high concentrations of corticosteroids; includes increased amounts of glycogen in the hepatocytes (liver cells) and increased levels of enzymes produced by liver cells.

stimulus (plural *stimuli*) something that elicits a response.

strangles a disease of puppies that causes severe swelling of the face and oozing skin inflammation.

stratum basale the base layer of the skin that gives rise to all others; attached to the basement membrane zone.

stratum corneum the fully keratinized outermost layer of the skin; horny layer.

stratum spinosum the layers of the skin between the stratum basale and stratum corneum, composed of keratinocytes in the processes of becoming keratinized.

subcutaneous under the skin.

submandibular lymph nodes lymph nodes located at the base of the lower jaw.

symmetric lupoid onychodystrophy an immune-mediated disease affecting the germinal cells of the claw; results in separation and sloughing of the claws.

systemic referring to a body-wide condition or to a drug that, given orally or by injection, acts on the entire body.

tapeworm a flat intestinal parasite of the class Cestoda; includes a mouth that attaches to the intestinal wall and a segmented body.

tartar dental plaque that has hardened into a more solid substance.

T cells see *lymphocytes*.

telogen the resting stage of the hair growth cycle—the hair is not growing and is easily removed from the follicle.

thyroglobulin a protein containing the precursors of thyroid hormones; stored in the colloid within the thyroid gland.

thyroiditis inflammation of the thyroid gland, usually by infiltrating lymphocytes.

thyroxine a hormone produced by the thyroid gland; also known as levothyroxine, tetraiodothyronine, and T_4.

tick blood-sucking members of the family Ixodidae or Argasidae; important pests of birds and mammals and transmitters of many diseases.

tick paralysis flaccid paralysis (inability to move) caused by toxins of several species of ticks; toxins interfere with nerve transmission.

tolerance the ability to endure or be less responsive to a stimulus, especially over a period of continued exposure.

topical referring to a local effect or to a drug that is applied to a local area, often the skin.

toxicity the state of being poisoned.

trichogram microscopic examination of hairs that have been plucked; can be used to distinguish between anagen and telogen hairs and to check hairs for breakage and other abnormalities.

tularemia a disease caused by *Francisella tularensis*; usually transmitted from rodents to people or other animals by the bites of ticks or flies.

tumor a swelling (tumefaction).

tympanic bulla the bone surrounding the middle ear cavity.

tympanic membrane the eardrum.

ulcer a sore in the skin or a mucous membrane resulting from loss of tissue, usually with inflammation.

ultrasonography the location, measurement, or delineation of deep structures within the body by measuring the reflection or transmission of high-frequency or ultrasonic waves; also called *ultrasound examination*, *echography*, and *sonography*.

ultraviolet radiation damaging rays from the sun.

urinalysis laboratory testing of urine; can be used to detect disorders involving the kidneys, urinary tract infections, and some metabolic diseases.

vasculitis inflammation of the arteries and veins; caused by a variety of diseases and toxic conditions.

vector (the Latin word for "carrier") an organism, such as a mosquito or tick, that transmits microorganisms that cause disease.

vesicle a fluid-filled blister in the skin less than 1 cm wide.

video-otoscope fiberoptic instrument that produces magnified images of the ear canal and eardrum.

vitiligo presence of nonpigmented white patches of various sizes in otherwise normal skin; epidermal melanocytes are lost in the depigmented areas by an autoimmune process.

Western blot a procedure used to identify specific antigens, antibodies, or other proteins in serum.

West Nile virus infection   a potentially serious infection spread by mosquitoes; affects the central nervous system, causing signs that may include headaches (in people), fever, weakness, and, in severe cases, paralysis and death.

white blood cells   cells formed in the bone marrow and lymphoid tissues that circulate in the blood and are also found in body tissues. Involved in the destruction of foreign substances and organisms that invade the body; also called *leukocytes*; include granulocytes (neutrophils, eosinophils, and basophils), lymphocytes, and monocytes.

yeast   a general term for an organism that belongs to the true fungi (family Saccharomycetaceae). True fungi usually have little or no mycelium and reproduce by budding; *Malassezia* is a yeast that frequently colonizes the skin and ear canals of pets.

zinc-responsive dermatosis   skin disease that improves when the animal is given zinc supplements.

Credits

Page 2   Courtesy Dr. Jennifer Matousek
Page 4   Courtesy DVM Pharmaceuticals, Inc., Miami
Page 9   Courtesy Sandra Grable
Page 72 *(top)*   Courtesy Dr. Warren Anderson
Page 142   Courtesy DVM Pharmaceuticals, Inc., Miami
Page 149   Courtesy Dr. Warren Anderson
Page 153   Courtesy DVM Pharmaceuticals, Inc., Miami
Page 161   Courtesy Erwin Small, DVM
Page 163   Courtesy DVM Pharmaceuticals, Inc., Miami
Page 184   Courtesy Dr. Donna Angarano
Page 210   Courtesy Dr. Erwin Small
Page 218   Courtesy Dr. Erwin Small
Page 219   Courtesy Dr. Jennifer Matousek
Page 222   Courtesy Dr. Jennifer Matousek
Page 229   Courtesy Dr. Warren Anderson
Page 295 *(top)*   Courtesy Dr. Warren Anderson
            (bottom)   Courtesy Dr. Jennifer Matousek
Page 296   Courtesy Dr. Adam Patterson
Page 309   Courtesy Dr. Rod AW Rosychuk. In Campbell KL: *Small Animal Dermatology Secrets*, St Louis, 2004, Hanley & Belfus
Page 319   Courtesy Dr. Adam Patterson
Page 323 *(bottom)*   Courtesy Dr. Warren Anderson
Page 335   Courtesy Dr. Warren Anderson
Page 349   Gotthelf LN: *Small Animal Ear Diseases*, ed 2, St Louis, 2005, Saunders.
Page 380   Campbell KL: *Small Animal Dermatology Secrets*, St Louis, 2004, Hanley & Belfus
Page 391 *(top)*   Campbell KL: *Small Animal Dermatology Secrets*, St Louis, 2004, Hanley & Belfus

Index

A

Abdominal drooping, in Cushing's disease, 185
Abdominal ultrasonography, in Cushing's disease, 187
Ablation, in ear surgery, 367
Abscess, subcutaneous, 138
Acantholysis, in phemigus diseases, 258
Acantholytic keratinocytes, 126, 258
Acanthosis nigricans, 284-285, 285f
Acetate tape, in parasitic examination, 46-47
Acid fast staining, in cytological examination, 52
Acids, fatty. *See* Fatty acids.
Acne, 131-133, 132f, 228
Acral lick dermatitis, 314-322, 315f, 316f, 319f
Acral mutilation syndrome, 285-286, 286f
Acrochordons, in keratoses, 372
Acrodermatitis, lethal, 300, 301f
Acromegaly
   in mucinosis, 302
   in pituitary dwarfism, 216
ACTH stimulation test, in Cushing's disease, 187-189
Actinic keratoses, 336, 371-372, 372f
Acute moist dermatitis, 119-121, 119f, 121f
Addisonian crisis, in Cushing's disease, 190
Adenitis, sebaceous, 44, 306-308, 307f, 342
Adenoma, sebaceous gland, 340
Adhesion molecules, intercellular , in pemphigus vulgaris, 264
Adnexa
   in immune-mediated diseases, 257
   production of, as skin function, 2
Adrenal-dependent hyperadrenocorticism, 183
Adrenal disorders, 182-194, 184f, 185f
Adult-onset generalized demodicosis, 150, 152
Adult-onset growth hormone deficiency, 216-217
Adulticides, in flea control, 145-147
ALD. *See* Acral lick dermatitis.
Allergens
   characteristics of, 73-75
   danders as, 74t, 78-79
   defined, 66
   drugs as, 114-115, 115f
   in earflap diseases, 337-338
   environmental, 80-81
   house dust as, 79, 80f
   insects as, 74t, 80-81
   in *Malassezia* dermatitis, 245
   molds as, 78
   pollens as, 76-78
   seasonality of, 72-73
Allergen-specific immunotherapy, in atropy, 88t, 98-99
Allergy(ies). *See also* Atopy.
   bathing techniques in, 16
   in cats, 65f, 71-72, 70f, 72f
   contact, 99-101, 100f
   defined, 66

Allergy(ies)—cont'd
  diagnosis of, 45
  in dogs, 68-70, 69f
  in earflap diseases, 337-338
  food, 103-111
  in granulomas, 371
  itching from, 63
  in otitis externa, 349-350
  parasite-related, 111-114, 112f, 113f
  testing for, 53-54
Alopecia
  bilaterally symmetrical, 197-198, 213
  canine recurrent flank, 222-223, 223f
  color mutant, 287
  diagnosis of, 56, 61-62, 62f
  ear, 335
  in endocrine diseases, 181
  feline endocrine, 213-214
  feline paraneoplastic, 390-391
  growth hormone-responsive, 216-217
  in hyperestrogenism, 209
  in hyperthyroidism, 206
  hormone testing for, 54
  pattern baldness in, 303, 303f
  psychogenic, 322-327, 323f, 324f, 326f
  in ringworm, 226
  seasonal flank, 222-223, 223f
Alopecia areata, 340
Alopecia X, 217-221, 218f, 219f, 222f
Alpha-interferon, in canine oral papillomatosis, 373
Alternaria, as allergen, 78
Amblyomma tick, 169
American dog tick, 169
Amitraz, antiparasitic use of, 38t
Amphotericin B, in systemic mycoses, 250
Amyloidosis, in plasma cell pododermatitis, 275
Anaerobic bacteria, in subcutaneous abscess, 138
Anagen hair, in alopecia, 62
Anagen phase, of hair cycle, 7-8
Anal licking, 330, 331f
Anal sac
  anatomy of, 10-11
  bathing techniques in, 16
  impacted
    in anal licking, 330
    in psychogenic alopecia, 322
  tumors of, 390
Analgesics
  in acute moist dermatitis, 120
  in total ear canal ablation, 368
Anatomic factors, in otitis externa, 344
Anemia, in hypothyroidism, 201
Anestrus, in hypothyroidism, 200
Anorexia, in ringworm, 239
Anipryl, in Cushing's disease, 193
Anoplura lice, 170
Antibacterial agents, in ear medications, 361
Antibacterial shampoos, 24
Antibodies
  IgE, 66
  in immune-mediated diseases, 257
  in ringworm, 231

Antibody-antigen complexes, in immune-mediated vasculitis, 273-274, 340
Antidepressants, in atropy, 90
Antifungal agents, in ringworm, 235t
Antifungal shampoos, 25, 246
Antigen(s)
  defined, 66
  in immune-mediated diseases, 257
  in systemic mycoses, 253
Antigen-antibody complexes. See Antibody-antigen complexes.
Antihistamines, in atopy, 87t, 89, 90
Antimicrobial drugs
  in bacterial infections, 117
  in granulomas, 371
Antimicrobial functions, of skin, 3-4
Antiparasitic shampoos, 25
Antipruritic shampoos, 25
Antiseborrheic shampoos, 23-24
  in acanthosis nigricans, 284
  in ichthyosis, 297
Antiseptic agents, in ear cleaning, 358
Anxiety, in obsessive-compulsive disorder, 311
Anxiolytic drugs, in acral lick dermatitis, 320
Apocrine cystadenomatosis, 341
Apocrine glands
  in Cushing's disease, 183
  cysts of, 341
  defined, 10
  protective function of, 2
  tumors of, 378
Armpit. See Axillae.
Arrector pili muscle, 8
Aspergillus, as allergen, 78
Aspirates, fine-needle, in fungi examination, 48-49
Assay, canine TSH, in hypothyroidism, 202-203
Asthenia, cutaneous, 293-294, 295f
Astringents
  in acute moist dermatitis, 120
  in ear cleaning, 358
  in Malassezia dermatitis, 246
  in otitis externa, 346
Asymptomatic carriers, of ringworm, 230
Atopic dermatitis, in earflap diseases, 337-338
Atopy, 67-68, 74t. See also Allergy(ies).
  in acanthosis nigricans, 285
  in acral lick dermatitis, 316
  defined, 67
  diagnosis of, 81-85
  inheritance of, 67-68
  management of, 85-99
  in otitis externa, 349
Atrophy
  in Cushing's disease, 185
  idiopathic thyroid gland, 197
Aural hematomas, 342
Auricular chondrosis, 340
Autoantibodies
  in immune-mediated diseases, 257
  in lymphocytic thyroiditis, 197
Autoimmune disease, immunologic testing for, 55
Awns, plant, in otitis externa, 349, 349f

Axillae
  in acanthosis nigricans, 284
  in dog atopy, 68
Azathioprine
  in dermatomyositis, 293
  in immune-mediated disease, 281

B

Bacteria, examination for, 51-52. *See also specific infections.*
Bald thigh syndrome, idiopathic, of Greyhounds, 303, 303f
Baldness, pattern, 303, 303f
Band, coronary, defined, 12
Barrier, enclosing, as skin function, 1
Basal cell tumors, 376
Basement-membrane zone, 5-6, 272
Bathing, 15-18, 16f
  of cats, 26-30, 29f
  of dogs, 26
Behavior modification, in acral lick dermatitis, 318. *See also*
    Psychogenic skin diseases.
Benign neoplasms, 369. *See also* Tumors.
Benzoyl peroxide shampoos, in *Malassezia* dermatitis, 246
Bilaterally symmetrical alopecia, 197-198, 213
Biochemical profile, in Cushing's disease, 186
Biopsies, skin. *See* Skin, biopsies of.
Biting, of tail, 327
Biting lice, 170
Black hair follicular dysplasia, 287-288, 288f
Blackheads. *See* Comedones.
Blastomyces dermatitidis, in systemic mycoses, 249
Blood count, complete. *See* Complete blood count.
Blood sugar, in Cushing's disease, 186-187
Blood tests, specialized, in immunologic testing, 55
Blood-clotting powder, in grooming, 14
Blot, Western, analysis of, in identifying allergens, 84
Blue Doberman syndrome, 287
Body suit,in atropy, 95, 95f
Borrelia burgdorferi tick, 169
Breed predisposition, 44
Brown dog tick, 168-169
Brushing, in grooming, 14
Bullae
  defined, 57t
  in interdigital pyoderma, 136
  lateral, osteotomy of, 367-368
  tympanic, in otitis media, 365
Bullous pemphigoid, 272-273, 273f, 340

C

Calcification, of ear canal, 344
Calcinosis, 57t
Calcinosis circumscripta, in acral lick dermatitis, 315
Calcinosis cutis
  in Cushing's disease, 183
  hormone testing for, 54
Calculus, in periodontal disease, 31
Cancer, defined, 369. *See also* Tumors.
Canine demodicosis, 148-152, 149f, 150f
Canine leproid granulomas syndrome, 338
Canine leprosy, 338

Canine oral papillomatosis, 373, 373f
Canine recurrent flank alopecia, 222-223, 223f
Canine scabies, 155-160, 156f
Canine TSH assay, in hypothyroidism, 202-203
"Canker", 255
Carbaryl, antiparasitic use of, 35t
Carcinoma. *See also* Tumor(s).
  sebaceous gland, 377
  squamous cell, 340, 375, 375f
Carriers
  of feline cowpox virus, 339
  of ringworm, 230
Castration-responsive dermatosis, 213
Casts, in sebaceous adenitis, 306, 342
Catheter, in otitis media, 365
Cationic surfactant hair conditioners, 30
CBC. *See* Complete blood count.
Cells, mast. *See* Mast cells.
Cellulitis, juvenile. *See* Puppy strangles.
Cerumen
  composition of, 11
  in otitis externa, 346
  in primary seborrhea, 304
Ceruminal gland tumors, 380
Ceruminolytic agents
  in ear cleaning products, 358, 359t
  n otitis externa, 346
Cheyletiella spp., in otitis externa, 348
Cheyletiellosis, 162-164, 163f
Chiggers, 164-165, 348
Chin pyoderma, 131-133, 132f
Chitin, in ringworm, 240
Chlorambucil, in immune-mediated disease, 281
Chlorpyrifos, antiparasitic use of, 35t
Chondrosis, auricular, 340
Circumanal gland tumors, 379-380, 380f
Cladosporium, as allergen, 78
Claws. *See* Nails.
Cleaning, of ears, 357-360, 357f
Coat conditioner, medicated, 31
Coccidioides immitis, in systemic mycoses, 249, 254
Coccidiomycosis, 254
Cockroach eggs, as allergen, 80
Colitis, anal licking in, 330
Collagen fibers, 6, 294
Collar, Elizabethan. *See* Elizabethan collar.
Collarette, epidermal, 59t
Color mutant alopecia, 287
Color-mutant hair dysplasia, in alopecia, 62
Comedo, 57t
Comedones
  in Cushing's disease, 183
  in feline acne, 132
Common deer tick, 169
Complete blood count
  in Cushing's disease, 185
  in immunologic testing, 55
Computed tomography scans, in Cushing's disease, 187
Conditioners, hair, 30-31, 87t
Conformational factors, in otitis externa, 344
Congenital skin diseases. *See* Hereditary skin diseases.

Connective tissue
   in Ehlers-Danlos syndrome, 293-294
   flexibility of, 2
   soft tissue sarcomas of, 383
Contact allergies, 99-101, 100f
Corneum, stratum. *See* Stratum corneum.
Cornifying epitheliomas, intracutaneous, 379
Coronary band, 12
Cortex, 7
Corticosteroids
   in acanthosis nigricans, 284
   in acral lick dermatitis, 318
   in acute moist dermatitis, 120
   in atropy, 88t, 89-94
   in bullous pemphigoid, 273
   in dermatomyositis, 292
   in immune-mediated disease, 280
   in otitis externa, 347
   in pemphigus erythematosus, 264
   in pemphigus follaceus, 261
   in ringworm, 231
   in sterile nodular panniculitis, 276
   in uveodermatological syndrome, 278
Cotton linters, as allergen, 80
Cottonseed, as allergen, 80
Cowpox virus, feline, 339
Crest, ungual, 12
Crisis, Addisonian, in Cushing's disease, 190
Crust, 59t
Cryosurgery
   in acral lick dermatitis, 319
   in earflap lesions, 336
Cryptorchidism, in hyperestrogenism, 209
Cryptococcus neoformans, in systemic mycoses, 249, 252-253, 253f
CT scans. *See* Computed tomography scans.
CTCL. *See* Cutaneous T-cell lymphoma.
Culture and sensitivity testing, in otitis media, 365
Culture and susceptibility testing, in staphylococcal pyoderma, 130-131
Curvularia, *as allergen,* 78
Cushing's disease, 182-194, 184f, 185f
   in acanthosis nigricans, 285
   diagnosis of, 44-45
   in earflap lesions, 339
   hormone testing for, 54
   iatrogenic, 183, 280
   paraneoplastic skin disease as, 391
Cutaneous asthenia, 293-294, 295f
Cutaneous histiocytomas, 385, 385f
Cutaneous horns, in keratoses, 371
Cutaneous papillomas, 373
Cutaneous T-cell lymphoma, 341, 386-387, 387f
Cutaneous tags, in keratoses, 372
Cuterebra *larvae, 172-173*
Cuticle, defined, 7
Cyclosporine, in atropy, 88t, 92
Cyst(s), 370
   in apocrine gland, 341
   defined, 57t
   in perianal fistula disease, 135

Cystadenomatosis, apocrine, 341
Cytological examination
    in acanthosis nigricans, 284
    in acral lick dermatitis, 315
    in basal cell tumors, 376
    defined, 51-52
    in *Malassezia* dermatitis, 245
    in skin fold pyoderma, 122-123
Cytoplegic solution, in uveodermatological syndrome, 278

D
Danders, as allergen, 74t, 78-79
Dandruff, walking, 162-164, 163f
Declawing, in symmetric lupoid onychodystrophy, 272
Decontamination, environmental, in ringworm, 233-234
Deep pyoderma, 136-138, 137f
Deer tick, common, 169
Definitive diagnosis, 42
Degranulation, 66
Dental care, 31-32
Demodex canis, 47, 336
Demodex cati 47, 152-153, 336, 348
Demodex gatoi, 47, 153, 336, 348
Demodicosis
    in acral lick dermatitis, 315
    canine, 148-152, 149f, 150f
    in earflap lesions, 336
    feline, 152-155, 153f, 154f
    in feline endocrine alopecia, 214
    generalized, 44, 54, 150, 152
    in German Shepherd Dog pyoderma, 134
    in hypothyroidism, 198
    juvenile-onset, 44
    in pemphigus follaceus, 260
    symptoms of, 124-125
L-Deprenyl, in Cushing's disease, 193
Dermacentor ticks, 169
Dermal hemangiosarcoma, 384
Dermal papilla, 7
Dermal tumors, 381-384, 381f, 382f, 383f
Dermatitis
    in acanthosis nigricans, 285
    acral lick, 314-322, 315f, 316f, 319f
    acute moist, 119-121, 119f, 121f
    atopic, in earflap diseases, 337-338
    flea-bite, 112, 112, 134f
    idiopathic facial, 298, 299f
    Malassezia, 241-248, 243f, 244f
    miliary, 71, 144
        in ringworm, 228, 229f
    psychogenic, in cats, 322-327, 323f, 324f, 326f
    pyotraumatic, 119-121, 119f, 121f
    rhabditic, 176-177
Dermatological examination, 46
Dermatomyositis, 44, 291-293, 292f, 293f, 335
Dermatoparaxis, 293-294, 295f
Dermatophagoides mites, in house dust, 79, 80f
Dermatophyte test medium, 50-51, 51f

Dermatophytes
   as allergen, 114
   in alopecia, 62
   examination for, 49, 324
   shampoos for, 25
Dermaphytosis, 225-241, 226f, 227f, 228f, 229f
   diagnosis of, 49
   in earflap lesions, 338
   in feline endocrine alopecia, 214
   in pemphigus follaceus, 259-260
   symptoms of, 124-125
Dermatosis
   castration-responsive, 213
   estrogen-responsive, 212
   testosterone-responsive, 212-213
   zinc-responsive, 260, 308-310, 309f, 342
Dermis
   in Cushing's disease, 183
   cysts in, 370
   deep pyoderma of, 136-137
Desensitization, in pet allergies, 82
Dexamethasone suppression test, in Cushing's disease, 189
Dewclaws, trimming of, 33
Diagnosis. *See also* Physical examination.
   approaches to, 42
   history-taking in, 42-45
   testing in
      allergy, 53-54
      hormone, 54
      immunologic, 54-55
   treatment trials in, 55-56
Diets
   elimination, in diagnosing food allergies 105
   protein
      hydrolyzed, 108-110
      novel, 105, 107t
   restrictive, 54
Diff-Quick stains, in cytological examination, 52
Differential diagnosis, 42
Direct impression smear, 52
Dirty face syndrome, 298, 299f
Discoid lupus erythematosus, 266-268, 267f, 339
DM. *See* Dermatomyositis.
Dopamine
   in Cushing's disease, 193
   in psychogenic alopecia, 326
Dosing, pulse, in ringworm, 239-240
Doxycycline
   in immune-mediated disease, 280
   in plasma cell pododermatitis, 276
Dracunculiasis, 178-179
Drooping, abdominal, in Cushing's disease, 185
Drugs. *See also specific drugs.*
   as allergen, 114-115, 115f
   psychoactive, in acral lick dermatitis, 320-322
Dry shampoos, 23
Drying agents, in ear cleaning products, 358, 359t
DTM. *See* Dermatophyte test medium
Dust, house. *See* House dust.
Dwarfism
   in hypothyroidism, 200
   pituitary, 215-216, 216f

Dysplasia
    black hair follicular, 287-288, 288f
    color-mutant hair, 62, 287, 287f
    follicular, 297

E

Ear diseases, 11, 32, 63. *See also* Otitis *entries.*
    allergic, 337-338
    diagnosis of, 352-357, 356f
    ear cleaning in, 357-360, 357f
    in earflap, 334-343, 335f, 337f, 338f, 341f, 342f, 343f
    environmental, 335-336
    hereditary, 335
    parasitic, 336-337
    surgery for, 367-368
Ear mites, 47, 165-167, 347
Ear swabs, in parasitic examination, 47
Earwax. *See* Cerumen.
EB. *See* Epidermolysis bullosa.
Ectoparasites. *See also* Parasites.
    in acral lick dermatitis, 316
    control of, 34-39
    diagnosis of, 45
    in otitis externa, 348
    shampoos for, 23-24
EDS. *See* Ehlers-Danlos syndrome.
Effect, summation, in atopy, 86-87
Effector cells, in ringworm, 231
Ehlers-Danlos syndrome, 293-294, 295f
Elastin fibers, 6
Electron microscopy, in Ehlers-Danlos syndrome, 294
Electrophoresis, urine, in immunologic testing, 55
Elimination diet, in diagnosing food allergies, 105
ELISA. *See* Enzyme-linked immunosorbent assay.
Elizabethan collar
    in acral lick dermatitis, 320
    in acute moist dermatitis, 120
    in atropy, 95, 95f
    in Malassezia furfur, 95, 95f
Emollients
    in ear medications, 361
    in hair conditioners, 30-31
Enclosing barrier, as skin function, 1
Endemic organisms, in fungal infections, 248-249
Endocrine alopecia, feline, 213-214
Endocrine-related skin diseases
    Cushing's disease as, 182-194, 184f, 185f
    of earflap, 339
    hormone testing for, 54
    thyroid, 194-208
Endorphins
    in obsessive-compulsive disorder, 312-314
    in psychogenic alopecia, 326
Enilconazole
    in *Malassezia* dermatitis, 247
    in ringworm, 234
Environmental allergies. *See* Atopy.
Environmental decontamination, in ringworm, 233-234
Environmental diseases, of earflap, 335-336
Enzyme-linked immunosorbent assay, in identifying allergens, 84-85
Enzymes, proteolytic, in ear discharge, 357
Eosinophilic granuloma. *See* Granuloma, eosinophilic.

Eosinophilic placques, in cat allergies, 71
Eosinophils, defined, 71-72
Epicoccum, as allergen, 78
Epidermal collarette, 59t
Epidermal turnover time, 5
Epidermis
  defined, 5
  shampoos for, 23
Epidermolysis bullosa, 295-296, 296f
Epinephrine, in muscle contraction, 8
Epithelial cells
  in cysts, 370
  tumors of, 372-374, 373f, 374f
Epitheliomas, intracutaneous cornifying, 379
Epitrichial sweat glands, 10
Erosion, 59t
Erythema
  in cutaneous T-cell lymphoma, 387
  discoid, 266-268, 267f
  in interdigital pyoderma, 136
  systemic, 268-270
Erythematosus, 335
  discoid lupus, 266-268, 267f, 350
  systemic lupus, 268-270, 350
Estrogen,in alopecia X, 220
Estrogen-responsive dermatosis, 212
Eustachian tube, in otitis externa, 352
Eutrombicula spp., in otitis externa, 348
Examination, physical. *See* Physical examination.
Excisional biopsy, 53
Excoriation, 101
Exfoliative skin disease, thymomas in, 391
Exudates
  in acute moist dermatitis, 119
  cytological examination for, 51-52
  in fungal infections, 248
  in *Malassezia* dermatitis, 243
Eye abnormalities, in hypothyroidism, 200

F

Facial dermatitis, idiopathic, 298, 299f
Facial nerve paralysis, in otitis media, 365
Familial predisposition, 67
Fatty acids
  omega-3
    in cutaneous T-cell lymphoma, 387
    in symmetric lupoid onychodystrophy, 271-272
  omega-6, in cutaneous T-cell lymphoma, 387
  supplements to, in atopy, 87t
Fecal flotation test, in parasitic examination, 47
Feeding trials, in diagnosing food allergies, 104-105
Felicola subrostratus lice, 171
Feline endocrine alopecia, 213-214
Feline cowpox virus, 339
Feline demodicosis, 152-155, 153f, 154f
Feline endocrine alopecia, 213-214
Feline fur mites, 161-162
Feline immunodeficiency virus, 138, 371
Feline leukemia virus,138, 371
Feline paraneoplastic alopecia, 390-391

Feline sarcoma virus, 383
Feline scabies, 160-161, 161f
Feline urologic syndrome, 327
FeSV. *See* Feline sarcoma virus.
Fibroepithelial polyps, in keratoses, 372
Fibroma, of connective tissue, 383
Fibrosarcoma, of connective tissue, 383
Film-forming hair conditioners, 30
Fine-needle aspiration
    in Cushing's disease, 187
    in fungi examination, 48-49
    in systemic mycoses, 253
Fipronil, 37t, 159
Fistula
    defined, 59t
    focal metatarsal, 134-135
    perianal, 135, 330
FIV. *See* Feline immunodeficiency virus.
Flank alopecia, seasonal , 222-223, 223f
Flare factor, in atropy, 89
Fleas
    in allergic dermatitis, 112, 112f
    in German Shepherd Dog pyoderma, 134
    in parasitic skin diseases, 142-147, 142f, 143f
Flexibility, as skin function, 2
Flies, 173-174, 173f
"Florida leeches", 255
Flotation, fecal, in parasitic examination, 47
Focal metatarsal fistulation, 134-135
Follicles, hair. See Hair follicles.
Follicular casts, in sebaceous adenitis, 306, 342
Follicular dysplasia, 297, 335
    black hair , 287-288, 288f
Follicular mange, 148-152, 149f, 150f
Folliculitis, 57t, 133
Food allergies, 103-111, 134
Foreign bodies, in otitis externa, 349
Free T_4, in hypothyroidism, 201-202
Frontline Spray, in sarcoptic mange, 159
Fungal hyphae, in alopecia, 62
Fungal infection
    examination for, 48-51, 48f, 49f, 50f
    ringworm as, 225-241, 226f, 227f, 228f, 229f
    shampoos for, 25
    subcutaneous and systemic, 248-254, 250f, 251f, 253f
    yeast, 241-248, 243f, 244f
Fungoides, mycosis, 341, 386-387, 387f
Fur mites, feline, 161-162
Furunculosis, 59t, 133, 227
FUS. *See* Feline urologic syndrome.

G
Generalized demodicosis, 54, 150
German Shepherd Dog pyoderma, 133-135, 134f
Glucocorticoids, in plasma cell pododermatitis, 276
Glycogen deposits, in Cushing's disease, 185
Gram's staining, in cytological examination, 52
Granuloma
    canine leproid, 338
    defined, 370-371
    eosinophilic, 71-72, 275

Granuloma—cont'd
    in feline acne, 132
    in plasma cell pododermatitis, 275
    in psychogenic alopecia, 324
  in feline acne, 132
  lick, 314-322, 315f, 316f, 319f
Grass allergens, 74t, 77
Griseofulvin, 236-239, 247
Groin
  in Cushing's disease, 183
  in *Malassezia* dermatitis, 243
  tumors of, 378
Grooming, 13-15, 15f
Ground substance, 5-6, 302
Growing hair, in alopecia, 62
Growth hormone, in alopecia X, 220
Growth hormone-responsive alopecia, 216-217
Gulf Coast tick, 169
Gynecomastia, in hyperestrogenism, 209

H

Hair
  composition and growth of, 7-9, 8f, 9f
  conditioners for, 30-31, 87t
  tactile, 9, 9f
Hair follicles
  bacteria in, 117
  defined, 7
  grooming of, 14
  in ringworm, 227
  tumors of, 378-379
Hair loss. *See* Alopecia.
Hair root, 7
Hair shaft, 7
Hand-stripping, in grooming, 14
Harvest mites, 164-165
Hay fever, ragweed in, 77
Heart rate, in hypothyroidism, 200
Helminthosporium, as allergen, 78
Hemangioma, 340-341, 384
Hemangiopericytoma, 384
Hemangiosarcoma, 341, 384
Hematomas
  aural, in earflaps, 342
  in sterile nodular panniculitis, 276
Hemostat, in diagnosing alopecia, 56, 61-62
Hemostatic powder, in grooming, 14
Hepatopathy, steroid, in Cushing's disease, 185, 280
Hereditary skin diseases
  acanthosis nigricans as, 284-285, 285f
  acral mutilation syndrome as, 285-286, 286f
  black hair follicular dysplasia as, 287-288, 288f
  color mutant alopecia as, 287
  congenital hypotrichosis as, 289-290, 291f, 335
  dermatomyositis as, 44, 291-293, 292f, 293f
  of earflap, 335
  Ehlers-Danlos syndrome as, 293-294, 295f
  epidermolysis bullosa as, 295-296, 296f
  follicular dysplasia as, 297, 335
  ichthyosis as, 297, 298f
  idiopathic facial dermatitis as, 298, 299f

Hereditary skin diseases—cont'd
  lethal acrodermatitis as, 300, 301f
  mucinosis as, 302, 302f
  pattern baldness as, 303, 303f
  primary seborrhea as, 304-306, 305f
  puppy strangles as, 138-140, 139f, 140f, 299, 300f, 341
  sebaceous adenitis as, 44, 306-308, 307f
Heterodoxus spiniger lice, 171
Histamine, 66
Histiocyte, 385
Histiocytomas
  in acral lick dermatitis, 315
  cutaneous, 385, 385f
  in earflap, 340
Histiocytosis, systemic, 386, 386f
Histoplasma capsulatum, in systemic mycoses, 249, 251-252
Histopathology
  defined, 53
  of nail diseases, 64
History-taking, in diagnosis, 42-45
Hookworms, 177, 178f
Hormonal ear flap lesions, 339
Hormone-related skin diseases. *See* Endocrine-related skin diseases.
Hormone testing, in diagnosis, 54
Horner's syndrome, in otitis media, 365
Horns, cutaneous, in keratoses, 371
Hot spots, 119-121, 119f, 121f
House dust
  as allergen, 79, 80f
  mite in, control of, 96-97
Humectants, 31, 308
Hydrolyzed protein diet, in diagnosing food allergies, 108-110
Hyperadrenocorticism. *See* Cushing's disease.
Hyperandrogenism, 211-212, 211f
Hyperestrogenism, 209-211, 210f
Hyperkeratosis, 60t
Hyperpigmentation
  in contact allergies, 101
  defined, 60t
  in *Malassezia* dermatitis, 243
Hyperplasia
  ear canal, 343-344
  nodular sebaceous, 377
  in otitis externa, 352
  tail gland, 211
Hypersensitivity
  in contact allergies, 99-100
  mosquito-bite, 338
Hyperthyroidism, 45, 205-208, 324
Hyphae, fungal, in alopecia, 62
Hypoallergenic diet, in diagnosing food allergies, 105
Hypodermis, 6
Hyposomatotropism, 216-217
Hypothyroidism, 195-205, 199f
  in acanthosis nigricans, 285
  of earflap, 339
  in German Shepherd Dog pyoderma, 134
  hormone testing for, 54
  in mucinosis, 302
  in pituitary dwarfism, 216
Hypotrichosis, congenital, 289-290, 291f, 335

I

Iatrogenic Cushing's disease, 183, 280
Iatrogenic factors, in otitis externa, 347
Ichthyosis, 297, 298f
Idiopathic bald thigh syndrome of Greyhounds, 303, 303f
Idiopathic facial dermatitis, 298, 299f
Idiopathic thyroid gland atrophy, 197
IDIs. *See* Insect development inhibitors.
IDSTs. *See* Intradermal skin tests.
IgE antibodies. *See* Immunoglobulin E antibodies
IgE-specific antigen, 66
Imaging
    magnetic resonance, in Cushing's disease, 187
    nuclear, in hyperthyroidism, 207
Imidacloprid, antiparasitic use of, 37t
Immune complexes, in immune-mediated vasculitis, 273-274
Immune-mediated diseases
    bullous pemphigoid as, 272-273, 273f, 340
    discoid lupus erythematosus as, 266-268, 267f, 339
    focal metatarsal fistulation as, 134-135, 335
    follicular dysplasia as, 297
    immunologic testing for, 55
    lupus as, 266
    medications for, 279-281
    in otitis externa, 350
    paraneoplastic pemphigus as, 265-266
    pemphigus erythematosus as, 263-264, 263f
    pemphigus follaceus as, 258-262, 259f, 260f, 261f, 262f, 339
    pemphigus vulgaris as, 264-265, 265f
    plasma cell pododermatitis as, 275-276, 275f
    sterile nodular panniculitis as, 276
    symmetric lupoid onychodystrophy as, 270-272, 271f
    systemic lupus erythematosus as, 268-270
    uveodermatological syndrome as, 277-278, 277f, 278f
    vasculitis as, 273-274, 274f, 340
Immune response, 66
Immune system
    bacteria in, 117
    defined, 66
    in otitis externa, 347
    in ringworm, 226
Immunodeficiencies, 134, 347
Immunoglobulin E antibodies, 66, 245
Immunoglobulin quantitation, in immunologic testing, 55
Immunologic deficiencies, immunologic testing for, 54
Immunologic testing, in diagnosis, 54-55
Immunosuppression
    in bullous pemphigoid, 273
    in systemic mycoses, 252
Immunosurveillance, as skin function, 3
Immunotherapy
    allergen-specific, in atropy, 88t, 98-99
    in pet allergies, 82
Impression smear
    in acute moist dermatitis, 120
    defined, 52
    in systemic mycoses, 253
Indolent ulcers, in cat allergies, 71
Infectious ear flap lesions, 338-339

Inflammation
    in acanthosis nigricans, 284
    in acute moist dermatitis, 120
    in cysts, 370
    defined, 66
    itching from, 63
    in psychogenic alopecia, 322
    in yeast infection, 242
Infundibular keratinizing acanthomas, 379
Inguinal region. *See* Groin.
Inner ear infections. *See* Otitis interna.
Insect allergens, 74t, 80-81
Insect development inhibitors, in flea control, 145-147
Intercellular adhesion molecules, in pemphigus vulgaris, 264
Interdigital pyoderma, 136
Interstitial cell tumors, in hyperandrogenism, 211-212
Intertrigo, 122-123, 121f, 123f, 124f
Intracutaneous cornifying epitheliomas, 379
Intradermal skin tests, in identifying allergens, 83-84, 324
Iodides, in fungal infections, 248
Itching. *See* Pruritus.
Itraconazole
    in coccidiomycosis, 254
    in *Malassezia* dermatitis, 247
    in ringworm, 239-240
    in systemic mycoses, 250
Ivermectin, antiparasitic use of, 39t
Ixodes ticks, 169

J
Juvenile cellulitis. *See* Puppy strangles.
Juvenile-onset generalized demodicosis, 44, 54, 150, 152
Juvenile pyoderma. *See* Puppy strangles.

K
Kapok, as allergen, 80
Keratin
    in Cushing's disease, 183
    in cysts, 370
    in feline acne, 132
Keratinization defects
    in alopecia, 335
    bathing techniques in, 16
    ichthyosis as, 297, 298f
    in otitis externa, 350
    primary, 304-306, 305f
    shampoos for, 23-24
Keratinizing acanthomas, infundibular, 379
Keratinocytes
    acantholytic, 126
    in epithelial cell tumors, 372
    in phemigus diseases, 258
Keratoacanthomas, 379
Keratolytic activity, of antiseborrheic shampoos, 24
Keratoplastic activity, of antiseborrheic shampoos, 24
Keratosebaceous casts, in sebaceous adenitis, 306
Keratoses, actinic, 336, 371-372, 372f
Ketoconazole
    in alopecia X, 219
    in Cushing's disease, 193

Ketoconazole—cont'd
  in *Malassezia* dermatitis, 247
  in ringworm, 239
  in systemic mycoses, 250

L

Lagenidiosis, 255
Lagenidium infections, 254-256, 256f
Lamp, Wood's, in diagnosis, 49
Langerhans cells, in epithelial cell tumors, 372
Larvae, *Cuterebra*, 172-173
Laser surgery
  in acral lick dermatitis, 318-319
  in canine oral papillomatosis, 373
  in earflap lesions, 336
Lateral bulla osteotomy, 367-368
Lateral wall resection, in ear surgery, 367
LBO. *See* Lateral bulla osteotomy.
Leishmaniasis, in feline cowpox virus, 339
Leproid granulomas, canine, 338
Leprosy, canine, 338
Lesions, skin. *See* Skin, lesions of.
Lethal acrodermatitis, 300, 301f
Lethargy, in hypothyroidism, 200
Levothyroxine, in hypothyroidism, 203-205
Libido, in hypothyroidism, 200
Lice, 170-172, 337
Lichenification
  in contact allergies, 10
  defined, 60
  in *Malassezia* dermatitis, 242
Lick granuloma, 314-322, 315f, 316f, 319f
Licking
  anal, 330, 331f
  foot, 329, 329f
Lime-sulfur solution
  in *Malassezia* dermatitis, 246-247
  in ringworm, 234
  in sarcoptic mange, 158
D-Limonene, antiparasitic use of, 36t
Linognathus setosus, 171
Linters, cotton, as allergen, 80
Lipomas, 389-390
Lone Star tick, 169
Lufenuron
  antiparasitic use of, 38t
  in flea control, 146-147
  in ringworm, 240
Lupoid onychodystrophy, symmetric, 64, 230, 270-272, 271f
Lupus, 266
Lupus erythematosus. *See* Erythematosus.
Lyme disease, 169
Lymph nodes, submandibular, of earflap, 341
Lymphocyte(s)
  in atropy, 92
  in Cushing's disease, 186
  in cutaneous T-cell lymphoma, 387
  defined, 385
  in immune-mediated diseases, 257, 340
  protective function of, 3
Lymphocyte blastogenesis test, in immunologic testing, 55

Lymphocyte thyroiditis, 195-197, 203
Lymphohistiocytic tumors, 385-388, 385f, 386f, 387f
Lymphoma, cutaneous T-cell, 341, 386-387, 387f
Lynxacarus radosky, in feline fur mites, 161-162

M

Maceration, 122, 346
Macroconidia, 50-51, 51f
Macrophages
    defined, 385
    in granulomas, 370-371
    in sterile nodular panniculitis, 276
Macule, 57t
Magnetic resonance imaging, in Cushing's disease, 187
Malassezia dermatitis, 241-248, 243f, 244f
Malassezia furfur
    as allergen, 114
    Elizabethan collar in, 95, 95f
    in human dandruff, 24
    infection from, 241-248, 243f, 244f
    shampoos for, 25
Malassezia pachydermatis, 241, 338, 351
Malignant neoplasms, 369. *See also* Tumors.
Mallophaga lice, 170
Mange
    follicular, 148-152, 149f, 150f
    notoedric, 160-161, 161f
    red, 148-152, 149f, 150f
    sarcoptic, 55, 155-160, 156f
Masses, examination of, 52
Mast cells
    defined, 66
    tumor of, 341, 381-382, 381f, 382f
McKenzie toothbrush screening procedure, in ringworm, 230,
        240-241
MCT. *See* Mast cells, tumor of.
Medicated coat conditioners, 31
Medium, dermatophyte test, 50-51, 51f
Medulla, 7
Melanin
    in alopecia, 62
    in black hair follicular dysplasia, 287-288
    in immune-mediated diseases, 257
    in uveodermatological syndrome, 277
Melanocytes
    defined, 5
    in epithelial cell tumors, 372
    in skin pigmentation, 3
Melatonin
    in alopecia, 219, 223
    in estrogen-responsive dermatosis, 212
    in pattern baldness, 303
Mental retardation, in hypothyroidism, 200
Merkel cell tumors, 372, 376
Metabolic diseases, in otitis externa, 347
Metabolic epidermal; necrosis, 270-271
Metastases, defined, 369. *See also* Tumors.
Metatarsal fistulation, focal, 134-135
Methoprene, 38t, 147
Methylcarbamate, antiparasitic use of, 35t
Milbemycin, antiparasitic use of, 39t

Microbiology culture and susceptibility test, in cytological examination, 52
Microscopy, electron, in Ehlers-Danlos syndrome, 294
Microsporum canis, 49
    in ringworm, 226, 229f, 232-233
Microsporum gypseum, in ringworm, 226, 228, 241
Middle ear infections. *See* Otitis media.
Miliary dermatitis, 71, 144, 230
    in ringworm, 228, 229f
Mites
    ear, 47, 165-167, 347
    feline fur, 161-162
    harvest, 164-165
    in house dust, 79, 80f
Miticides, in sarcoptic mange, 159
Mitotane
    in alopecia X, 219-220
    in Cushing's disease, 192-193
Moist dermatitis, acute, 119-121, 119f, 121f
Moisture, excessive, in otitis externa, 346
Molds
    as allergens, 75t, 77
    control of, 97-98
Molecules, intercellular adhesion, in pemphigus vulgaris, 264
Monocytes
    in Cushing's disease, 186
    defined, 385
Mosquitoes, 174-176,175f
Mosquito bite allergies, 113,113f
MRI. *See* Magnetic resonance imaging.
Mucinosis, 302, 302f
Mucor, *as allergen*, 78
Mupirocin cream, in skin fold pyoderma, 123
Mutilation syndrome, acral, 285-286, 286f
Mycobacteria, in earflap lesions, 338
Mycobacterium lepraemurium, 338
Mycoses, subcutaneous, 248
Mycosis fungoides, 341, 386-387, 387f
Myiasis, 174
Myringotomy, in otitis media, 365
Myxomas, 384
Myxosarcomas, 384

N
Nails
    anatomy of, 12
    care of, 32-34
    diseases of, 64
    in ringworm, 228
Nasopharyngeal polyps, 347, 364
Necrosis
    in immune-mediated diseases, 340
    metabolic epidermal, 270-271
    in ringworm, 239
Neoplasms, defined, 369. *See also* Tumors.
Neoplastic factors, in itching, 63
Nerve paralysis, facial, in otitis media, 365
Neuroendocrine cell tumors, 376
Neurogenic factors, in itching, 63
Neurological signs, in otitis media, 364-365
Neuroma, tail dock, 327

Neutrophils
  in Cushing's disease, 186
  in phemigus diseases, 258
  in pyogranulomas, 371
  protective function of, 3
  in ringworm, 227, 231
  in sterile nodular panniculitis, 276
  in systemic mycoses, 252
Niacinamide, 276, 279-280
Nitenpyram, antiparasitic use of, 37t
Nodular panniculitis, sterile, 276
Nodules
  in interdigital pyoderma, 136
  non-neoplastic, 370
  in systemic mycoses, 249, 252
Nongrowing hair, in alopecia, 62
Non-neoplastic skin masses, 370-372, 371f
Notoedres cati
  in earflap lesions, 336
  examination for, 47
  in otitis externa, 348
Notoedric mange, 160-161, 161f
Novel protein diet, in diagnosing food allergies, 105, 107t
Nuclear imaging, in hyperthyroidism, 207

O

Obesity, in hypothyroidism, 200
Obsessive-compulsive disorder, 25, 311-314, 311f
Obstructive ear disease, in otitis externa, 347
Occlusive agents, in ear medications, 361
Otobius ticks, 170
Oil-producing glands. *See* Sebaceous glands.
Omega-3 fatty acids
  in cutaneous T-cell lymphoma, 387
  in symmetric lupoid onychodystrophy, 271-272
Omega-6 fatty acids, in cutaneous T-cell lymphoma, 387
Oncologists, defined, 370. *See also* Tumors.
Oncology, defined, 370. *See also* Tumors.
Onychectomy, in symmetric lupoid onychodystrophy, 272
Onychodystrophy, symmetric lupoid, 64, 230, 270-272, 271f
Oomycete infections, 255
Oral papillomatosis, canine, 373, 373f
Orthopedic Foundation for Animals, thyroid registry of, 203
Osteoporosis, in Cushing's disease, 185-186
Otitis externa
  causes of
    perpetuating, 351-352
    predisposing, 344-347, 344f
    primary, 347-351
  clinical signs of, 343-344
  diagnosis of, 352-357, 356f
  in hypothyroidism, 198-200
  long-term management of, 363-364
  in *Malassezia* dermatitis, 243, 338-339
  in pemphigus foliaceus, 258
  treatment of, 360-362
Otitis interna, 365-367, 366f
Otitis media, 364-365, 364f
  in otitis externa, 351-352
Otobius megnini, 170, 348
Otodectes cynotis, 47, 165-167, 347

Otoscope, in otitis externa, 347
Ototoxicity, in otitis interna, 366
Outer ear infections. *See* Otitis externa.

P

PAD. *See* Psychogenic alopecia and dermatitis in cats.
Panniculitis, sterile nodular, 276
Papilla, dermal, 7
Papillomas, 372-374, 373f, 374f
Papillomatosis, canine oral, 373, 373f
Papillomavirus
    feline, 374
    in keratoses, 371
Papules
    in cat allergies, 71
    in contact allergies, 101
    in cutaneous T-cell lymphoma, 387
    defined, 58t
    in earflap lesions, 336
    in interdigital pyoderma, 136
    multiple pigmented, 374
    in otitis externa, 347-348
    in papillomas, 373
    in ringworm, 226
    in systemic mycoses, 252
Parakeratosis
    in lethal acrodermatitis, 300
    in zinc-responsive dermatosis, 308
Paralysis
    facial nerve, in otitis media, 365
    tick, 169
Paraneoplastic pemphigus, 265-266
Paraneoplastic skin diseases, tumors in, 390-392, 391f, 392
Parasites. *See also* Ectoparasites.
    allergies to, 111-114, 112f, 113f
    in earflap lesions, 336-337, 337f
    examination for, 46-47
    itching from, 63
    in skin and hair coat, 14
Paronychia, 243, 259, 329
Pasteurella multocida, in subcutaneous abscess, 138
Patch, defined, 58t
Pathologist, defined, 53
Pattern baldness, 303, 303f
Pediatric skin diseases. *See* Hereditary skin diseases.
Pediculosis, 170-172
Pelodera strongyloides, 47, 176-177
Pemphigoid, bullous, 272-273, 273f, 340
Pemphigus, paraneoplastic, 265-266
Pemphigus erythematosus, 263-264, 263f
    immune-mediated, 339
    in otitis externa, 350
Pemphigus follaceus, 258-262, 259f, 260f, 261f, 262f, 329
    as allergen, 114
    immune-mediated, 339
    in otitis externa, 350
    symptoms of, 124-125
Pemphigus vulgaris, 264-265, 265f
Penetrance, in dermatomyositis, 291
Penicillium, as allergen, 78

Pentoxifylline
  in contact allergies, 101
  in dermatomyositis, 292
  in immune-mediated disease, 274, 280
  in sterile nodular panniculitis, 276
  in symmetric lupoid onychodystrophy, 272
Perianal fistula, 135, 330
Perianal gland tumors, 379-380, 380f
Perineum,in acanthosis nigricans, 284
Periodontal disease, 31-32
Permethrin, antiparasitic use of, 36t
Perpetuating causes, of otitis externa, 351-352
Phoma, as allergen, 78
Phosmet, antiparasitic use of, 35t
Photoperiod, 8
PHSO. *See* Primary hereditary seborrhea oleosa.
Physical examination. *See also* Diagnosis.
  for bacteria, 51-52
  dermatological, 46
  for fungi, 48-51, 48f, 49f, 50f
  for masses, 52
  for parasites, 46-47
  skin biopsies in, 53
  for yeasts, 48-51, 48f, 49f, 50f
Phytates, in zinc-responsive dermatosis, 308
Pigmentation, as skin function, 3
Piloerection, in temperature regulation, 3
Pinna, anatomy of, 11
Pituitary-dependent hyperadrenocorticism, 182-183
Pituitary dwarfism, 215-216, 216f
Pityrosporum ovale, in human dandruff, 24
Pityrosporum pachydermatis, 241
Plant awns, in otitis externa, 349, 349f
Planum nasale, in ichthyosis, 297
Plaques
  defined, 58t
  in earflap lesions, 336
  eosinophilic, in cat allergies, 71
  multiple pigmented, 374
  in papillomas, 373
  in periodontal disease, 31
Plasma cells
  in auricular chondrosis, 340
  in pododermatitis, 275-276, 275f
Plasmacytoma, 387-388
Platelet count, in Cushing's disease, 186
Plucking, in grooming, 14
Pododemodicosis, foot licking in, 329
Pododermatitis, 136
  plasma cell, 275-276, 275f
Pollens
  as allergens, 76-78
  control of, 98
Polyphagia, in Cushing's disease, 185
Polyps
  fibroepithelial, in keratoses, 372
  in otitis externa, 347
  in otitis media, 364
  in systemic mycoses, 252
Polyuria, in Cushing's disease, 185

Porphyrins, in dog atopy, 69
Powder, hemostatic, in grooming, 14
Predisposing causes, of otitis externa, 344-347, 344f
Predisposition
    breed, 44
    familial, 67
Prednisolone, in atropy, 91
Prednisone, in atropy, 91
Primary acanthosis nigricans, 284
Primary hereditary seborrhea oleosa, 305-306
Primary keratinization defects, 304-306, 305f
Primary seborrhea, 304-306, 305f
Profile, biochemical. See Biochemical profile.
Protection, as skin function, 2
Protein-based hair conditioners, 30
Protein diet
    hydrolyzed, 108-110
    novel, 105, 107t
Proteolytic enzymes, in ear discharge, 357
Proteus mirabilis, in otitis externa, 351
Pruritic threshold, in atopy, 87-89
Pruritus
    in cutaneous T-cell lymphoma, 387
    cyclosporine in, 92
    shampoos for, 25
    symptoms of, 62-63
Pseudo-Cushing's disease, 216-217
Pseudomonas aeruginosa, in otitis externa, 351
Psychoactive drugs, in acral lick dermatitis, 320-322
Psychogenic alopecia and dermatitis, 322-327, 323f, 324f, 326f
Psychogenic skin diseases
    acral lick dermatitis as, 314-322, 315f, 316f, 319f
    flank sucking as, 328
    foot licking as, 329, 329f
    obsessive-compulsive disorders as, 311-314, 311f
    self-nursing as, 328
    tail sucking and biting as, 327
Pullularia, as allergen, 78
Pulse dosing, in ringworm, 239-240
Puppy strangles, 138-140, 139f, 140f, 299, 300f, 341
Purulent discharge
    in acute moist dermatitis, 119
    in pemphigus follaceus, 258
    in systemic mycoses, 249
Pustules
    defined, 58t
    in interdigital pyoderma, 136
    in phemigus diseases, 258
    in ringworm, 226
Pyoderma
    in acral lick dermatitis, 316
    bacteria I, 117-118
    chin, 131-133, 132f
    deep, 136-138, 137f
    German Shepherd Dog, 133-135, 134f
    interdigital, 136
    juvenile, 138-140, 139f, 140f, 299, 300f, 341
    in mucinosis, 302
    in pemphigus follaceus, 259
    skin fold, 122-123, 121f, 123f, 124f
    staphylococcal, 124-131,124f, 125f, 126f, 230

Pyogranuloma, in interdigital pyoderma, 136
Pyotraumatic dermatitis, 119-121, 119f, 121f
Pyrethrins, antiparasitic use of, 36t
Pyriproxyfen, antiparasitic use of, 38t
Pythiosis, 255
Pythium insidiosum, 254-256, 256f

Q

Quantitation, immunoglobulin, in immunologic testing, 55

R

Radiation therapy. *See also* Tumors.
  in Cushing's disease, 190
  defined, 370
  in earflap, 335-336
  in pemphigus erythematosus, 264
Radioallergosorbent test, in identifying allergens, 84-85
Ragweed, in hay fever, 77
RAST. *See* Radioallergosorbent test.
Red mange, 148-152, 149f, 150f
Regulation, of temperature as skin function, 2-3
Relative risk, in diagnosis, 44
Resection, lateral wall, in ear surgery, 367
Restrictive diet trial, 54, 105
Retinoids
  in earflap lesions, 336
  in ichthyosis, 297
  synthetic, in sebaceous cell carcinomas, 377
Revolution. *See* Selamectin.
Rhabditic dermatitis, 176-177
Rhabditis strongyloides, 176-177
Rhipicephalus sanguineus ticks, 168-169
Rhizopus, as allergen, 78
Ringworm. *See* Dermaphytosis
Risk, relative, in diagnosis, 44
Rocky Mountain spotted fever, 169
Rodent ulcers, in cat allergies, 71
Rotenone, antiparasitic use of, 36t
Rubber puppy disease, 293-294, 295f

S

Sac, anal. *See* Anal sac.
Sarcomas, soft tissue, 383-384, 383f
Sarcoptes scabiei
  in earflap lesions, 336
  examination for, 47
  in otitis externa, 348
Sarcoptic mange, 55, 155-160, 156f
Scabicide, in treatment trials, 55
Scabies
  canine, 155-160, 156f
  feline, 160-161, 161f
Scale, 60t
Scar, 60t
Seasonal flank alopecia, 222-223, 223f
Seasonality, of allergens, 72-73
Sebaceous adenitis, 44, 306-308, 307f, 342
Sebaceous glands
  bathing techniques for, 15-16
  carcinomas of, 377

Sebaceous glands–cont'd
    in cysts, 370
    in immune-mediated diseases, 257
    protective functions of, 2
    tumors of, 376-377, 377f
Seborrhea
    bathing techniques in, 16
    in hyperestrogenism, 210
    in *Malassezia* dermatitis, 243
    in pemphigus follaceus, 260
    in pituitary dwarfism, 216
    primary, 304-306, 305f
    shampoos for, 23-24
    vitamin A-responsive, 305
Seborrhea oleosa
    in hyperandrogenism, 211
    in primary seborrhea, 304
Sebum
    in Cushing's disease, 183
    defined, 9
    in otitis externa, 350
    in ringworm, 236
Selamectin, 37t, 159
Selenium sulfide, in *Malassezia* dermatitis, 246
Self-nursing, 328
Semicircular canals, 11
Sensory function, of skin, 3
Serpiginous lesions, in sebaceous adenitis, 306
Sertoli cell tumors, in hyperestrogenism, 209, 210f, 391-392
Serum, in cysts, 370
Serum allergy tests, 83-85, 105
Sex hormone disorders
    estrogen-responsive dermatosis as, 212
    hyperandrogenism as, 211-212, 211f
    hyperestrogenism as, 209-211, 210f
Shampoos, 17, 18-25
    in acanthosis nigricans, 284
    in atopy, 87t
    in color mutant alopecia, 287
    in ichthyosis, 297
    in sebaceous adenitis, 306
    in staphylococcal pyoderma, 129
Show cut, in nail care, 33
Signalment, in diagnosis, 42
Skin
    biopsies of, 53
        in chin pyoderma, 131
        in immunologic testing, 55
    functions of, 1-4, 2f
    glands of, 9-10
    lesions of
        primary, 56, 57t, 58t
        secondary, 56, 59t, 60t
    structure of, 4-6, 4f, 6f
Skin fold pyoderma, 122-123, 121f, 123f, 124f
Skin gland tumors, 376-380, 377f, 378f, 380f
Skin tests, intradermal, in identifying allergens, 83-84
SLE. *See* Systemic lupus erythematosus
Sloughing, in spiders, 179
Smear, impression. *See* Impression smear.
Smoke, tobacco, as allergen, 80

Soft tissue sarcomas, 383-384, 383f
Spiders, 179, 179f
Spinous ear tick, 170, 348
Spores
   as allergen, 78
   in alopecia, 62
   in ringworm, 230
Sporotrichosis, 248
Spots, hot, 119-121, 119f, 121f
Sprays, in acute moist dermatitis, 120
Squamous cell carcinoma, 340, 375, 375f
Staphage Lysate, in staphylococcal pyoderma, 130
Staphylococcal pyoderma, 124-131,124f, 125f, 126f
   in German Shepherd Dogs, 133
   in *Malassezia* dermatitis, 247-248
Staphylococci, 138, 241
Staphylococcus, as allergen, 114
Staphylococcus intermedius, in pyoderma, 117
Stemphylium, as allergen, 78
Stenosis, of ear canal, 343-344
Stereotypic behaviors, in obsessive-compulsive disorder, 311
Sterile nodular panniculitis, 276
Steroid hepatopathy, in Cushing's disease, 185, 280
Storage, as skin function, 3
Strangles, puppy, 138-140, 139f, 140f, 299, 300f
Stratum basale
   basal cell tumors of, 376
   defined, 5
   in pemphigus vulgaris, 264
Stratum corneum
   in lethal acrodermatitis, 300
   in nail diseases, 64
   in otitis externa, 346
   in pyoderma, 117
   in ringworm, 225
   in skin diseases, 4, 5
Streptococci, in subcutaneous abscess, 138
Stressors, in acral lick dermatitis, 318
Stud tail, 10
Subcutaneous abscess, 138
Subcutaneous fungal infections, 248-254, 250f, 251f, 253f
Subcutaneous hemangiosarcoma, 384
Subcutaneous tissue, 6, 383
Submandibular lymph nodes, of earflap, 341
Substance, ground, 5-6
Sucking, of tail, 327
Sucking lice, 170
Suit, body, in atropy, 95, 95f
Sulfur, antiparasitic use of, 39t
Summation effect, in atopy, 86-87
Supplements, fatty acid, in atopy, 87t
Surgery. *See* Cryosurgery; Laser surgery
Swabs, ear, in parasitic examination, 47
"Swamp cancer", 255
Sweat glands
   protective functions of, 2
   tumors of, 378, 378f
Symmetric lupoid onychodystrophy, 64, 230, 270-272, 271f
Synthetic retinoids, in sebaceous cell carcinomas, 377
Systemic fungal infections, 248-254, 250f, 251f, 253f
Systemic histiocytosis, 386, 386f

Systemic lupus erythematosus, 268-270, 340
Systemic medications, in fungal infections, 237t, 238t

T

T-cell lymphoma, cutaneous, 341, 386-387, 387f
T_4 concentrations, in hypothyroidism, 201-202
Tacrolimus, in immune-mediated vasculitis, 274
Tactile hairs, 9, 9f
Tags, cutaneous, in keratoses, 372
Tail
   biting of, 327
   glands of, 10
   stud, 10
   sucking of, 327
Tail-dock neuroma, 327
Tape, acetate, in parasitic examination, 46-47
Tapeworm infestation, anal licking in, 330
Tartar, in periodontal disease, 31
TECA. *See* Total ear canal ablation.
Telangiectasis, 58t
Telogen hair, in alopecia, 62
Telogen phase, of hair cycle, 8
Terbinafine
   in *Malassezia* dermatitis, 247
   in ringworm, 240
Testosterone, in alopecia X, 220
Testosterone-responsive dermatosis, 212-213
Testing, diagnostic. *See* Diagnosis, testing in.
Tetracycline, 276, 279-280
Thermoregulation, as skin function, 2-3, 8
Threshold, pruritic, in atopy, 87-89
Thymomas, 391
Thyroid disorders, 194-208
Thyroid hormone replacement therapy, 203-205
Thyroid radionuclide uptake, in hyperthyroidism, 207
Thyroiditis, lymphocytic, 195-197, 203
Thyrotoxicosis. *See* Hyperthyroidism.
Tick paralysis, 169
Ticks, 14, 167-170
   in earflap, 337
   in otitis externa, 348
Tissue death. *See* Necrosis
Tobacco smoke, as allergen, 80
Toothbrush culture, in ringworm, 230, 240-241
Total ear canal ablation, 367, 368f
Transmissible venereal tumor, 390
Tree allergens, 75t, 76-77
Trauma, in otitis externa, 351
Trental, in dermatomyositis, 292
Trial feedings, 104-105
Trichodectes canis lice, 170
Trichogram, in diagnosing alopecia, 56, 61-62
Trichophyton mentagrophytes, in ringworm, 226, 241
Trilostane
   in alopecia X, 219
   in Cushing's disease, 193
Trombiculiasis, 164-165
TSH assay, canine, in hypothyroidism, 202-203
Tularemia, 169

Tumor(s)
  anal sac, 390
  basal cell, 376
  ceruminal gland, 380
  circumanal gland, 379-380, 380f
  defined, 58t, 369
  dermal, 381-384, 381f, 382f, 383f
  earflap, 336, 340-341
  epithelial cell, 372-374, 373f, 374f
  general characteristics of, 369t
  interstitial cell, 211-212
  lipomas as, 389-390
  lymphohistiocytic, 385-388, 385f, 386f, 387f
  mast cell, 341,381-382, 381f, 382f
  non-neoplastic, 370-372, 371f
  in paraneoplastic skin diseases, 390-392, 391f, 392
  perianal gland, 379-380, 380f
  sebaceous gland, 376-377, 377f
  Sertoli cell, 209, 210f
  skin gland and hair follicle, 376-380, 377f, 378f, 380f
  soft tissue sarcoma as, 383-384, 383f
  thymomas as, 391
  transmissible venereal, 390
Turnover time, epidermal, 5
TVT. See Transmissible venereal tumor.
Tympanic bullae, in otitis media, 365

U
Ulcer
  in acral lick dermatitis, 314
  defined, 60t
  in epidermolysis bullosa, 296
  indolent, in cat allergies, 71
  in interdigital pyoderma, 136
  in pemphigus follaceus, 258
  in squamous cell carcinoma, 375
  in systemic mycoses, 249
Ultrasonography, abdominal, in Cushing's disease, 187
Ultraviolet radiation,in pemphigus erythematosus, 264
Ungual crest, 12
Urinalysis, in Cushing's disease, 186
Urine electrophoresis, in immunologic testing, 55
Uveodermatological syndrome, 277-278, 277f, 278f

V
Vasculitis
  immune-mediated, 273-274, 274f, 340
  in ringworm, 239
  in symmetric lupoid onychodystrophy, 270
Vasoconstriction, in temperature regulation, 2
Vasodilation, in temperature regulation, 2
Venereal tumor, transmissible, 390
Vertical canal ablation, in ear surgery, 367
Vesicles
  defined, 58t
  in epidermolysis bullosa, 296
  in phemigus diseases, 258
Vibrissae, 9, 9f
Video-otoscope, in otitis externa, 347

Vitamin A-responsive seborrhea, 305
Vitamin D production, as skin function, 3
Vitamin E
   in immune-mediated disease, 280
   in pemphigus erythematosus, 264

W
Walking dandruff, 162-164, 163f
Warts, 372-374, 373f, 374f
Weed allergens, 75t, 77-78
Western blot analysis, in identifying allergens, 84
Wheal, 58t
Whiskers, 9, 9f
White blood cells. *See* Neutrophils.
Wood's lamp, in diagnosis, 49
Worms, 178-179

Y
Yeasts
   in acanthosis nigricans, 284
   in dog atopy, 68
   examination for, 48-51, 48f, 49f, 50f
   in hypothyroidism, 198
   infection from, 241-248, 243f, 244f
   in otitis externa, 346, 351

Z
Zinc-responsive dermatosis, 260, 308-310, 309f, 342
Zone, basement-membrane, 5-6